THERAPEUTIC EXERCISE IN DEVELOPMENTAL DISABILITIES

SECOND EDITION

Therapeutic Exercise In Developmental Disabilities

◆

Second Edition

Edited By
Barbara H. Connolly, Ed.D., P.T.
Patricia C. Montgomery, Ph.D., P.T.

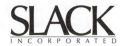

SLACK
INCORPORATED

An innovative information, education and management company
6900 Grove Road • Thorofare, NJ 08086

Publisher: John H. Bond
Editorial Director: Amy E. Drummond
Editorial Assistant: William J. Green
Cover Illustration: Karen Lively

The procedures and practices described in this book should be implemented in a manner consistent with the professional standards set for the circumstances that apply in each specific situation. Every effort has been made to confirm the accuracy of the information presented and to correctly relate generally accepted practices. The author, editor, and publisher cannot accept responsibility for errors or exclusions or for the outcome of the application of the material presented herein. There is no expressed or implied warranty of this book or information imparted by it.

This book was previously published by Chattanooga Group, Inc., Hixson, TN

Printed in the United States of America.

ISBN 1-55642-555-4

Published by: SLACK Incorporated
                6900 Grove Road
                Thorofare, NJ 08086 USA
                Telephone: 856-848-1000
                Fax: 856-853-5991
                www.slackbooks.com

Contact SLACK Incorporated for more information about other books in this field or about the availability of our books from distributors outside the United States.

Authorization to photocopy items for internal or personal use, or the internal or personal use of specific clients, is granted by SLACK Incorporated, provided that the appropriate fee is paid directly to Copyright Clearance Center, 222 Rosewood Drive, Danvers, MA 01923 USA, 978-750-8400. Prior to photocopying items for educational classroom use, please contact the CCC at the address above. Please reference Account Number 9106324 for SLACK Incorporated's Professional Book Division.

For further information on CCC, check CCC Online at the following address: http://www.copyright.com.

Last digit is print number: 10 9 8 7 6 5 4 3 2 1

PREFACE

◆

Physical therapy in pediatrics has expanded over the past decade and has been identified as one of the areas of specialization in physical therapy. Although texts on therapeutic exercise in pediatrics have been published, they have been aimed generally at the physical therapist with pediatric experience. Some texts emphasize specific theoretical frameworks (i.e., neurodevelopmental theory — NDT) or specific diagnostic categories (i.e., cerebral palsy). A textbook which provides a framework for assessment and treatment of children with developmental disabilities is needed for both the physical therapy student and for inexperienced practitioners. The purpose of this text is to integrate theory, assessment, and treatment using functional outcomes and a problem solving approach. Case studies of four children representing common developmental disabilities encountered by the physical therapist in pediatrics were chosen as the mechanism for applying the problem solving approach. We hope that this text is valuable to the student and the clinician and, in turn, to the children they treat.

BIOGRAPHICAL SKETCHES

◆

EDITORS: THERAPEUTIC EXERCISE IN DEVELOPMENTAL DISABILITIES

BARBARA CONNOLLY
is an Associate Professor and Chairman of the Department of Rehabilitation Sciences at the University of Tennessee, Memphis. She currently holds an adjunct clinical appointment at the University of Indianapolis and has held adjunct appointments at numerous other Universities in the past. Dr. Connolly has lectured throughout the United States and has published extensively on topics dealing with children with developmental delays and specific learning disabilities. Dr. Connolly continues to be active clinically through private practice and consultations with early intervention programs, school systems, and state facilities for persons with mental disabilities. She received a B.S. in physical therapy from the University of Florida, an M.Ed. in special education and an Ed.D. in curriculum and instruction from Memphis State University.

PATRICIA MONTGOMERY
received a B.S. in physical therapy from the University of Oklahoma, an M.A. in educational psychology, and a Ph.D. in child psychology from the University of Minnesota. Dr. Montgomery has a private practice in pediatric physical therapy in the Minneapolis-St. Paul area and holds academic appointments in the physical therapy programs at the University of Minnesota, Minneapolis, Hahneman University, Philadelphia, and the University of Tennessee, Memphis. Dr. Montgomery is the author of several books and articles in the area of pediatrics and she is actively involved in presenting continuing education workshops for developmental therapists in the United States and internationally.

AUTHORS/CHAPTERS

ANN VANSANT
is an Associate Professor in the Department of Physical Therapy at Temple University, Philadelphia. She received her B.S. in physical therapy from Russell Sage College, an M.S. in physical therapy from Virginia Commonwealth University and a Ph.D. in physical education - motor development from the University of Wisconsin-Madison. Dr. VanSant has given numerous continuing education workshops related to physical therapy for children and adults with neurologic dysfunction. She is actively involved in research designed to describe developmental change in movement patterns across the human lifespan.

CAROLYN FITERMAN
received her B.S. and M.S. in physical therapy from the University of Minnesota. She received training in neurodevelopmental theory from the Bobaths in London. Ms. Fiterman has worked in a variety of clinical settings including a University-affiliated facility, a therapeutic preschool, a public school, and an acute care children's hospital. She has also served as a consultant in a state hospital for the mentally retarded and coordinated a neonatal intensive care unit follow-up clinic for five years.

MEREDITH HINDS HARRIS
is an Associate Professor in the Department of Physical Therapy at Northeastern University and a research associate at Boston University School of Medicine, Department of Pediatrics at Boston City Hospital, Boston, MA. She received her B.S. in physical therapy from the University of Connecticut, an M.S. from Hunter College, New York, and an Ed.D. from Teachers College of Columbia University in special education. She has published several articles and teaches continuing education workshops on motor deficits in children with HIV infection. She is a consultant to several early intervention and pediatric rehabilitation centers and continues her research and clinical practice with children affected by substance abuse and HIV infection.

REBECCA PORTER
is an Associate Professor and Director of the Graduate Program in Physical Therapy at Indiana University. She has a private physical therapy practice, presents continuing education workshops, and has published in the area of neurologic physical therapy. Dr. Porter received a B.S. in physical therapy, an M.S. in allied health education, and a Ph.D. in medical neurobiology from Indiana University.

JANET STERNAT
received her B.S. degree in physical therapy from the University of Wisconsin. Further certification and training include workshops in neurodevelopmental treatment, sensory integration, Feldenkrais, and joint mobilization. She is currently in private practice in pediatric physical therapy in western Wisconsin and Minnesota. Ms. Sternat also is a preceptor in the Physical Therapy Program at the University of Wisconsin - LaCrosse and Madison and St. Scholastica, Duluth, MN. She is involved in workshop training for therapists and paraprofessionals serving pediatric clientele.

SUSAN EFFGEN
is the Director of Pediatric Physical Therapy and Associate Professor of Orthopedic Surgery & Rehabilitation at Hahnemann University, Philadelphia. She received her B.S. in physical therapy from Sargent College of Allied Health Professions at Boston University, her MMSc in pediatric physical therapy from Emory University, and a Ph.D. in special education from Georgia State University. She started her research in postural control in 1974. She has taught at several universities and is co-founder of the Adaptive Learning Center for Infants and Children, Inc., Atlanta, Georgia.

RONA ALEXANDER
is a speech-language pathologist who specializes in the assessment and treatment of oral-motor and respiratory-phonatory-sound production functioning in infants and children with neuromotor involvement. She maintains a private practice, serves as a part time staff member in the Speech-Language Pathology and Audiology Department at the Children's Hospital of Wisconsin in Milwaukee, Wisconsin, and conducts continuing education workshops. Dr. Alexander teaches in basic 8-week N.D.T. courses and in advanced N.D.T. courses. She has contributed chapters to numerous publications in the areas of speech-language and pediatric assessment and habilitation. Dr. Alexander received a B.A. in speech pathology and audiology from Indiana University, an M.A. in speech pathology from New York University, and a Ph.D. in speech pathology from the University of Illinois at Urbana-Champaign.

JANET WILSON
received a B.S. and Certificate in physical therapy from the University of Michigan and an M.A. in College Teaching from the University of North Carolina (UNC) at Chapel Hill. She is an Adjunct Associate Professor in Physical Therapy at UNC and has a private practice in pediatrics in Hillsborough, NC. Ms. Wilson is the physical therapy consultant and Vice President of Kaye Products, Inc., adaptive equipment for children. She teaches continuing education workshops on various topics related to children with CNS dysfunction and has published in the area of cerebral palsy and related topics.

REGI BOEHME

received her B.S. in occupational therapy from Western Michigan University and is a certified occupational therapy instructor in neurodevelopmental treatment. She is currently in private practice in Milwaukee, Wisconsin and a clinic consultant to the Department of Orthopedic Surgery at the Medical College of Wisconsin. Mrs. Boehme has lectured extensively throughout North America on topics related to treatment of children and adults with neurologic impairments.

WENDY TADA

is an Assistant Professor in the Hawaii University Affiliated Program, University of Hawaii. Dr. Tada received her masters degree in physical therapy from Stanford University, her masters degree in public health from San Diego State University, and her Ph.D. in psychology from the University of California, San Diego.

SUSAN HARRIS

is an Associate Professor in the School of Rehabilitation Medicine at the University of British Columbia in Vancouver, B.C., Canada and an Adjunct Associate Professor in the Department of Orthopaedic Surgery & Rehabilitation at Hahnemann University in Philadelphia. In 1989, she was elected a Catherine Worthingham Fellow of the APTA. She currently serves on the Editorial Board of Physical Therapy as well as several other editorial boards. Her research interests include early diagnosis of cerebral palsy as well as the efficacy of early intervention strategies for infants and young children with developmental disabilities. She has published more then 70 articles and chapters, including several research articles involving the use of single subject design. Dr. Harris received a B.S. in physical therapy from Russell Sage College and a Ph.D. in special education from the University of Washington.

JOANELL BOHMERT

received her B.S. and M.S. in physical therapy from the University of Minnesota. She has extensive experience in public schools and currently is employed by Anoka-Hennepin Independent School District 11 in Minnesota. She is co-owner of Creative Solutions, which provides private consultation on special education issues. She currently is chair of the Practice Committee, for the Section on Pediatrics, American Physical Therapy Association.

TABLE OF CONTENTS

CHAPTER 1

CONCEPTS OF NEURAL ORGANIZATION AND MOVEMENT

Ann F. Van Sant, Ph.D., PT

◆

INTRODUCTION

Physical therapists apply principles of motor control, motor learning, and motor development when designing treatment programs for children with motor disabilities. Having studied these foundation sciences, therapists consciously or unconsciously subscribe to theories of how the nervous system is organized, and how individuals learn and develop motor skills. Theories then are used clinically to 1) select assessment tools that identify a child's impairments and disabilities, 2) set treatment objectives, and 3) plan and sequence treatment activities. In this chapter, new concepts of motor control and development are explored that are currently affecting the types of evaluations and treatment that physical therapists use with children. Later, in Chapter 3, concepts of motor learning are explored and applied to the treatment of children.

MOTOR CONTROL

The term motor control refers to processes of the brain and spinal cord that govern posture and movement. Therapists have gained their understanding of these control processes through courses in neurophysiology. Neurophysiologists commonly focused their

research on the neurophysiology of animal movement. Often their work focused on the chemical or electrical activity of single nerve cells or nuclei in order to understand the organization of spinal motor mechanisms and mechanisms of "higher control" which are mediated by various brain structures. These control processes typically occur in extremely short time periods, often in fractions of seconds. It should be recognized that while human posture and movement comprise behaviors that we can easily observe, the processes of motor control in people are not observable directly. This is because the functions of the brain and spinal cord are, even in this world of high technology, relatively hidden from view. As therapists, we have a long history of observing human movement, and much of what is known about patients' motor control is due to careful observation of posture and movement.

Neuroanatomists and neurophysiologists have studied the spatial (geographical) and temporal characteristics of central nervous system (CNS) organization. They sought specifically to understand which brain structures were involved in various postures and movements and how these structures contributed to motor control. The scientific interest in motor control is spreading and now includes a broader range of disciplines, including behavioral scientists who, like physical therapists, observe motor behavior and then apply inductive reasoning to make conclusions about "central processes" that underlie motor activity. The contributions of these behavioral scientists are beginning to greatly enrich our understanding of motor control.

We know that processes of motor control are not random. This is because postures and movements appear well organized. In fact, postures and movements are comprised of well defined patterns of action, and it is these action patterns that behavioral scientists and physical therapists can see and study to better understand the invisible internal control processes mediated by neural structures.

MOTOR DEVELOPMENT

In contrast to motor control, motor development refers to the processes of change in motor behavior that occur over relatively extended time periods. Typically these extended time periods are measured in units that reflect "age." The formal study of motor development originated in behavioral sciences, specifically psychology and clinical medicine. Yet psychologists and physicians were influenced strongly by the biological scientists who studied how the CNS controlled movement and thus there is affinity and overlap in classical thought about how the motor system develops and is controlled.[1]

Motor development, age related change in motor behavior, results from internal and external influences and often has been attributed to processes such as maturation, growth, or learning. From our background in biological science we, as physical therapists, acquire respect for the influences of growth and maturation which are commonly thought to be biological processes. On the other hand, we know that developmental change can be affected by environmental or external influences, such as learning or one's culture. Controversies and debate over which changes in motor behavior are due to maturation and which are due to learning are as old as developmental science.

More recently, maturation-learning or nature-nurture controversies have led to the recognition that interactions between internal and external influences cause developmental change. Yet, the ongoing controversies are an important force which have enabled a greater understanding of the intimate relationship of the individual to the world around him.

Debates over whether change in motor behavior is due to external influences, such as those brought about

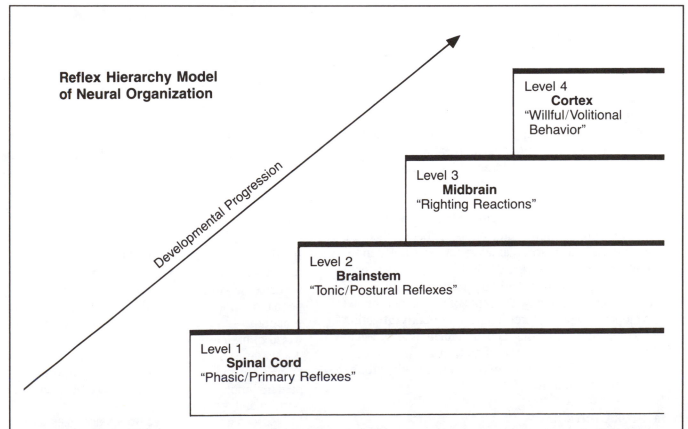

FIGURE 1. *The reflex hierarchy represents a traditional model of neural organization and development. A staircase of levels of neuro-anatomical structures and reflexive behaviors is surmounted with volitional behavior felt to be controlled in the cerebral cortex. Neuromotor development proceeds from Level 1 up to Level 4. Tests of reflexes and reactions help the therapist determine the child's level of neuromotor development.*

by a physical therapy program, or to maturational influences will continue. Through debate and research designed to settle these arguments, the process of motor development will be further understood and therapists will know better how to affect positive change in children's motor abilities.

Physical therapists observe motor behavior and use theories, models, and principles of motor control and development to help interpret their observations. Treatment programs then are designed based on a "model" or theoretical understanding of how the neuromotor system is organized and develops. This process rests on the premise that motor behavior is a reflection of CNS function. The accuracy of observations of a child's behavior and the models of neuromotor organization and development that are used to interpret these observations are critical. Let's examine how a model of neural organization and development affects what therapists think and do.

If the CNS is envisioned in a traditional way, as a hierarchy consisting of levels of reflexive responses (Figure 1) which ultimately is controlled at the highest level by volitional activity, then evaluation procedures consistent with this model will include reflex tests to determine the level of central nervous system function. If neuromotor development is envisioned as moving from reflexive to volitional control, then our reflexive test also may be used to interpret how far up the developmental staircase a child has progressed. The hierarchy of reflexes, derived principally from research in the basic neurosciences, is one model that is used to understand neuromotor development. This model has been commonly used by physical therapists to evaluate and interpret infants' and childrens' motor behavior in terms of "levels of neural organization and development."

The developmental reflex hierarchy also can be used to plan and sequence treatment. Having determined the "level of neurodevelopmental function" the goal of treatment is to progress the child to successively higher levels of reflexes and reactions. Motor tasks representing these higher levels become the progressive sequence of treatment activities. This example is used here only as a means of understanding how models and concepts of neural organization and development affect what a physical therapist thinks and does. Models and theories are somewhat simplified abstract representations of some more complex process. They are neither right nor wrong, true or false. Rather, theories and models should be judged by their usefulness in helping us 1) understand how the CNS is organized and develops, 2) design effective treatment procedures, and 3) predict how patients respond to treatment.

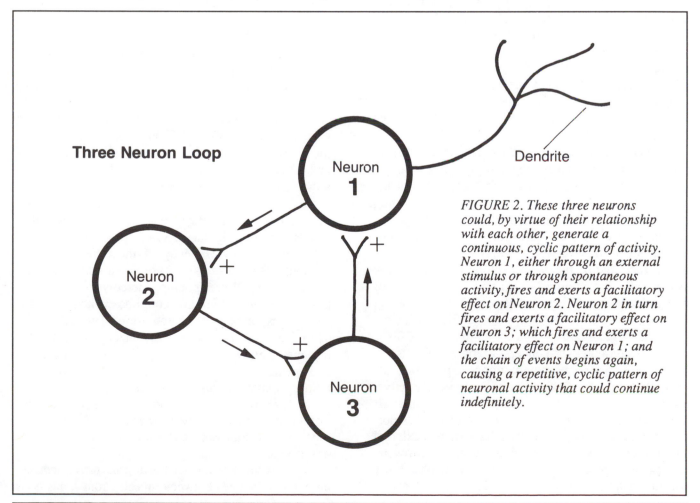

Three Neuron Loop

Neuron **1**

Dendrite

Neuron **2**

Neuron **3**

FIGURE 2. These three neurons could, by virtue of their relationship with each other, generate a continuous, cyclic pattern of activity. Neuron 1, either through an external stimulus or through spontaneous activity, fires and exerts a facilitatory effect on Neuron 2. Neuron 2 in turn fires and exerts a facilitatory effect on Neuron 3; which fires and exerts a facilitatory effect on Neuron 1; and the chain of events begins again, causing a repetitive, cyclic pattern of neuronal activity that could continue indefinitely.

In the past, brain function was modeled as a telephone switch-board with an operator sitting in the brain making connections between one brain region and another. The telephone switchboard model is now virtually forgotten and the computer serves as the "model" that helps us understand how the CNS functions. Because the variety of processes that can be represented, explained, and understood is greater when using a computer model of neural function than when using a telephone switchboard model, the computer model of the brain is currently quite popular. Models are simply tools for understanding and only should be judged relative to their accuracy and usefulness for illustrating how the CNS functions and responds to different influences. It is important to remember that models are not real. The brain is not a computer, but a computer can be used to illustrate various aspects of brain function. In the sections that follow, some newer concepts and models of neuromotor organization and development are presented that hold promise for an even more thorough understanding of the motor behaviors observed in children.

NEURAL ORGANIZATION AND DEVELOPMENT
THE ACTIVE ORGANISM CONCEPT

The CNS traditionally has been viewed as a system of reflexes arranged in a hierarchy of complexity with volitional processes dominating or controlling the reflexive base.[2] The parallel model of development portrays the infant as a passive, purely reflexive being, acting solely in response to the environment. Only when the cerebral cortex becomes mature and exerts its control over lower level reflexes is volitional behavior possible. This concept of the infant can be considered a "passive organism" concept.

Recently there has been an increasing tendency to recognize the active role of the CNS in the creation and control of body actions. From the "active organism" perspective the CNS is viewed as capable of anticipating the demands of the environment and planning ahead. We have regarded the CNS as the passive recipient of stimuli for so long, in accord with the reflex model of neural functioning, that we forget the CNS is a living system, and that activity is a primary characteristic of living things. The processes of planning, originating, and controlling motor acts require an active CNS. How can this active organism concept be modeled? This is where the computer and concepts of logical circuits can be helpful to portray neuromotor control processes. To understand how the CNS might be continuously active, a simple three neuron loop may be used to illustrate. If three neurons are arranged in a circle or loop as portrayed in Figure 2, it can be seen that either an external stimulus or the spontaneous firing of a single neuron, be it accidental or not, could create continuous activity within the loop. An ongoing cyclic pattern of neural

activity arises as an emergent property of the little system of three neurons.

Computer programmers make use of such "loop" concepts to instruct computers to complete repetitive functions. Recently loops such as this one have been employed by neuroscientists in models used to illustrate rhythmic repetitive neuromotor functions, such as the gait cycle, the suck-swallow of infant feeding, and other motor phenomena that were previously regarded as a simple chaining together of reflexes.[3,4]

With neuroscientists offering a plausible explanation for ongoing active processes within the CNS, the study of spontaneous behavior in infants has become of increasing interest for developmentalists.[5,6,7] Spontaneous, non-reflexive behaviors, previously ignored in scientific study, have become a focus for researchers interested in neurodevelopmental processes.

The active organism concept has caused therapists to question the traditional reflex hierarchy model. Physical therapists influenced by the view of the CNS as a passive mechanism developed models of evaluation and treatment consistent with this perspective. As our models are changing so are our evaluation and treatment procedures. Therapists are relying less on reflex tests to determine developmental "levels" of neural organization and control and are more often documenting motor behaviors that are self-generated by their patients.

THE CONCEPT OF A MOTOR PATTERN

In the past, the reflex was considered the fundamental unit of neuromotor behavior. That is, the reflex was regarded as the simplest form of movement and the foundation for all other forms of action. A reflex relies on an outside agent or force, called the stimulus, to generate motor behavior. Though easy to understand, the reflex is of limited usefulness in explaining movements that are not initiated by external stimuli. Neither volitional or spontaneous movements are dependent on external agents for their initiation. For this reason the reflex is not a useful concept if we wish to explain either spontaneous or voluntary action.

Despite the insufficiency of the reflex theory in explaining spontaneous and volitional movement, the reflex was useful in explaining stereotyped patterns of posture and movement that could be evoked with specific types of sensory stimulation. The reflex, by definition, encompasses a well organized patterned motor response. Reflex responses involve consistent temporal and spatial relationships among muscle groups. In a reflex, even the simplest stretch reflex, muscles are controlled in relation to one another (agonists to antagonists) and produce observable behaviors. These stable relationships among muscle groups are termed postural or movement "patterns." (See Chapter 8)

The concept of patterns of posture and movement, the observable linkages between muscle groups, has been long accepted by therapists.[8,9,10] These postural and movement patterns, however, commonly have been linked to specific stimuli, such as the flexor withdrawal response pattern associated with a noxious stimulus applied to the sole of the foot or tonic neck response patterns bound to specific movements of the neck.

These response patterns, dissociated or uncoupled from the stimuli that produce them, are examples of motor patterns. A motor pattern is simply the neural representation of a posture or movement that underlies action. The motor pattern specifies distinct temporal and spatial relationships between muscles. The concept of a motor pattern has a decided advantage over the concept of a reflex because the motor pattern is more versatile. The motor pattern need not be bound to a specific sensory stimulus. A motor pattern could be brought into action either by sensory stimuli or by internal processes within the CNS. When one considers the motor pattern as a basic unit of neuromotor organization rather than the reflex, it is possible to explain why, for example, there are so many different stimuli that can be used to evoke a specific movement pattern from an infant; or why a child with hemiplegia demonstrates the same movement pattern during both volitional effort and in response to a variety of sensory stimuli.

The motor pattern has been offered as a concept that represents the CNS's solution to the problem of controlling a multitude of muscles and joints throughout the body.[11,12,13] From a biomechanical perspective, the human body can be modeled as a series of rigid segments (such as an arm or a forearm) connected by joint structures that both permit and restrict motion between the links. In determining the number of degrees of freedom or possible cardinal plane movement combinations, beginning proximally at the shoulder girdle and moving distally to the terminal phalanx of a finger, it becomes obvious that the brain faces an enormous task to control so many possible movement combinations. By establishing functional linkages between groups of muscles, motor control becomes simplified. The terms "motor patterns," "motor synergies," and "coordinative structures" have been used to refer to the functional units of neuromotor organization that assure that the CNS need not construct motor acts anew each time there is a need or desire to move.

Milani-Comparetti,[14] a developmentalist, suggested that the motor pattern was the underlying neural basis for spontaneous action of fetuses observed through ultrasonography. When movements were first observed in the developing fetus, he was unable to identify stimuli that could be triggering the actions. Fetal movements appeared spontaneous, being generated by the CNS. According to Milani-Comparetti, it was later in the course of prenatal development that a link between sensory stimuli and the movements became evident. He termed the initial spontaneous actions "primary motor patterns" (PMPs). Later in fetal development, "primary automatisms" appeared. Primary automatisms were linkages between sensory stimuli and PMPs, and represented adaptations to the environment. Thus, the fetus was primarily active and secondarily responsive to the surrounding environment.

How are motor patterns formed? The traditional explanation has been that some motor patterns are "hard-wired" or pre-programmed genetically. Basic flexor and extensor motor patterns that are incorporated into the classic flexor and extensor reflex responses (flexor withdrawal and extensor thrust) commonly have been considered inherent motor patterns. These flexor and extensor movement patterns seem to be incorporated into the reflexive response to a variety of stimuli. Further spontaneous kicking movements of infants are in some ways similar to reflexive primary stepping movements.[15] As researchers begin to study infants' motor behavior from this viewpoint, motor patterns other than those characterized as reflexive responses, have received increasing attention.

Milani-Comparetti believed that a full complement of movement patterns are available and used appropriately in functional contexts prior to birth.[14] He reported that the fetus demonstrates a great repertoire of motor behaviors in utero: changing position; reaching, grasping, moving, releasing the umbilical cord when it brushes against the face; and moving into position in the birth canal in preparation for birth.

Why then do the motor abilities of the newborn seem so limited? Why should a fetus be considered so competent and a newborn appear so helpless? A plausible answer lies in the vast difference in the natural environments of the fetus and the newborn. Milani-Comparetti observed fetuses in utero, surrounded by amniotic fluid, and not experiencing the effects of gravity.[14] The prenatal and post-natal environments are drastically different. The newborn is experiencing the full force of gravity for the first time.

FEEDBACK AND ITS EFFECT ON A HIERARCHY OF MOTOR CONTROL

The newer concepts for understanding neuromotor function include motor patterns and the active organism that was modeled using a circular arrangement of neurons. In the circular arrangement, feedback is a fundamental property of the small system of neurons. Feedback is a very important aspect of a circular system of neurons. Its importance to motor control is likely only superseded by its importance in motor learning (see Chapter 3). Motor acts must be adaptable if favorable outcomes are to occur and feedback allows this adaptation. The process of modifying motor behavior to assure a more successful outcome requires that the results of actions be relayed back to the CNS. Feedback from lower centers of the CNS provide higher centers with information needed to plan subsequent actions.

Models of neural organization without feedback loops are termed "open systems" and are characterized by a single direction of transfer of information, input to output (Figure 3).[16] "Closed systems," on the other hand, are those that incorporate the concept of feedback and therefore provide the CNS control over actions that are to come. Feedback contributes to this control by providing the system with information regarding the results of action. Knowledge of the results of past action are needed in order to generate a modified action.

Although the idea of feedback is not new,[17] the effects of feedback loops on the traditional reflexive hierarchical model of neuromotor organization have not been fully recognized. Feedback loops, particularly those that link lower levels to the uppermost levels of a hierarchy, challenge the concept of hierarchical control. If information from lower levels is relayed to the top level of the control hierarchy (for example the cerebral cortex), and, as a result of this feedback, actions are modified, then what level of the system is really in control? (Figure 4) If an interneuron in the spinal cord provides information to the cortex concerning the state of a motor neuron and this information is used in modifying a subsequent motor act, then are not the interneuron and the motor neuron sharing in the control process? Can a model that provides feedback from the lowest to the highest level of control truly be hierarchical? Where does control reside in such a model? I would suggest that a "distributed control" model of neuromotor control can help resolve this dilemma.

THE CONCEPT OF DISTRIBUTED CONTROL

Rather than envisioning a fixed hierarchy with a top level devoid of feedback controlling motor behavior, consider a less rigid model that enables sharing of the control function as an alternative.[18,19] Indeed, the CNS increasingly is being modeled as a flexible complex of systems and subsystems that share information in the process of controlling motor behavior.[20] This is termed "distributed control." In a distributed control model, the "controller" varies.[18] A sub-system with the most relevant information concerning the status of the individual in the context of the situation would assume control. The sub-system would be given control as a function of both the individual's state and the environmental situation in which the individual is functioning. With systems and subsystems in the CNS sharing information, consensus can be reached concerning which system might best serve as the primary controller at a specific point in time.

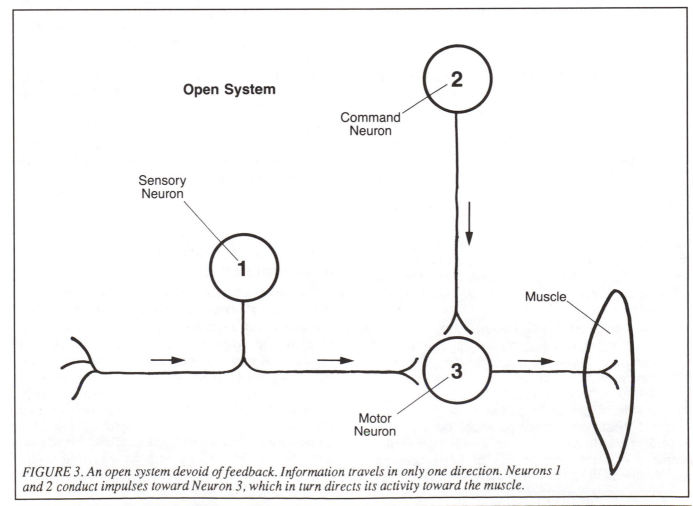

FIGURE 3. An open system devoid of feedback. Information travels in only one direction. Neurons 1 and 2 conduct impulses toward Neuron 3, which in turn directs its activity toward the muscle.

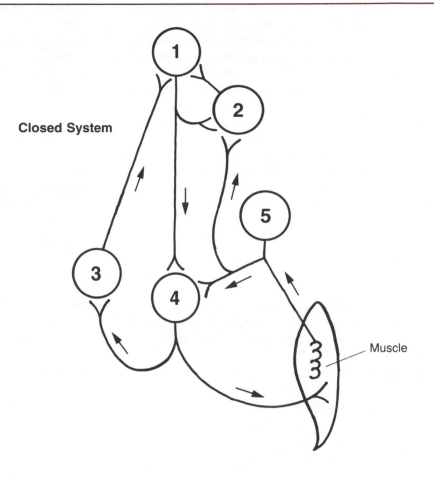

FIGURE 4. A closed-loop system with multiple feedback loops. Although Neuron 1 appears to be at the top of the hierarchy, and thus in command of the system, it is apparent on closer analysis that there is no hierarchy in this organizational arrangement of neurons. By inspecting Neurons 1 to 4, it is easy to see that each of these elements could conceivably be under control of at least one other neuron: Neuron 1 receives information from Neurons 2 and 3; Neuron 2 receives information from Neurons 1 and 5; and so on. Only Neuron 5 appears to be outside the sphere of other neurons. Neuron 5 is indirectly affected by the activity in Neuron 4.

Closed System

Muscle

COMPARING THE RESULTS OF ACTION WITH INTENTION AND ITS EFFECT ON MOTOR CONTROL

Not only is feedback an integral element of motor control but the capacity to compare the intended and the actual result of neuromotor activity is also necessary. Only through a process of comparison can unsuccessful actions be changed. Without feedback and comparison between intended and resultant actions, the CNS is destined to either repeat the same patterns without modification or to be totally dependent upon someone in the external environment to affect change in motor behavior. When the CNS is afforded the capacity to compare intention with outcome, an element of control is removed from the environment and the individual becomes less dependent on the external world for the correction of behavior. The individual need not wait for an external source to provide a correcting stimulus in order to change motor behavior. This awarding of control to the individual is profoundly influencing physical therapy. Therapists increasingly are recognizing the very active role patients must play in correcting their own behavior. They are encouraging patients to form their own judgements about how well they performed and helping them modify their motor behavior based on comparisons of self-generated feedback with the intended outcome. Children are capable of judging and correcting their actions and can be encouraged to do so.

The traditional concept of the infant as a reflexive being has kept us from fully recognizing the infant's ability to initiate and to continue action until a goal is attained: be it fussing until fed or changed, or swiping at an object until contacting it. This capability rests on the use of feedback to judge the result of action. Thus, it appears that even young infants have the basic organizational elements of motor control. These include the ability to initiate action, motor patterns that can be both self-initiated and brought into action in response to appropriate sensory conditions, and feedback processes to modify and adapt motor patterns in order to get along successfully in this world. With these basic elements of neuromotor organization in place, the infant is quite ready to begin to conquer the effects of gravity.

MEMORY

A fifth concept considered necessary for motor control is "memory." Successful motor acts include elements of pre-planning. For example, to be successful in a wheelchair transfer to a toilet, a child must position the chair in expectation of the activity that will follow, such as opening a door to a bathroom stall. The child must adjust the distance between his body and the door handle to successfully reach and pull the door open. The child needs to anticipate the arc of the door as it is opened. From where does this capacity to anticipate or predict the outcome of action arise? The ability to plan successful action is based in previous experiences. While practice usually is considered to be the reason for success, practice is more than just repeating an act over and over again. The key to the child's future motor success is the ability to use the results of one act to make the next motor act more successful. Key information related to the solution of the motor problem must be used in order to be successful in a situation not previously encountered. Commonly the theoretical construct of "memory" is used to explain how an individual benefits from prior experience. It has been theorized that practice permits the formation of memory structures [21,22] that can be used in novel situations. Storing the exact solution for every problem encountered would not enable transfer of motor abilities to a novel situation. What has been proposed is that general rules or "schema" [21] that specify the relationships among the conditions surrounding performance, the intended action, and the results of the action are stored in memory. These schema enable the individual to solve novel motor problems.

In summary, integral elements of motor control include: the CNS as a fundamentally active agent with the capacity to generate action; motor patterns as the fundamental unit of neuromotor behavior; the processes of feedback and comparison of intention and result which enable the modification of action; a distributed control system that delegates the control of behavior to the most appropriate subsystem; and memory structures such as schema that permit transfer of skills to new situations.

CURRENT ISSUES AND TRENDS IN MOTOR CONTROL AND MOTOR DEVELOPMENT THEORIES

A recent trend in motor control and development theories is embodied in the emergence of "dynamical systems theories" of control and development. [23,24,25,26] These theories have arisen from systems theory, particularly dynamical systems that operate in accord with the laws of thermodynamics. A good introduction to the basic theory of dynamical systems can be obtained by reading the popular book *Chaos: Making A New Science*. [27] Two dynamical systems theories are discussed below: Dynamical Pattern Theory, a theory of motor control, and Dynamical Action Theory, a theory of motor development.

DYNAMICAL PATTERN THEORY

"Dynamical Pattern Theory" developed by Kelso and his colleagues [22,24] proposes that there are general principles of motor coordination that can be used to explain the motor behavior of a variety of animal forms, including man. The theory includes two main ideas: "order parameters" and "control parameters." Order parameters are variables that incorporate the action of many of a systems subunits and can be used to characterize coordinated behavior of the system. For example, the timing of action between the two limbs during walking could be considered an order parameter. One might plot the position of the right and left feet with respect to each other to characterize a coordinated walking pattern. In fact, plotting of common kinematic variables such as positions, velocities, and accelerations across components of a coordinated system is a typical practice among dynamical system theory researchers. The convention of characterizing coordination through the so called order parameters is beginning to lead to quantitative measures of motor coordination. Such measures may be used in the future by therapists to evaluate their patients' coordination and to document the effect of therapy designed to change a patient's motor coordination. [28]

Dynamic Pattern Theory predicts that order parameters can be distinguished if one can identify variables or factors that can institute changes in patterns of action. Variables that initiate change in order parameters are termed "control parameters". For example, there are a variety of movement patterns that are used to rise to standing from the floor. [29] We have found that body weight influences movement patterns used to perform this task. [30] A recent investigation demonstrated that adding extra weight to individuals will cause the movement patterns to undergo qualitative change. [31] According to dynamical pattern theory, an order parameter for this task should change value when there is change from one form of rising to another. The change in an order parameter results when some critical value of a control parameter, proposed to be weight in this example, is reached.

Thelen has extended dynamical systems theory to motor development. [25,32] A basic assumption of Thelen's theory is that biological organisms are complex multidimensional systems. No single subsytem is more important in determining behavior than any other subsystem. In previous theories the CNS held a preeminent role in the determination of behavior. According to dynamical systems theory of motor development, organized behavior is an emergent property of the complex set of subsystems that constitute the individual, the environments surrounding the individual, and the task to be performed. Behavioral patterns represent a compression of the many degrees of freedom and infinite number of possible forms of action.

Thelen and her co-workers have studied the development of stepping and kicking in infants while exploring the reaches of dynamical systems theory. [33] According to reflexive theory, primary stepping behavior of infants disappears as a result of cortical maturation which enables inhibitory influences to be exerted over the spinal stepping reflex. Thelen and her colleagues in an elegant series of studies demonstrated that rather than cortical maturation, increasing weight of the lower limbs might be the reason why babies stopped stepping. [32]

Some behavioral patterns are more common than others. In dynamical systems terms these patterns are called attractors. Attractors are preferred patterns of the system. Attractors are further described as having deep or shallow attractor wells. Deep attractor wells can be used to portray behavior that is quite stable and relatively difficult to change. Shallow attractor wells are characteristic of behaviors that are easily changed.

Developmental change is brought about by control parameters reaching critical values that bring the system to a period of instability. During developmental transitions from one stable attractor state to another, individuals are particularly sensitive to control variables. During phase transitions very small influences can have very large effects on behavior. Transitions from one phase to another have been likened to a ball being balanced at the top of a hill. Just a slight puff of wind might determine the developmental outcome. A large effect that results from such a small change in a control parameter is a characteristic of non-linear dynamical systems. It is suggested that therapists be sensitive to phase transitions in their patients and try to discover the control parameter that is driving the system to new forms of behavior.

Previously, therapists tended to look for all explanations of developmental change in the CNS. Dynamical systems theory makes us aware of the role of many elements of the complex system of the child, the child's environment, and the motor tasks the child is required to perform. In dynamical systems theory terminology the CNS was the control parameter. Thelen's discovery that movement patterns of infants may vary as a function of the child's weight brings a whole host of interesting concepts to the forefront. As physical therapists we know that postural and movement patterns vary with age across childhood. One explanation for this observation is that the physical size of the body is changing with age and, therefore, motor patterns may reflect an appropriate, but temporary solution in the face of changing body dimensions. Thus, motor patterns used to accomplish a task, such as rising to stand, might vary not only as a result of practice, but also as a result of the relative size of different body segments. As the child grows and changes in relative body proportions, different motor patterns may serve as the most appropriate solution to the same task. As an example, envision a small three or four year old, who when asked to sit on the bed must first climb up on the mattress using both arms and legs to accomplish the task. That same child grown to adolescence, may sit on the bed directly from standing. Given that the bed has remained a stable object in the environ-

ment of the child, why have the movement patterns changed? It is difficult to deny that the older child by virtue of size alone is able to sit on the bed. The younger child, although he may have a motor pattern for sitting down, is confronted with a mattress of a relative height that does not allow sitting directly from standing. Variability in motor patterns may be brought about through changes in the relative size of an individual with respect to the environment. Yet, variability in motor patterns is not solely due to growth of an individual.

Children who are developing normally appear to vary their motor patterns for the sheer joy of the experience, and to learn about their bodies and their environments. Given that a child is able to throw an object, he experiments with throwing far, accurately, and as hard as possible. He throws not only balls, but anything that is throwable: books, food, a stool, and so forth. As a result of all this throwing, he learns of his body and his world. He learns about books, their weight, how they tend to open when thrown, and why books are not to be thrown. Food, although throwable, spatters about and also is not supposed to be thrown. Should he attempt to throw a stool, he discovers stools are not throwable, at least not when you are small. Several things result from all this throwing. The child learns to vary the throwing pattern to accommodate the objects, learns of the size, weight, and consistency of the objects, and learns socially acceptable behaviors, such as don't throw in the house. Young children also learn about their environment and their motor abilities by using an object to accomplish a variety of tasks.

For example, a large ball can be used to sit on, lie on, push, kick, roll, hug, and even stand on. Thus, an object can be used for purposes not necessarily in the mind of the inventor. The most popular toys are those that can be put to a variety of uses, and the most boring are those that can be used for but one activity. Think of the versatility of something as simple as a cooking pot. The young child plays for hours with containers or things that serve as containers, such as boxes, pots, bags, and pocketbooks. Things get put in, dumped, poured, thrown, and kicked into and out of these containers. Again, the child learns of the world about him and of his motor abilities in that world. This is where the rules relating the child's body to the environment are acquired. The young child initiates and varies the task out of curiosity and joy in seeing the effect of his actions on the world around him.

We must recognize that different phases in the human life span are characterized by different motor behaviors, different environments, and different demands on the neuromotor system. Infancy seems to be a period when fundamental laws about the body and the physical world are discovered. Early childhood is a time for expansion of motor abilities within the environment. Various forms of locomotion are acquired, such as running, hopping, skipping, jumping, riding tricycles, skating, and riding bicycles.

In addition, some degree of accuracy in fine motor tasks is demanded of children when they begin school. They must manage their clothes, draw, cut and paste, and begin to print letters and numbers. Children of school age begin to participate in games with other children that require the application of fundamental movements such as throwing, running, and catching. Children begin to acquire fine motor skills, particularly those that require control of small objects or tools, such as pencils, rulers, screw drivers, needles, and thread. Through motor abilities, children come to know their unique competencies. As children grow and develop, they participate in team or individual sports, select hobbies that enable achievement, and develop pride in their physical abilities. During this period, the ability to discriminate kinesthetic and visual cues and to modify behaviors become more discrete. The generalizability of motor activity appears to decrease. In late childhood, individuals tend to learn what they practice and attempt to improve. Spending hours with a joystick in front of a videoscreen will likely result in improved performance only in tasks that require speed and accuracy in control of a visual blip by means of a joystick. Eye-hand coordination will not improve in general. The videogame addict will not become a better pitcher or catcher in softball as a result of hours in front of the television. The motor patterns used for the latter tasks are entirely different than those required by the videogame. Having learned the rules of using the eyes to direct and control the path of the upper extremity during late infancy and early childhood, later childhood seems the time for taking pride in the degree of discrimination and subsequent control over very specific movement patterns. Over the course of infancy, childhood, and adolescence, sensory and motor subsystems develop at different rates and share in the control of motor behavior at different times. Likewise, the environments in which children function are changing with time. The relatively protected environments of infancy provided by the home or infant day care facility gradually are replaced by the nursery and school that require increasing responsibility and independence of children.

APPLICATION OF THE NEWER CONCEPTS OF MOTOR CONTROL AND MOTOR DEVELOPMENT TO THE EVALUATION AND TREATMENT OF CHILDREN

Having presented newer concepts of neuromotor control and development, the logical next step is to indicate how these ideas can be applied to the evaluation and treatment of the child with motor dysfunction. Evaluation of the child should incorporate the concepts presented in the first part of this chapter. We need to evaluate motor patterns, the child's spontaneous motor activity, and activity evoked by sensory stimuli or objects in the environment. We need to evaluate the child's ability to modify his motor behavior based on both external and internal feedback. We need to assess the child's ability to remember the rules for solving a motor problem. Finally, we should assess the environment, or environments, in which the child is expected to function.

As is frequently the case, concepts arising in the basic sciences lead to changes in clinical practice. As we explore the usefulness of the information embodied in these new models and ideas, concepts are refined, and standard evaluation procedures and treatment principles may be developed.

As a physical therapist, I attempt to help the child become motorically independent, capable of controlling and caring for his own body. I encourage the child to develop those processes that enable adaptation to changing environments. I teach not just motor skills, but how to learn motor skills. I am careful not to overly structure therapy sessions so that I totally direct and control the child's actions. I do not enforce adult standards of performance on the motor patterns used to achieve tasks nor do I unnecessarily restrict the tasks and objects to which motor patterns are applied. I no longer view the infant or child as passively waiting for my stimulation to develop and learn. I look for the inherent ability of each child to produce motor patterns spontaneously, as well as in response to my manipulations. I examine the child's environment for "control parameters" that might be influencing behavior. I attempt to foster in each child self-control as well as responsiveness to external demands.

I look for variability in the child's actions. It has been argued that variability in motor patterns is the essence of normalcy. Indeed, stereotypic motor behavior is a well recognized sign of pathology. For the child with cerebral palsy, one of the most significant findings of motor pathology is the lack of variability in motor behavior. That is, the same motor patterns are used repeatedly across a great variety of tasks. Variability in the child's motor behaviors needs to be fostered in therapy. To do this I am less prescriptive about which specific movement patterns the child uses to accomplish a motor task. No single "right" or "normal" way to move generalizes to all situations. Encouraging the child to explore movement options within a specific task enables the formation of rules that can be applied in future situations. I encourage the child to explore objects in the environment and how they can be used. Stairs can be used for so many different tasks, such as climbing, sitting, jumping, and sliding. Within each of these tasks, stairs afford a multitude of movement patterns, including climbing on hands and knees, climbing on hands and feet, standing on two feet, sitting with feet on the step below, or sitting sideways on the stair with legs extended. The child will explore these options if given the opportunity and encouragement.

Having recognized that different motor abilities are exhibited at different ages, I attempt to select age appropriate tasks. I realize that by school age, the child is expected to have acquired independence in mobility and basic elements of self care. I do my best to see that these expectations are met. I encourage the school age child to select tasks of interest and importance to him and encourage him to share in the responsibility for improving his motor performance and caring for his body.

I keep in mind that each child may be influenced by my attitude about his motor abilities. If a child's motor performance is judged against my standard of normalcy, and if the child's performance never meets my standard, the child may infer failure through my feedback. The child may eventually become totally dependent on external standards for judging his motor performance and, as a result, lose the desire and ability to acquire skills on his own. He may, therefore, never seek the experience of setting ever increasing demands on himself for the sheer pleasure of working to meet those demands. Thus, I encourage the school age child to participate in setting goals for treatment so that he might increasingly become an active, responsible, and competent individual. ❏

SUGGESTED READINGS

1. Anokhin PD: Systemogenesis as a general regulator of brain development. Prog Br Res 9:54-86, 1964
2. Arbib MA: The Metaphorical Brain: An Introduction to Cybernetics as Artificial Intelligence and Brain Theory. New York, NY, Wiley-Interscience 1972
3. Bruner JS: Organization of early skilled action. Child Dev 44:1-11, 1973
4. Eckert HM: A concept of force-energy in human development. Phys Ther 45:213-218, 1965
5. Frank LK: The cultural patterning of child development. In Falkner F (ed): Human Development. Philadelphia, PA, WB Saunders, 1966, pp 411-432
6. Holt K (ed): Movement and Child Development, Clinics in Developmental Medicine. No. 55. Philadelphia, PA, JB Lippincott, 1975
7. Hunt JMcV: Environmental programming to foster competence and prevent mental retardation in infancy. In Walsh RN, Greenough WT (eds): Advances in Behavioral Biology: Environments as Therapy for Brain Dysfunction. New York, NY, Plenum Press, 1976, vol 17, pp 201-255
8. Ianniruberto A, Tajani E: Ultrasonographic study of fetal movements. Sem Perinat 5:175-181, 1981
9. Kugler PN, Kelso JAS, Turvey MT: On the control and coordination of naturally developing systems. In Kelso JAS, Clarke JE (eds): The Development of Movement Control and Coordination. New York, NY, John Wiley & Sons, 1982, pp 5-78
10. Oppenheim RW: Ontogenetic adaptations and retrogressive processes in the development of the nervous system and behaviour: A neuroembryological perspective. In Connolly KJ, Prechtl HFR (eds): Maturation and Development: Biological and Psychological Perspectives, Clinics in Developmental Medicine, No. 77/78. Philadelphia PA, JB Lippincott, 1981, pp 73-109
11. Prechtl HFR (ed): Continuity of Neural Function from Prenatal to Postnatal Life, Clinics in Developmental Medicine, No. 94. Philadelphia, PA, JB Lippincott, 1984
12. Roberton MA, Halverson LE: Developing Children - Their Changing Movement: A Guide for Teachers. Philadelphia, PA, Lea & Febiger, 1984
13. Shephard RJ: Physical Activity and Growth. Chicago, IL, Yearbook Medical Publishers, 1982
14. Young JZ: Programs of the Brain. New York, NY, Oxford University Press, 1978

REFERENCES

1. McGraw MB: The Neuromuscular Maturation of the Human Infant. New York NY, Hafner Publishing Co, 1966
2. Wyke B: The neurologic basis of movement: A developmental review. In Holt KS (ed): Clinics in Developmental Medicine: Movement and Child Development. Philadelphia, PA, JB Lippincott, 1975, no 55, pp 19-33
3. Delcomyn F: Neural basis of rhythmic behavior in animals. Science 210:492-498, 1980
4. Grillner S, Wallen P: Central pattern generators for locomotion, with special reference to vertebrates. Ann Rev Neurosci 8:233-261, 1985
5. Connolly KJ: Maturation and ontogeny of motor skills. In Connolly KJ, Prechtl HFR (eds): Maturation and Development: Biological and Psychological Perspectives. Clinics in Developmental Medicine. No 77/78. Philadelphia, PA, JB Lippincott, 1981, pp 216-230
6. Prechtl HFR: The study of neural development as a perspective of clinical problems. In Connolly KJ, Prechtl HFR (eds): Maturation and Development: Biological and Psychological Perspective, Clinics in Developmental Medicine, No. 77/78. Philadelphia, PA, JB Lippincott, 1981, pp 198-215
7. Thelen E: Rhythmical stereotypes in normal human infants. Animal Behavior 27:699-715, 1979
8. Bobath B: Abnormal Postural Reflex Activity Caused by Brain Lesions, ed 3. Rockville, MD, Aspen Systems, 1985
9. Knott M, Voss DE: Proprioceptive Neuromuscular Facilitation: Patterns and Techniques, ed 2. New York, NY, Harper & Row, 1968
10. Stockmeyer SA: An interpretation of the approach of Rood to the treatment of neuromuscular dysfunction. Am J Phys Med 46:900-956, 1967
11. Bernstein N: The coordination and regulation of movement. New York, NY, Pergamon Press, 1967
12. Easton TA: On the normal use of reflexes. Am Sci 60:591-599. 1972
13. Kelso JAS (ed): Human Motor Behavior: An Introduction. Hillsdale, NJ, Lawrence Erlbaum Associates, 1982
14. Milani-Comparetti A: The neurophysiologic and clinical implications of studies on fetal motor behavior. Sem Perinat 5:183-189, 1981
15. Kamm K, Thelen E, Jensen J: A dynamical systems approach to motor development. Phys Ther 70:763-775, 1990
16. Stelmach GE: Motor control and motor learning: The closed-loop perspective. In Kelso JAS (ed): Human Motor Behavior: An Introduction. Hillsdale, NJ, Lawrence Erlbaum Associates, 1982, pp 93-115
17. Smith KU: Cybernetic foundations for rehabilitation. Am J Phys Med 46:379-467, 1967
18. Davis WJ: Organizational concepts in the central motor networks of invertebrates. In Herman RL, et al (eds): Advances in Behavioral Biology: Neural Control of Locomotion. New York, NY, Plenum Press, 1976, vol. 18, pp 265-292
19. Kilmer WL, McCollough WS, Blum J: A model of the vertebrate central command system. Int J Man-Machine Studies 1:279-309, 1969
20. Brooks VB: The Neural Basis of Motor Control. New York: Oxford University Press, 1986, pp 18-37
21. Adams JA: A closed loop theory of motor learning. J Motor Beh 3:149, 1971
22. Schmidt RA: A schema theory of discrete motor skill learning. Psy Rev 82, 225-260, 1975
23. Kelso JAS, Tuller B: A dynamical basis for action systems. In Gazzaniga MS, (ed): Handbook of Cognitive Neuroscience. New York, NY: Plenum Press, 1984, pp 321-356
24. Kugler PN, Turley MT: Information, Natural Law, and the Self-Assembly of Rhythmic Movements. Hillsdale, NJ: Lawrence Erlbaum Associates Inc, 1987
25. Schoner G, Kelso JAS: Dynamic pattern generation in behavioral and neural systems. Science 239:1513-1520, 1988
26. Thelen E, Kelso JAS, Fogel A: Self-organizing systems and infant motor development. Dev Rev 7:39-65, 1987
27. Gleick G: Chaos: Making a New Science. New York, NY: Penguin Press, 1987
28. Scholtz JP: Dynamic pattern theory — Some implications for therapeutics. Phys Ther 70:827-843, 1990
29. VanSant AF: Rising from a supine position to erect stance: description of adult movement and a developmental hypothesis. Phys Ther 68:185-192, 1988
30. VanSant AF, Sabourin PT, Luehring SK, et al: Relationships among age, gender, body dimensions and movement patterns in a righting task. Poster presentation at the 64th Annual Conference of the American Physical Therapy Association; June 11-15, 1989, Nashville, TN
31. Dehadrai LB: The effect of three levels of weight on the movement patterns used to rise from supine to standing. Philadelphia, PA: Temple University, 1991, Master's thesis
32. Thelen E: Dynamical approaches to the development of behavior. In Kelso JAS, Mandell AJ, Schelsinger ME, (eds): Dynamical Patterns in Complex Systems. Singapore, Republic of Singapore: World Scientific Publishing Co Pte Ltd, 1989, pp 348-362
33. Thelen E, Fisher DM: Newborn stepping: an explanation for a disappearing reflex. Dev Psy 18:760-775, 1982

CHAPTER 2

TESTS AND ASSESSMENT

Barbara H. Connolly, Ed.D., PT

◆

Testing has become an integral part of developmental therapists' practice. This trend has occurred due to several factors, such as the need for standardized testing for placement of children with disabilities in the appropriate classroom, the setting of criteria for therapy services in some school systems (e.g. 1.5 standard deviations below the mean), and the need for documenting efficacy of treatment. Testing using standardized or non-standardized tools is but a small part of the larger process known as assessment. Assessment of a child involves more than merely the administration of a test and is qualitative as well as quantitative.

Factors to be considered when assessing a child include current life circumstances, health history, developmental history, and extrapersonal interactions as well as other factors. Current life circumstances relate to the child's current health. If the child is not feeling well during the assessment, the examiner may not get an accurate picture of the child's abilities. Likewise, if the examiner is unaware of the attitudes and values of the child's immediate family, an inaccurate picture may be obtained. The family who values excellence in gross motor performance is more likely to have a child involved in motor activities than the family who values

excellence in fine motor activities. The acculturation of the child would also play a major role in the assessment. If the child has never seen a yellow tennis ball, but has seen yellow apples, he is apt to try to eat the ball rather than toss it.

The child's health history is an important factor in the acquisition of certain motor skills. The child who has had poor health or nutrition is apt to be delayed in the acquisition of skills such as sitting, creeping, and walking. Delays in overall development may be seen if the child has a history of repeated hospitalizations.

Examination of the child's developmental history is important in determining the child's past rate of achievement of developmental milestones and in deciding what performance might be expected in the future. Even with the best intervention, the child who progressed only 2 months in gross motor skills during a 12 month period may not progress 12 additional months during the next 12 month period. The developmental history also allows the therapist to identify events that might have had profound effects on the child, either physically or psychologically.

Extrapersonal interactions to be considered during the assessment include the reaction of the child to the

---

Therapeutic Exercise In Developmental Disabilities   *15*

examiner and the conditions under which the child is observed. Some children do not perform well because they refuse to separate from the parent or they refuse to cooperate with the examiner. Other children are able to perform well under all circumstances and with any examiner. Some children will perform in a familiar surrounding, such as the home, but refuse to cooperate in the school or clinical setting. The interpretation of the child's performance, particularly if these extrapersonal interactions are operating must be tentative.

PURPOSES OF ASSESSMENT

Assessment may be done for screening, placement of the child into an appropriate therapy program, program planning, program evaluation, or assessment of individual progress. Tests such as the Denver Developmental Screening Test or the Bruininks Oseretsky Test of Motor Proficiency may be administered to large groups of children to determine which children need further evaluation of their developmental skills. Norm referenced tests, those standardized on groups of individuals, must be used in the screening process to determine if a child's performance is typical of a child of a similar age. Norm referenced tests also should be used when using assessment as a means of determining the appropriate placement of the child in a special service. Norm referenced tests allow the examiner to determine the exact developmental age of the child and to compare the child's performance to the performance typically expected.

Program planning is an important aspect of managing the child with a disability. The therapist must assess the level of the child's current functioning and then plan activities that will help the child progress in his abilities. A criterion referenced test, one that measures a child's development of particular skills in terms of absolute levels of mastery, may be very appropriate for such program planning. Items on the criterion referenced tests may be linked directly to specific instructional objectives and therefore facilitate the writing of behavioral objectives for the child. The use of selective items from a norm referenced test to develop behavioral objectives should be discouraged since this may lead to "teaching the test" and developing splinter skills. Assessment of the child's progress using the same criterion referenced test used for program planning is appropriate since the examiner wishes to determine if the child has achieved mastery of certain skills. Norm referenced tests may be used but the tests should be used only once or twice yearly so that "teaching the test" does not occur. Overall program evaluation may be an important purpose of assessment. If one is comparing a new method of teaching gross or fine motor skills with a current method, assessment of the children in each group using a norm referenced test would be imperative. The thera-

pist would need to be able to compare the overall performance of each group with their peers as established by the norm referenced tests.

NORM REFERENCED VERSUS CRITERION REFERENCED TESTS

The purposes of norm referenced and criterion referenced tests were described briefly in the preceding section. More delineation, however, needs to be made between the two types of tests. As previously stated, norm referenced tests have standards or reference points which represent average performances derived from a representative group. Criterion referenced tests have reference points which may not be dependent on a reference group. In other words, with criterion referenced tests, the child is competing against himself, not a reference group. Norm referenced tests may not overlap with actual objectives of instruction, whereas, criterion referenced tests are directly referenced to the objectives of instruction. Therefore, norm referenced tests may not be as sensitive to the effects of instruction as criterion referenced tests.

Norm referenced tests must meet minimal standards of reliability and validity before being widely accepted. As with other tests, tests of motor abilities should be both reliable and valid. Reliability refers to the consistency between measurements in a series. Types of test reliability include alternate forms, inter-rater, split-half, and test-retest. Alternate forms reliability assesses the relationship of scores by an individual on two parallel forms of the test. The Miller Analogy Tests are a good example of alternate form reliability in which scores obtained by the same individual on the two forms of the test are highly correlated. Inter-rater reliability examines the relationship between items passed and failed between two independent observers. Split-half reliability is the measure of internal consistency of a test. The test is split into two halves and the scores obtained on the two halves by the individual are correlated. Test-retest reliability refers to the relationship of an individual's score on the first administration of the test to his score on the second administration. Test-retest reliability scores may be adversely affected by practice or memory. Validity is the extent to which a test measures what it purports to measure. For example, the Bruininks Oseretsky Test of Motor Proficiency is valid for measuring gross and fine motor proficiency, but not developmental reflexes or muscle tone. Three types of validity, construct, content, and criterion, are used to assess the viability of a test. Construct validity examines the theory or hypothetical constructs underlying the test. For example, the Gesell Developmental Schedules are based on the theory that children with motor delays can be identified using the scales. Content validity refers to test appropriateness, or how well the content of the test samples the subject matter or behaviors about which conclusions are to be drawn. The specific items on the test must be representative of the behaviors to be assessed. Construct and content validity are not determined using single measures of correlation but are determined by examining the results of the tests. Criterion related validity is measured by examining concurrent validity and predictive validity. Concurrent validity represents the relationship of the performance on the test with performance on another well reputed test. Predictive validity examines the relationship of the test to some actual behavior of which the test is supposed to be predictive. For example, delays on the Gesell Scales of Development should be predictive of future delays.

NEWBORN DEVELOPMENTAL AND SCREENING ASSESSMENTS

Neurological Assessment of the Preterm and Full Term Infant.

The Neurological Assessment of the Preterm and the Full Term Infant was developed by Dubowitz and Dubowitz to be suitable for use by staff without expertise in neonatal neurology, to be used with preterm and full term infants, administered in a short period of time, and repeated as the infant matures.[1] The repeatability of the test is important to the examiner because this allows comparison of the preterm infant after birth with newborn infants of corresponding postmenstrual age. The test documents deviations in neurologic signs and their eventual resolution.

Test items are drawn from the assessment tools of Saint-Anne Dargassies,[2] Prechtl,[3] Parmelee,[4] and Brazelton.[5] Scoring of the items is done on a five-point ordinal scale. All of the items do not have to be administered with each child and no single total score is achieved. The pattern of responses, however, is examined and compared with case histories described in the test manual. No reliability information is reported on the scale by the authors. Concurrent validity was determined by comparing the results on the scale with ultrasound scans used to detect intraventricular bleeds. The results revealed that 24 of 31 infants born at less than 36 weeks gestation with ultrasound evidence of a bleed had three or more abnormal clinical signs out of six items administered, as compared with only 2 of 37 infants of the same gestational age without evidence of intraventricular bleeds.[1] Of the 37 infants without evidence of intraventricular bleeds, 21 had no abnormal clinical signs as compared with only 1 of the 31 infants with documented bleeds. No studies on predictive abilities of this test are currently available.

Brazelton Neonatal Behavioral Assessment Scale

The Brazelton Neonatal Behavioral Assessment Scale (BNBAS) was developed by Brazelton in 1973 as a behavioral scale for infants from birth to the approximate postterm age of 1 month.[5] A second edition of the BNBAS was published in 1984.[6] (Figure 1) Changes made in the original version of the BNBAS will be included where appropriate in the following description of the scale. The BNBAS is not considered a neurologic assessment, although it contains some neurologic items as outlined by Prechtl. Prechtl, however, stated that the BNBAS reflex items are inadequate to assess neural intactness or impairment. He also stated that the assessment of the reflexes used in the BNBAS is not the same as what he originally described.[7] The BNBAS includes assessment of the infant's state of consciousness as an important element. The infant's use of state to maintain control of his reactions to environmental and internal stimuli is thought to be an important mechanism reflecting the infant's potential for organization of sensory input. For each of the behavioral items, the appropriate state of consciousness for testing is indicated. State specifications are delineated for several of the test items in the second edition.

The original BNBAS contained 26 biobehavioral items and 20 reflex items. The revised BNBAS contains 27 biobehavioral items with decrement in response to inanimate visual and auditory stimuli added to the 26 original items. Items on the BNBAS were developed to assess the neonate's ability to organize states of consciousness, habituate reactions to disturbing events, attend to and process simple and complex environmental events, control motor activity and postural tone, and perform integrated motor acts. Nine new optional supplementary items are included in the second edition. The supplemental items are needed when applying the concepts of behavioral organization to preterm or fragile infants and address the quality of alert responsiveness, cost of attention, examiner persistence, general irritability of the neonate, robustness and endurance, regulatory capacity, state regulation, balance of muscle tone, and reinforcement value of the infant's behavior. The supplemental items were prompted by ideas from the Assessment of Preterm Infant Behavioral Scale[8] and the BNBAS with Kansas supplements (BNBAS-K).[9] Each of the biobehavioral items is scored individually according to the criteria given in the test manual. The mean score for each item is based on the behavior exhibited by an average full term (7 pounds), normal, Caucasian infant with an APGAR of no less than 7 at one minute and 8 at five minutes and whose mother did not have more than 100 mg of barbiturates for pain or 50 mg of other sedative drugs as premedication in the 4 hours prior to delivery. The initial test is done ideally on the

Behavioral and Neurological Assessment Scale

Infant's name

Sex		Age	
Mother's age		Father's age	

Examiner(s)

Conditions of examination:

Birthweight

Time examined

Time last fed

Type of delivery

Length of labor

Type, amount and timing of medication given mother

Initial state: observe 2 minutes

1	2	3	4	5	6
deep	light	drowsy	alert	active	crying

Predominant states (mark two)

| 1 | 2 | 3 | 4 | 5 | 6 |

Date		Hour	
Born			

Father's S.E.S.

Apparent race

Place of examination

Date of examination

Length

Head circ.

Type of feeding

Apgar

Birth order

Anesthesia?

Abnormalities of labor

Elicited Responses

	O*	L	M	H	A†
Plantar grasp		1	2	3	
Hand grasp		1	2	3	
Ankle clonus		1	2	3	
Babinski		1	2	3	
Standing		1	2	3	
Automatic walking		1	2	3	
Placing		1	2	3	
Incurvation		1	2	3	
Crawling		1	2	3	
Glabella		1	2	3	
Tonic deviation of head and eyes		1	2	3	
Nystagmus		1	2	3	
Tonic neck reflex		1	2	3	
Moro		1	2	3	
Rooting (intensity)		1	2	3	
Sucking (intensity)		1	2	3	
Passive movement		1	2	3	
Arms R		1	2	3	
L		1	2	3	
Legs R		1	2	3	
L		1	2	3	

O* = response not elicited (omitted)
A† = asymmetry

Descriptive paragraph (optional)

Attractive	0	1	2	3
Interfering variables	0	1	2	3
Need for stimulation	0	1	2	3

What activity does he use to quiet self?

hand to mouth

sucking with nothing in mouth

locking onto visual or auditory stimuli

postural changes

state change for no observable reason

COMMENTS:

Behavior Scoring Sheet

Initial state

Predominant state

Scale (Note State)	1	2	3	4	5	6	7	8	9
1. Response decrement to light (1,2)									
2. Response decrement to rattle (1,2)									
3. Response decrement to bell (1,2)									
4. Response decrement to tactile stimulation of foot (1,2)									
5. Orientation—inanimate visual (4,5)									
6. Orientation—inanimate auditory (4,5)									
7. Orientation—inanimate visual and auditory (4,5)									
8. Orientation—animate visual (4,5)									
9. Orientation—animate auditory (4,5)									
10. Orientation—animate visual and auditory (4,5)									
11. Alertness (4 only)									
12. General tonus (4,5)									
13. Motor maturity (4,5)									
14. Pull-to-sit (4,5)									
15. Cuddliness (4,5)									
16. Defensive movements (3,4,5)									
17. Consolability (6 to 5,4,3,2)									
18. Peak of excitement (all states)									
19. Rapidity of build-up (from 1,2 to 6)									
20. Irritability (all awake states)									
21. Activity (3,4,5)									
22. Tremulousness (all states)									
23. Startle (3,4,5,6)									
24. Lability of skin color (from 1 to 6)									
25. Lability of states (all states)									
26. Self-quieting activity (6,5 to 4,3,2,1)									
27. Hand-to-mouth facility (all states)									
28. Smiles (all states)									
29. Alert responsiveness (4 only)									
30. Cost of attention (3,4,5)									
31. Examiner persistence (all states)									
32. General irritability (5,6)									
33. Robustness and endurance (all states)									
34. Regulatory capacity (all states)									
35. State regulation (all states)									
36. Balance of motor tone (all states)									
37. Reinforcement value of infant's behavior (all states)									

FIGURE 1. *Scoring sheet from the Brazelton Neonatal Behavioral Assessment Scale — 2nd Edition. From: Brazelton TB: Neonatal Behavioral Assessment Scale. ed. 2. Philadelphia, PA, JB Lippincott, 1984. — Reprinted by permission*

third day after birth since the infant may be disorganized during the first 48 hours.[5] The scoring of the infant's performance is different from many other standardized assessment procedures in that the scores are based on the best, not the average performance. The clinical uses for the BNAS that have been advocated are: screening infants for behavioral or motor problems, educating parents about the infant's development and behavior, assessing what impact the infant's behavior will have on parent-infant bonding, planning behavioral or motor interventions, providing a behavioral and motor baseline, and objectively monitoring the medical status of infants with neurologic insults.[5]

Reliability studies on the BNBAS are limited. Inter-rater reliability is stated to be high if one completes training at one of the six training sites (Boston, Chapel Hill, Portland, Seattle, San Francisco, and Lawrence, Kansas). Sameroff and colleagues found low test-retest relationships between days 2 and 3 in a group of full term infants.[10] Test-retest reliabilities, however, may be affected by changes in the infant's chronological age, behavioral state, and internal physiologic state. Brazelton stated that the testing outcome may be dependent on physiologic variables such as hunger, nutrition, degree of hydration, and time within the wake/sleep cycle.[5]

Predictive validity of the BNBAS as reported by Brazelton is not well researched. In an investigation by Tronick and Brazelton involving 53 children, the BNBAS was found to be superior to a standard neurologic examination given during the neonatal period.[11] The BNBAS also has been used to predict mental and motor scores on the Bayley Scales of Infant Behavior with correlation scores of .67 to .80.[6] Bakow and colleagues reported good correlations between the BNBAS items of alertness, motor maturity, tremulousness, habituation, and self quieting with infant temperament at 4 months.[12] Since the ability to detect developmental changes during the neonatal period is an important attribute of any assessment instrument, the prognostic value of the BNBAS may be enhanced by repeated testing of the infant.

SCREENING INSTRUMENTS

Denver Developmental Screening Test

The Denver Developmental Screening Test (DDST) was developed in 1967 by Frankenburg and Dodds to identify developmental delays in infants and young children.[13] The test was standardized on 1036 normal children in the Denver area using a cross section of the population. The authors stated that the test can be used with children throughout the United States even though the standardization was done using a limited number of children in only one geographic location. The test was designed to be administered to children from birth to six years of age. The test is administered with ease and speed and lends itself to serial evaluations of the children on the same scoring sheet. As a developmental screening device, it is valuable in screening asymptomatic children for possible problems, in confirming clinical suspicions with an objective measure, and in monitoring high risk children. The DDST, however, should never be substituted for a diagnostic evaluation or a physical examination.

The test relies on the observations of what a child can and cannot do and on reports by a parent. Only those test items identified by an "R" on the score sheet can be passed by report of the parent. Direct observation should be used whenever possible. For the younger child, testing may occur while he sits on the parent's lap. The materials needed for testing are included in the test kit and are used to insure that the test remains standardized. A skein of red wool, box of raisins, rattle with a narrow handle, small bottle with a 5/8 inch opening, bell, tennis ball, and 8 one-inch cubical colored counting blocks are included in the test materials. (Figure 2) The steps in administering the test include determining the child's chronological age and drawing a vertical line on the score sheet to represent his age. For preterm infants, the corrected age must be used on the score sheet. All items on the test through which the age line passes should be administered. Additionally, the examiner should be certain that the child has several passes to the left of any failure on the test. All four categories, Personal-Social, Fine Motor - Adaptive, Language, and Gross Motor, should be assessed for each child. Each of the items in the four categories are designated by a bar which is located under the age scale to indicate the ages at which 25%, 50%, 75%, and 90% of the standardization population performed the particular test item. Failure to perform an item passed by 90% of children of the same age should be considered significant. Several failures in any category are considered abnormal. Each individual item should be scored (P) for pass, (F) for fail, (R) for refuse, or (NO) for no opportunity to administer. A delay is any item failed which is completely to the left of the age line. Validity, stability and reliability of the original DDST were established by the authors on more than 20,000 children.[14-15] A deterrent to use of the test was thought to be the time required to screen each child. To alleviate this problem, the revised Denver Developmental Screening Test was developed in 1981.[16] The revised edition also allows for a more accurate portrayal of the dynamic process of development over time. Both the original and revised DDST should be viewed as tapping only a limited number of developmental skills and should not be viewed as identifying all children who may eventually have a developmental problem. Since development is an ongoing dynamic process, periodic rescreening of the child is highly recommended.

Milani-Comparetti Motor Developmental Screening Test

The Milani-Comparetti Motor Developmental Screening Test originally was developed by two Italian child neurologists, Milani-Comparetti and Gidoni, in 1964 and published in 1967.[17] The test was further adapted by Meyer's Children's Rehabilitation Institute and published in a slightly different format in 1978.[18] The adaptation will be described in this section. (Figure 3)

The purpose of the test is to evaluate motor development in relation to the emergence and disappearance of primitive reflexes and the sequential development of higher patterns of movement and postural control.[18] Information from the test allows for the documentation of developmental delays hypothesized to be the result of central nervous system dysfunction in children from birth to about two years of age.

The test manual has complete instructions for standardization of administration. Although training seminars are not necessary, therapists should follow the exact procedures as outlined in the test manual. The manual provides information on two types of scoring: the type originally suggested by Milani-Comparetti and Gidoni and the type suggested by the Meyer's Children's Rehabilitation Institute. The individual test items are to be graded pass (either by direct observation or by parental report if the child is uncooperative) or fail. The graphic scoring chart allows ease of understanding at a glance if the child is scoring above or below his age line. No special equipment is needed for the testing except for a tilt board. A regular table and mat are needed.

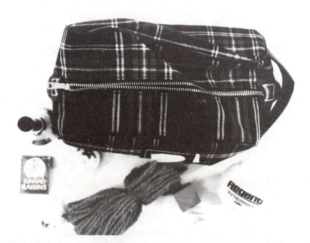

FIGURE 2. Testing kit for the Denver Developmental Screening Test.

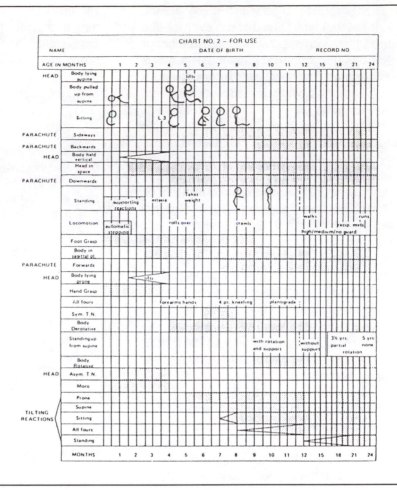

FIGURE 3. Scoring sheet for the Milani-Comparetti Motor Development Screening Test. From: Trembeth J: The Milani-Comparetti Motor Development Screening Test. Omaha, NE, University of Nebraska Medical Center Print Shop, 1978. — Reprinted by permission

The original Milani-Comparetti screening tool was developed based on clinical observations of normally and abnormally developing babies over a five year period.[17] Certain motor behaviors that were considered to be interrelated and which had a relationship between functional motor achievement and underlying structures of motor behaviors were included in the resulting testing instrument. Specific test items were included because they were able to document whether a particular motor response was emerging, present, or inhibited.

Data on standardization, reliability, and validity are limited on the Milani-Comparetti. This lack of information is a major weakness and may account for the test's limited use by therapists today. VanderLinden in a retrospective study, examined the predictive validity of the Milani-Comparetti for a small sample of fifteen high risk infants.[19] The analyses of the data revealed that the accuracy of the tool in predicting motor outcome in these infants at two and three years of age was low. VanderLinden suggested that the Milani-Comparetti be used primarily to document motor behavior in young children but not to classify the child as having a neuromotor disorder. Recently, Stuberg, White, Miedaner, and Dehne assessed the level of inter-rater and test-retest reliability of the Milani-Comparetti using sixty normal children between the ages of 1 through 16

months.[20] They reported that inter-rater percentage of agreement for the individual items on the test ranged from 79 to 98%. Test - retest agreement ranged from 80 to 100%. Therefore, acceptable inter-rater and test-retest reliabilities were found for all items on the assessment tool using normal children. No children with abnormal development, however, were used in the study and generalizability of the results to the clinical setting may be questioned. The major strengths of the test are in the ease and cost of administration.

Movement Assessment of Infants

Developed by Chandler, Swanson, and Andrews in 1975, the Movement Assessment of Infants (MAI) was created out of a need for a uniform approach to the evaluation of high risk infants.[21] Providing a detailed and systematic appraisal of motor behaviors during the first year of life, the MAI evaluates muscle tone, primitive reflexes, automatic reactions, and volitional movements and yields a record of the infant's observed behavior. The MAI has not been normed, instead a profile for normal motor behavior of a four month old infant has been developed. Children used in establishing the profile were Caucasian with only a few exceptions (Orientals). Apparently no blacks were included. Scores for each item on the MAI have been designated as normal or questionable for a four month old infant. When an infant receives a questionable score, a high risk point is given. High risk points are then totalled for each of the four sections and combined for a high risk score. The ratings of normal and questionable were determined by the authors on the basis of educational experience, review of the literature, and clinical pediatric experience. [19]

The value of the high risk score was studied using 35 infants at four months and then at twelve months of age. Twenty-seven of the children had normal movement at one year of age while eight were diagnosed as having cerebral palsy. Twenty-three children with normal movement received high risk scores of 0-7 at four months while six children with cerebral palsy received scores of 13-26. Four normal children and two with cerebral palsy received scores of 8-13. Therefore, if infants with high risk scores of eight or higher had been diagnosed as having cerebral palsy at four months, an incorrect identification of four children would have been made. No child with cerebral palsy, however, would have been incorrectly identified as normal. Three of the mid-range normal children received high risk points on the section on muscle tone due to low or variable tone.

Inter-rater reliability was assessed by the authors after development of the instrument and inter-rater reliabilities of 90 or above were stated to be regularly achieved. A more recent study, however, yielded an inter-rater reliability of 0.72 and a 0.76 test-retest reliability. [22] Haley et al examined item inter-rater and intra-rater reliability for each of the 65 individual items of the MAI using a sample of 53 high- and low-risk 4-month-old infants. [23] A sub-sample of 29 infants was assessed within one week of the initial test. Using percent agreement and the Kappa statistic, 2% of the items had Kappa coefficients with excellent inter-rater reliability and 58% had fair to good inter-rater reliability. Forty percent of the items had poor inter-rater reliability. Ten percent of the items had excellent intra-rater reliability, 42% had fair to good intra-rater reliability and 48% of the items had poor intra-rater reliability. These findings certainly distract from the reliability of use of certain items in the test as well as illustrating the need for revisions to the test items. Schneider, Lee, and Chasnoff expressed similar concerns about the use of the MAI in 1988. [24] In a sample of fifty 4-month-old infants, 30% of the infants were found to have total risk scores greater than seven which differed significantly from the 15% of infants used in the original Movement Assessment of Infants profile. Based on these findings, Schneider, Lee, and Chasnoff suggested that the current Movement Assessment of Infants profile may not reflect accurately normal motor behavior of healthy four month old infants and that more extensive data collection on healthy and high risk infants is warranted in order to develop an adequate profile. Darrah et al found that infants who were born at

less than 32 weeks gestation using the current MAI risk profile will likely accrue more high risk points than expected due to the variability of their responses. [25] They urged that caution be used in overdiagnosing these normal variations as abnormal responses in this group of high risk infants.

Bruininks Oseretsky Test of Motor Proficiency

The short form of the Bruininks Oseretsky Test of Motor Proficiency can be used for screening purposes, such as early identification of motor problems. Discussion on the use of the Bruininks Oseretsky will be included in the section on comprehensive developmental testing.

COMPREHENSIVE DEVELOPMENTAL TESTS

Bayley Scales of Infant Development

The Bayley Scales of Infant Development (BSID) is the product of several years of revisions, renorming, and expansions. The 1958-1960 version of the test drew heavily from three scales which are now out of print: the California First Year Mental Scale, the California Preschool Mental Scale, and the California Infant Scale of Motor Development. These three scales were reviewed, then deletions, modifications, or additions of other items were made. The first attempt at revising the scales was in 1958, but this version was unpublished and only covered the first 15 months of life. The second attempt resulted in the publishing of the test in 1960. The BSID was again revised, renormed, and expanded to its current form in 1969. [26] The 1958-1960 version of the mental and motor scales was administered to a national sample of 1400 children between the ages of 1 to 15 months and 160 children between the ages 18 and 30 months. A new revision of the test was published in 1969 and was normed on a national sample of 1262 normal children ranging in age from 2 to 30 months. [26] Both samples were controlled for sex, race, residence, and education of the head of the household and were selected according to the national proportions for these characteristics according to the 1960 U.S. Census of Population. In the most recent norming, the greatest discrepancy occurred in the residence variable with rural children tending to be under-represented. Additionally, the only significant difference between ethnic groups represented was the consistent tendency for black children to obtain slightly superior scores on the motor scale from 3 to 14 months of age. The Mental Scale of the BSID is designed to assess the following: sensory-perceptual acuities, discriminations, and the ability to respond to these; the early acquisition of "object constancy" and memory, learning and problem solving ability; vocalizations and the beginnings of verbal communication; and the early evidence of the ability to form generalizations and classifications. [26] All of these are thought to be the basis of abstract thinking. Scoring of the Mental Scale yields a Mental Development Index (MDI) for the child. The Motor Scale is designed to measure degree of control of the body, coordination of the large muscles, and finer manipulatory skills of the hands and fingers. Information from this scale is expressed as a Psychomotor Development Index (PDI). The mean standard score for each of the indexes for all age ranges is 100 with a standard deviation of 16 points. The indexes derived from the mental and motor scales have limited value in the prediction of later abilities, as the rates of development for any given child may be highly variable. The primary value of the scores is to provide a basis for establishing the child's current status and for instituting early corrective measures. In addition to the Mental and Motor Scales, the BSID contains an Infant Behavior Record which is to be completed after the other scales have been administered. The Infant Behavior Record helps assess the nature of the child's social and objective orientations toward his environment as expressed in attitudes, interests, emotional energy, activity, and tendencies to approach or withdraw from stimulation.

The test manual for the BSID provides in-depth explanations of how the test is to be administered. Additionally, all materials needed for administration of the test, except for facial tissues, stairs, walking board, and stopwatch are included in the test kit. Examiners using the BSID should be familiar with the BSID materials and procedures, be able to relate well and easily to mothers and children, and have a background in the theory of measurement and interpretation of test results. [26]

Scoring is done on each item and the activity is rated as passed, failed, omitted, refused, or reported by mother. Only those items noted as passed are credited in the scoring. In addition to the establishment of the MDI and PDI, the basal level (age level represented by the item preceding the earliest failure) and the ceiling level (age level represented by the highest success) should be reported for each child as a range of his abilities. In using the MDI, an intelligence quotient (IQ) should not be computed. [26] Reliability of the BSID has been measured through the use of split half, test-retest, and inter-rater studies. [26-27] Split half studies on the Mental Scale produced reliability coefficients of .81 to .93 with a median of .88. For the Motor scale, reliability coefficients of .68 to .92 with a median of 0.84 were obtained. The standard error of measurement (SEM), an estimation of the margin of error associated with the test score, also was used to assess reliability. The SEM obtained for the mental scores was 4.2 to 6.9. This score means that 2 out of 3 times the child is tested, his scores will fall between 4.2 to 6.9 points of the "true" MDI. For the Motor Scale, the SEM was 4.6 to 9.0. Werner and Bayley found that inter-rater reliability was 93.4 percent agreement and test-retest reliability was 75.3 percent agreement on the motor scales. [27] The validity of the Bayley Mental Scale was

assessed by comparing the scores of 120 children between the ages of 24 and 30 months with their scores on the Stanford Binet Intelligence Scale. [26] The correlation coefficient for the total group was .57 which indicated a substantial degree of agreement. [26] Ramey and associates found even higher correlations between the Bayley and the Stanford Binet for predictive validity in a group of subjects who attended day-care facilities and who were followed longitudinally from 6 to 8 months of age to 36 months. [28] Coryell et al examined the stability of the Bayley Motor Scale Scores during the first year of life by using a sample of 15 low risk and 8 high risk infants. [29] They reported that the "normal" infants did not change ranks over the six test ages of 2,3,4,8,12 and 24 or 36 months. Their scores, however, varied significantly from test to test. Scores of the infants with "non-normal" outcomes did not vary significantly from test to test. Other findings included inflation of scores at the 4 month level with many infants being identified as normal at 4 months who then later were identified as "non-normal". Based on the findings of this study, Coryell et al suggested that an individual child's scores at one time cannot be used to predict his or her score at another time and that serial testing may be essential for valid results.

Gesell Developmental Schedules

The Gesell Developmental Schedules is the oldest and probably the most widely used developmental tool. Most other developmental tests have either been directly or indirectly modeled after the Gesell. The original scales were published in the 1940's after being normed on a small sample. [30] The newest revision of the scales was published in 1980 after a more extensive standardization process. [30] Both the original and present revision were designed to provide functional and clinical assessments of developmental skills in children from 1 to 72 months of age. The purpose of the scales is to provide behavioral assessments in the areas of adaptive, gross motor, fine motor, language, and personal social development in an attempt to identify even minor deviations in children and to determine the maturity and integrity of the CNS. [31] In addition to the assessment of skills, the scales include a developmental history and a neurologic screening. In the restandardization for the 1980 revision, all examinations were done between January 1975 and December 1977. The 927 children were drawn from the Albany, New York area and were between 4 weeks and 36 months of age. [30] The mean percentage of black children in the study was comparable to the national average, as was the mean education of the white mothers. The black mothers had a slightly higher mean educational level. Items from the original Gesell, the Bayley Scales of Infant Development, the Uzgiris-Hunt and the Receptive and Expressive Language (REEL),

```
Program in Physical Therapy              Name: _____
Department of Rehabilitation Sciences    Unit No: _____
The University of Tennessee              BD: _____
  Center for the Health Sciences         Date of Evaluation _____
Memphis, Tennessee

Physical Therapy Evaluation              Gesell Motor Developmental Scale
```

4 WEEKS AGE LEVEL

SUPINE

1. Stares indefinitely (*8w) _____
2. Regards examiner; reduces activity (*8w) _____
3. Dangling ring, rattle Regards line of vision only (*8w) _____
4. Dangling ring, rattle follows to midline, not beyond (*8w) _____
5. Rattle, retains briefly (*8w) _____
6. ATNR predominates (*12w) _____
7. Hands Fisted (*12w) _____
8. Dangling ring, rattle Hands clenches on contact (*16w) _____

PRONE

9. Suspended in prone, head droops (*8w) _____
10. Prone placement, head rotates (*12w) _____
11. Prone placement, barely lifts head (*8w) _____
12. Hips held high (*8w) _____
13. Crawling movements of legs (*8w) _____

SITTING SUPPORTED

14. Complete head lag when pulled to sit (*20w) _____
15. Head sags forward (*8w) _____
16. Back evenly rounded (*16w) _____

8 WEEKS AGE LEVEL

SUPINE

1. Regards examiner recurrently (*12w) _____
2. Follows moving person _____
3. Dangling ring, rattle Delayed midline regard (*12w) _____
4. Dangling ring: Follows past midline (*16w) _____
5. Dangling ring: Follows vertically _____
6. Dangling ring: retains _____
7. Head midposition seen (*12w) _____

plus some newly developed items, were used in the development of the new scales. After item analysis the final scale contained a total of 489 items: 145 adaptive, 98 gross motor, 56 fine motor, 109 language, and 81 personal-social. The criteria for placement of the items at the specific age level included: behavior increased or decreased with age, behavior appeared at a particular age and then disappeared from the behavioral repertoire, and behavior distinguished between ages. [31] Changes that were noted in the revised scales included both changes in sequences and in ages of acquisition. In the adaptive area, the skills were achieved approximately 10% earlier by children in the sample and the sequences were changed in a few instances. In the gross motor area, the skills were attained approximately 17% earlier and the sequencing of skills was very different. For example, cruising at a rail was found to occur earlier than walking with both hands held and squatting in play occurred before walking alone. In the area of fine motor skills, the sequence remained essentially the same, but there was a slight acceleration of 5% in the acquisition of the skills. Some new items also were added for the 2 and 3 year levels. In the area of language, the acceleration of skills was approximately 12% with the addition of several new items and the separation of behaviors at different ages. In the area of personal social development, the acceleration of attainment was approximately 16% and most of the tested behaviors were shifted to lower age levels.

The child's performance is assessed by direct observation of the quality and integration of the five areas of development, as well as by parental interview. The scoring of the test allows for identifying established behaviors, emerging behaviors, and abnormal expression of behaviors. (Figure 4) A developmental age can be derived for each of the developmental areas, as well as a developmental age range which identifies basal and ceiling age levels. A developmental quotient (DQ) can be derived for each of the developmental areas by dividing the child's maturity age by the chronological age and multiplying the result by 100. Few reliability and validity studies have been done with the 1980 revision of the Gesell. An inter-rater reliability study using a sample of 48 children between 16 weeks to 21 months of age yielded overall percent agreement scores of 93.7, although the agreement varied from 88% in the fine motor to 97% in language. [31] On the previous versions of the scales, test-retest reliabilities were .82 but no information has been published on the present version. [32]

Predictive validity studies on previous versions of the scales suggested that the predictive value of the test was greatest for low scoring babies with neurologic or intellectual abnormalities. [33]

Peabody Developmental Motor Scales

The Peabody Developmental Motor Scales (PDMS), published in 1983, is an individually administered, standardized test that is designed to measure gross and fine motor skills of children from birth to 83 months of age. [34] Development of the scales began in 1969 as an attempt to develop a comprehensive sequence of gross and fine motor skills from which a relative developmental level of the child could be obtained and an instructional program planned. The scales originally were developed for deaf-blind children, thus items were prepared for this population. Field testing, both nationally and internationally, was done on test items in 1975. Feedback from field testing was used to change and improve test items and to change from a 5 point to a 3 point scoring system. A subsequent 1979 field test followed these revisions and was used in the standardization study conducted from December 1981 to April 1982. A stratified quota sampling was done to select ample representation of the U.S. population with factors such as geographical region, race, and sex being considered in the sampling. Communities selected as the testing sites met the respective region's rural-urban characteristics and included the entire range of the socio-economic status. Twenty states and 33 test administrators finally were selected for the standardization which included 617 children between the ages of 0-83 months. Testing was done either at home or at school.

The final version of the PDMS is divided into two components: the Gross Motor Scale and the Fine Motor Scale. The gross motor scale contains 170 items divided into 17 age levels with 10 items at each age level. The fine motor scale has 112 items divided into 16 age levels with 6 or 8 items at each age level. Additionally, the gross motor items are divided further into the skill categories of reflexes, balance, non-locomotion, locomotion, and propulsion of objects. Skill categories for fine motor items include grasping, hand use, eye hand coordination, and manual dexterity. For each item on the scales, the test manual describes the child's beginning position and the material needed for scoring. Each response is scored on a three point scale with 0 being unsuccessful, 1 being a clear resemblance to the item criterion but not fully met, and 2 being successful performance with the criterion met. With the information obtained on the test, the child's raw score for each scale and each skill category within the scale can be obtained. The raw score can then be converted into the following: age equivalent, developmental motor quotient, percentile ranking, and standard score. For each of the age levels, the mean motor quotient is 100 with a standard deviation of 15.

No special qualifications are required to use the PDMS. The examiner should read the manual and be familiar with the test before administering the scales.

Additionally, the examiner should administer the scale to normal children at least three times and should have 85 percent inter-rater reliability with an experienced examiner.[34] The scales were developed for use by teachers, physical therapists, occupational therapists, physical education teachers, and adaptive physical educators.

In addition to the assessment scales, the test kit contains activity cards which can be used in planning programs aimed at teaching the behaviors on the tests. The test kit contains about one half of the materials needed for the administration of the test.

Reliability of the test has been assessed by examination of test-retest and inter-rater reliability. Test-retest reliability was determined by the testing of 38 children from the normative sample a second time within one week of the initial testing. The children selected were approximately equally distributed across ages. Correlation coefficients of .95 and .80 were obtained for the gross and fine motor scales.[34] In a study on inter-rater reliability, coefficients of .97 and .94 were obtained for the gross and fine motor scales.[34]

Content validity of the scales was stated in the test manual to be intact since the test items were selected from established tests of motor development. Construct validity was addressed by determining significance of improvement in scores as a function of age. On both scales, gross and fine motor, significant differences occurred at each age level. An analysis of concurrent validity was done by comparing the mean standardized scores obtained by 104 children with identified motor problems to the results obtained by the normative sample. The standardized scores of the children with motor problems were significantly lower than the means of the normative scale except for the 0-5 months level.[34]

The strengths of the PDMS are that the test is standardized, extends from birth to 7 years, and has numerous test items at each age level. Additionally, inter-rater reliability and test-retest reliability are good to high. The test manual is detailed and most instructions in the manual are clear and explicit. The manual also gives suggestions for adapting the test items for children who may not understand the instructions as written. The tool also appears to be appropriate for children with disabilities. The major weaknesses of the PDMS are: the small normative sample (N = 617); criteria for the score of "1" are not explicit; all items at each age level must be administered before moving to the next level thus causing disruptions in the flow of the test; and the potential misuse of the activity cards. For many children, especially those with severe disabilities, the programs suggested on the activity cards may be inappropriate and may not address the child's motor problems. If so, inappropriate selection of motor activities may occur and splinter skills may be taught.

Bruininks Oseretsky Test of Motor Proficiency

The Bruininks Oseretsky Test of Motor Proficiency (BOTMP) was developed by Bruininks based on Doll's adaptation of the original Oseretsky Tests.[35] The purpose of the test is to assess gross and fine motor skills in children between the ages of 4.5 and 14.5 years and to assist in decision making about appropriate educational and therapeutic placement. The short form of the test can be used for screening for special purposes, such as early identification of developmental problems. The BOTMP was developed through a series of analytical studies. The original test was developed in 1973 with the test items being administered to 75 children. Following analysis of the results on this initial test, a second version was administered to 250 children between 5 to 14 years of age in the St. Paul - Minneapolis area. The children were selected randomly from schools which represented central city, suburbia, various socioeconomic and ethnic groups. The final version was written after analyzing the results of this second field test. The final items on the test were selected based on item difficulty, item discrimination, correlation between performance on an item and chronological age, and intercorrelations among items in the same content area. Eighteen items from the original Oseretsky and 28 new items were included on the final version. Standardization of the final version was done on 765 subjects who were representative of the 1970 United States census according to geographic region, community size, sex, and race. At least 38 children were assessed at each of the age levels of the test. The specific motor areas assessed by the subtests of the BOTMP are running speed and agility, balance, bilateral coordination, strength, upper limb coordination, response speed, visual motor control, and upper limb speed and dexterity. (Figure 5) Most equipment for the test is included in the test kit. The test instructions are written clearly and, although some instructions may be complex, substitutions of words that the individual child may understand are allowed. Certain items on the tests are identified for use as a short form and can be administered for screening. The complete battery typically takes 45-60 minutes to administer while the short form can be administered in 15-20 minutes.

Raw scores from each of the areas of assessment can be converted into point scores which may be further converted to standard scores. From the standard scores, one can calculate composite scores for gross and fine motor tasks. In addition, one can determine age levels of functioning in each of the specific areas. The manual reports that validity of the BOTMP is based on how well it assesses the constructs of motor development or proficiency.[35] Construct validity is stated to be present due to the statistical characteristics of the test. Scores of each subtest were found to be correlated significantly with the chronological age of the children in the stan-

BRUININKS-OSERETSKY TEST OF MOTOR PROFICIENCY / Robert H. Bruininks, Ph.D.

INDIVIDUAL RECORD FORM

COMPLETE BATTERY AND SHORT FORM

NAME _____ SEX: Boy ☐ Girl ☐ GRADE _____

SCHOOL/AGENCY _____ CITY _____ STATE _____

EXAMINER _____ REFERRED BY _____

PURPOSE OF TESTING _____

Arm Preference: *(circle one)*

    RIGHT   LEFT   MIXED

Leg Preference: *(circle one)*

    RIGHT   LEFT   MIXED

	Year	Month	Day
Date Tested	____	____	____
Date of Birth	____	____	____
Chronological Age	____	____	____

Complete Battery:

SUBTEST	POINT SCORE Maximum / Subject's	STANDARD SCORE Test (Table 23)	STANDARD SCORE Composite (Table 24)	PERCENTILE RANK (Table 25)	STANINE (Table 25)	OTHER _____
GROSS MOTOR SUBTESTS:						
1. Running Speed and Agility	15 ____	____				____
2. Balance	32 ____	____				____
3. Bilateral Coordination	20 ____	____				____
4. Strength	42 ____	____				____
GROSS MOTOR COMPOSITE		*[ ] SUM	[ ]	[ ]	[ ]	[ ]
5. Upper-Limb Coordination	21 ____	*[ ]				
FINE MOTOR SUBTESTS:						
6. Response Speed	17 ____	____				____
7. Visual-Motor Control	24 ____	____				____
8. Upper-Limb Speed and Dexterity	72 ____	____				____
FINE MOTOR COMPOSITE		*[ ] SUM	[ ]	[ ]	[ ]	[ ]
BATTERY COMPOSITE		*[ ] SUM	[ ]	[ ]	[ ]	[ ]

*To obtain Battery Composite: Add Gross Motor Composite, Subtest 5 Standard Score, and Fine Motor Composite. Check result by adding Standard Scores on Subtests 1-8.

Short Form:

	POINT SCORE Maximum / Subject's	STANDARD SCORE (Table 27)	PERCENTILE RANK (Table 27)	STANINE (Table 27)
SHORT FORM	98 ____	[ ]	[ ]	[ ]

DIRECTIONS

Complete Battery:

1. During test administration, record subject's response for each trial.

2. After test administration, convert performance on each item (item raw score) to a point score, using scale provided. For an item with more than one trial, choose best performance. Record item point score in *circle* to right of scale.

3. For each subtest, add item point scores; record total in circle provided at end of each subtest and in Test Score Summary section. Consult *Examiner's Manual* for norms tables.

Short Form:

1. Follow Steps 1 and 2 for Complete Battery, except record each point score in *box* to right of scale.

2. Add point scores for all 14 Short Form items and record total in Test Score Summary section. Consult *Examiner's Manual* for norms tables.

dardization group with correlations ranging from .57 to .86 with a median of .78. Validity was assessed by comparing the scores of normal children with the scores of children with either mental retardation or learning disabilities. Reliability for the BOTMP was assessed in three ways by the author. A test-retest study was done with 63 second graders and 63 sixth graders with the retest being given 7-12 days after the first test. The reliability coefficient for the Battery Composite was .89 for the second graders and .86 for the sixth graders. [35] Reliability also was measured by determining standard error of measurement (SEM) for the composites and for the subtests. In general, the SEM for the composites were 4 or 5 standard score points and the SEM for the subtests 2 to 3 standard score points. Finally, inter-rater reliability was determined using the eight items of the visual motor control subtest. For two separate groups of raters, the inter-rater reliability coefficients were found to be .98 and .90. [35]

SENSORIMOTOR TESTS

Miller Assessment of Preschoolers

The Miller Assessment of Preschoolers (MAP) was designed to identify children who exhibit mild to moderate developmental delays. The MAP was developed primarily for two purposes: to develop a short screening tool to identify those children who need further evaluation and to provide a comprehensive, clinical framework that would be useful in identifying the child's strengths and weaknesses as a basis for further intervention. [36]

The test is appropriate for children between the ages of 2 years 9 months to 5 years 8 months. The test was normed on a nationally randomly selected stratified sample of 600 normal preschool children and on a select sample of 60 children with preacademic problems. No children with physical or other identified disabilities were used in the sampling. The test edition used in the normative study contained 530 items, however, only 27 items and a series of structured observations were used in the final edition. The final edition of the test was standardized in all nine of the U.S. Census Bureau regions on a randomly selected sample of 1200 preschoolers with appropriate ratios according to sex, age, race, size of residential community, and socioeconomic factors.

The 27 test items are divided into five performance indices: foundations, coordination, verbal, nonverbal, and complex tasks. The test takes approximately 20-30 minutes to administer and score. A profile of the individual child's performance is derived by comparing the final scores to a table of Final Percentile Scores and a graphic profile of the child's abilities is obtained. Reliability studies were done using inter-rater and test-retest. [36] On a sample of 90 children, a test-retest study showed that the final score category of 81 percent of the children

remained stable over two testing sessions one to four weeks apart. The coefficient of internal consistency on the total sample was .79. An inter-rater reliability coefficient of .98 was obtained in a study involving 40 children and two examiners. [36]

Extensive validity studies have not been published on the MAP. According to the test manual, however, the MAP identified as "at risk" 80 percent of a sample of 80 children previously identified as having preacademic problems. [36]

DeGangi Berk Test of Sensory Integration

The DeGangi Berk Test of Sensory Integration (TSI), published in 1983, is designed for early identification of sensory integrative dysfunction in preschool children ages 3 to 5 years. [37] The authors state that young children who have sensory integrative problems may exhibit mild motor delays in the preschool years but not to the extent that they are referred for appropriate services. The reason why these children may remain undetected for sensory integrative problems appears due to a lack of measurement devices that are sensitive to the more subtle indicators of sensory integrative dysfunction. Therefore, the authors undertook the development of a standardized means of identifying activities that might be used to identify children who are either deficient or at risk in their sensory integrative abilities.

During the test development, the three subdomains of postural control, bilateral motor integration, and reflex integration were identified from the general domain of sensory integration as areas of assessment. A total of 73 test items were generated to represent these three subdomains. Many of the items were from the clinical observations portion of the Southern California Sensory Integration Tests. From these 73 test items, 36 items were selected for inclusion on the TSI. The 36 items were selected based on their ability to discriminate between groups of normal and delayed children and on their sensitivity to the developmental status of normal children.

Construct validity of the test was done by using two criterion groups of normal and delayed children. A total of 139 children, 101 normal and 38 delayed, representing ages three to five years and three ethnic groups (i.e. black, Hispanic, and white) were used. Results from administration of the original 73 items to these groups of children aided in determining item validity, decision validity, and test structure. The authors found that the total test scores could be used for screening decisions with better than 80% accuracy and a 9% false normal error rate. [37] The subtests of Postural Control and Bilateral Motor Integration were very accurate with false normal error rates below 7%. Based on the cutoff score used in the decision validity study, the test was found to be more effective in excluding normal children from a delayed population than including delayed children in a normal population.

Inter-rater reliability was assessed by using three different therapists and two independent samples of children which included a total of 33 children (26 normal and 7 delayed).[37] Inter-rater reliabilities of .80 to .88 were found for the Postural Control and Bilateral Motor Integration subtests. The reliability scores for the Reflex Integration subtest varied from .24 to .66. Therefore, the authors cautioned against using the Reflex Integration subtest alone in making diagnoses. Decision Consistency reliability was determined by using a sample of 29 children, 23 normal and 6 delayed, who were tested twice during a one week retest interval. Three observers conducted the testing. High levels of classification consistency were found for all three subtests and for the total test with reliability scores ranging from .79 to .93. Test-retest reliability information was obtained from the study on Decision Consistency reliability. The Test-Retest reliability coefficients ranged from .85 to .96 when each subtest, as well as the total test was considered.[37]

The test is comprised of 13 activities from which 36 scores are obtained. The 6 items used in the Postural Control subtests assess antigravity postures that are necessary for stabilization of the neck, trunk, upper extremities, and muscle cocontraction of the neck and upper extremities. The 5 activities in the Bilateral Motor Integration subtests assess bilateral motor coordination and components of laterality including trunk rotation and crossing midline. Rapid unilateral and bilateral hand movements, stability of the upper and lower extremities in bilateral symmetrical postures, and dissociation of trunk and arm movements also are evaluated. The 2 items included in the Reflex Integration subtest evaluate the asymmetrical and symmetrical tonic neck reflexes in the quadruped position and the presence of associated reactions of the upper extremities.

Each of the individual test items are weighted with point values ranging from 0 - 1 to 0 - 4. Criteria for the assigning of a point value are described in the test manual. Scores for Postural Control, Bilateral Motor Integration, and the Total Test are obtained from administration of the entire battery. These scores are then compared against "normed" scores for children between 3 - 4 years of age or 5 years of age. Based on these "normed" scores, an individual child's score may be interpreted as normal, at risk, or deficient. The authors stated that these results can be used for either screening or diagnosis, depending upon the needs of the child and examiner.

The strengths of the TSI are that the test is fun for the child and that administration of the test only takes about 30 minutes. Test materials are readily available from Western Psychological Services. The weaknesses of the TSI include the predominance of 3 - 4 year olds used in the construct and reliability studies. Further research

using larger sample sizes and more investigation of possible differential performance in terms of age, gender, and ethnicity should be undertaken according to the authors of the TSI. An additional problem is the use of the Reflex Integration subtests due to the low validity and reliability scores that were obtained. Even though the authors stated that the Reflex Integration subtests should not be used alone in making decision about an individual child's performance, these scores are used in determining the child's total test score.

Sensory Integration and Praxis Tests

The Sensory Integration and Praxis Tests published in 1989 represents an evolution of the Southern California Sensory Integration Test (SCSIT) and the Southern California Postrotary Nystagmus Test (SCPNT).[38-40] Ayres, during the 1960s and 1970s, performed numerous factor analyses on the subtests of the Southern California Sensory Integration Test.[41-44] Based on these factor analyses, several of the subtests from the SCSIT were not included on the new SIPT either due to their lack of clinical usefulness, the difficulty in administrating the subtest, or poor reliability in measurement of the function. Examples of subtests not included are double tactile stimuli and position in space. Several of the subtests from the SCSIT were changed to improve administration of the item and to improve reliability. Aspects of praxis that were thought to be most affected in developmental dyspraxia were added to the SIPT as new praxis subtests. In all, twelve of the subtests of the SCSIT and the SCPNT were included in the final version of the SIPT.

The seventeen subtests of the SIPT are categorized into four overlapping groups: Tactile and Vestibular-Proprioceptive Sensory Processing Tests; The Form and Space Perception and Visuomotor Coordination Tests; The Praxis Tests; and The Bilateral Integration and Sequencing Tests. Table 1 identifies the subtests that comprise the four groupings. The SIPT test materials and score sheets are available from Western Psychological Services.

The SIPT is individually administered with the entire test battery taking approximately two hours. The tests are then computer scored based on completed computer score sheets which are sent to Western Psychological Services for weighing of scores and determination of standard scores based on available norms. Certification in administration and interpretation of these tests is necessary for use of the test as a diagnostic tool.

In the development of the new subtests for the SIPT and in the revision of the SCSIT, field and pilot studies were done during the early 1980s. In these pilot studies, three criteria were used in the selection of the final tests and individual test items: the capability of each item to distinguish between dysfunctional and normal children; evidence of a logical association between items and

TABLE 1

TACTILE AND VESTIBULAR PROPRIOCEPTIVE SENSORY PROCESSING
 KINESTHESIA
 FINGER IDENTIFICATION
 GRAPHESTHESIA
 LOCALIZATION OF TACTILE STIMULI
 POSTROTARY NYSTAGMUS
 STANDING AND WALKING BALANCE

FORM AND SPACE PERCEPTION AND VISUOMOTOR COORDINATION
 SPACE VISUALIZATION
 FIGURE-GROUND PERCEPTION
 MANUAL FORM PERCEPTION
 MOTOR ACCURACY
 DESIGN COPYING
 CONSTRUCTIONAL PRAXIS

PRAXIS
 DESIGN COPYING
 CONSTRUCTIONAL PRAXIS
 POSTURAL PRAXIS
 PRAXIS ON VERBAL COMMAND
 SEQUENCING PRAXIS
 ORAL PRAXIS

BILATERAL INTEGRATION AND SEQUENCING
 ORAL PRAXIS
 SEQUENCING PRAXIS
 GRAPHESTHESIA
 STANDING AND WALKING BALANCE
 BILATERAL MOTOR COORDINATION
 SPACE VISUALIZATION CONTRALATERAL USE
 SPACE VISUALIZATION PREFERRED HAND USE

functions under assessment; and inter-rater / test-retest reliability.[38] Based on these pilot studies, the final version of the SIPT was comprised of tests designed to assess sensory perception and the processing of tactile, proprioceptive, vestibular, and visual input as well as several aspects of praxis.

The SIPT was normed using the 1980 U.S. Census to determine the appropriate representation of the U.S. population in the normative sample. The variables considered in selecting the sample were age, sex, ethnicity, type of community, and geographic location. The final normative sample was comprised of approximately 2,000 children, between the ages of 4 years 0 months to 8 years 11 months with an almost equal number of boys and girls. Children in the sample were evaluated by selected examiners who were trained on the administration and scoring of the SIPT and who were tested on their administration skills at workshops held around the U.S.

Preliminary analyses of the normative sample revealed significant age and sex differences on the SIPT tests. Therefore, separate norms were established for boys and girls in 12 age groups. Additionally, means and standard deviations were computed for each of the normative subgroups. Most of the individual tests of the SIPT also yielded subscores for time and accuracy.

Validity of the SIPT continues to be examined. Content validity was established according to Ayres through the work that led to the development of the SCSIT, the refinement of the SCSIT and through consultation with experts in the area of sensory integration.[38] Construct validity was examined through the use of numerous factor analyses conducted by Ayres and reported in the SIPT manual. Additionally, multiple discriminant analyses were used by Ayres with a matched sample of 352 children without dysfunction and children with sensory integrative problems. The weights for time and accuracy scores that adequately discriminated between the two groups of children were used in the final version of the test. In preliminary studies using the SIPT in various populations, each of the subtests of the SIPT discriminated between children without dysfunction and those with dysfunction at a statistically significant level (p<.01).[38] Construct validity has been further supported by Murray, Cermak, and O'Brien who studied 21 children with learning disabilities and 18 children without learning disabilities, aged 5 to 8 years to determine the relationship between form and space perception, constructional abilities, and clumsiness.[45] The children with learning disabilities in the study were further divided into two groups, clumsy and nonclumsy, based on their scores on a test of motor behaviors. All children in the study were assessed using six of the SIPT subtests that measure form and space perception and visual construction. Results indicated that both groups of learning disabled children scored lower than the non-learning disabled children on four of the six SIPT subtests (space

visualization, motor accuracy, design copying, and constructional praxis) at a significant level. Within the 2 learning disabled groups, the clumsy and nonclumsy children differed significantly from each other only on the Motor Accuracy and Design Copying subtests. The degree of clumsiness in the 12 children who were identified as clumsy was correlated significantly with three of the six subtests (Space Visualization, Motor Accuracy, and Design Copying).

Criterion related and predictive validity for the SIPT are currently under investigation. Murray, Cermak, and O'Brien's study comparing scores from the Test of Motor Impairment (TMI) and scores on subtests of the SIPT revealed that clumsy children identified on the TMI were also identified as clumsy by using the SIPT.[45-46] Additionally, McAtee and Mack reported that significant relationships (p=.05) were found between the SIPT Design Copy parameters of boundary, additions, segmentation, reversal, inversion and jogs and the visual subtests of the SCSIT (Space Visualization, Figure-Ground Perception, Position in Space, and Design Copying).[47]

Test - retest reliability coefficients for the 17 subtests of the SIPT were reported by Ayres as ranging from .48 to .93.[38] The praxis tests had the highest test-retest reliability, but reliabilities for most of the other tests were acceptable. Four of the tests had reliability coefficients below .70: Postrotary Nystagmus, Kinesthesia, Localization of Tactile Stimuli and Figure- Ground Perception. Ayres reported that the small sample size and the predominance of children with dysfunction in the test-retest reliability study, and the nature of the assessed neural functions in the SIPT may have affected the test-retest reliability of these subtests.[38] Inter-rater reliability studies for the SIPT revealed correlation coefficients for all of the major SIPT scores to be between .94 and .99 when trained examiners were used.[38]

STANDARDIZED ASSESSMENT OF INSTRUMENTAL DAILY LIVING SKILLS

The Pediatric Evaluation of Disability Inventory (PEDI)

The Pediatric Evaluation of Disability Inventory (PEDI) is a standardized assessment that uses parental reporting to determine a child's comprehensive level of function for children with disabilities ages 6 months to 7 years.[48] Part one of the inventory consists of the broad categories of self-care, mobility, and social function, with each having 13 - 15 items to be evaluated on a scale of 1 - 5. This part of the evaluation indicates the level at which the child can function without assistance. In part two, the same categories are evaluated based on the level of assistance and modifications that the child typically needs to function on a daily basis. A summary profile is determined.

Concurrent and construct validity of the PEDI have been examined by comparing outcomes of 20 children between the ages of 2 years and 8 years with arthritic conditions or spina bifida and 20 matched "normal" children using the PEDI and the Battell Developmental Inventory Screening Test (BDIST). [49] Concurrent validity was supported by moderately high Pearson product moment correlations ($r = .70 - .80$) when the scores on the PEDI and the BDIST were compared. The PEDI scores were found to be better discriminators of dysfunction than the BDIST with the children with disabilities, thus, supporting construct validity. Feldman, Haley, and Coryell stated that these results support further development and standardization of the PEDI as a clinical tool for assessment of functional abilities. [49]

SUMMARY

This overview of selected standardized and non-standardized tests should supply the developmental therapist with an understanding of the components of an acceptable test. The information given on each of the tests also should assist the therapist in the selection of the appropriate test for a given child in a given situation. The developmental therapist should be aware of other components of an assessment of a child in addition to the administration of a test and should use the information gathered from other parts of the assessment in the total evaluation of the child. ❏

References

1. Dubowitz L, Dubowitz V: The Neurological Examination of the Full Term Newborn Infant. Clinics in Developmental Medicine No. 79, Philadelphia, PA, J B Lippincott, 1981
2. Saint-Anne Dargassies S: Neurological Development in the Full Term and Premature Neonate. London, England, Excerta Medica, 1977
3. Prechtl HFR: The Neurological Examination of the Full Term Newborn Infant. Clinics in Developmental Medicine, No. 63, Philadelphia, PA, J B Lippincott, 1977
4. Parmelee AH, Michaelis R: Neurological examination of the Newborn. In Hellmuth J (ed): Exceptional Infant. Vol. 2: Studies in Abnormalities. London, England. Butterworths, 1971
5. Brazelton TB: Neonatal Behavioral Assessment Scale. Philadelphia, PA, JB Lippincott, 1973
6. Brazelton TB: Neonatal Behavioral Assessment Scale. ed 2. Philadelphia, PA, J B Lippincott, 1984
7. Prechtl HFR: Assessment methods for the newborn infant, A critical evaluation. In Stratton P, Chichest J (eds): Psychobiology of the Human Newborn. New York, NY, Wiley, 1982
8. Als H, Brazelton TB: A new model of assessing the behavioral organization in preterm and full term infants. J Am Acad Child Psychol 20: 239, 1981
9. Lancioni GE, Horowitz FD, Sullivan JW: The NBAS-K: A. A study of its stability and structure over the first month of life. Infant Behavior and Development 3:341-159, 1980
10. Sameroff AJ: Organization and stability of newborn behavior: a commentary on the Brazelton Neonatal Behavioral Assessment Scale. Monographs of the Society of Research in Child Development 43: 5 6, 1978
11. Tronick E, Brazelton TB: Clinical uses of the Brazelton Neonatal Behavior Assessment. In Friedlander BZ, Sterritt BM, Kirk GE (eds): Exceptional Infant: Assessment and Intervention. Vol. 3. New York, NY, Brunner/Mazel, 1975
12. Bakow H, Samaroff A, Kelly P, et al: Relation between newborn and mother-child interactions at four months. Paper presented at biennial meeting of the Society for Research in Child Development. Philadelphia, PA, 1973
13. Frankenburg WK, Dodds JB, Fandal AW, et al: Denver Developmental Screening Test: Reference manual. Denver, CO., University of Colorado Medical Center, 1975
14. Frankenburg WK, Camp BW, Van Natta PA: Validity of the Denver Developmental Screening Test. Child Development 42: 475, 1971
15. Frankenburg WK, Camp BW, Van Natta PA, DeMersseman JA, Voorhees SF: Reliability and stability of the Denver Developmental Screening Test. Child Development 42: 1315, 1971
16. Frankenburg WK, Fandal AW, Sciarillo W, Burgess D: The newly abbreviated and revised Denver Developmental Screening Test. Journal of Pediatrics 99: 995-999, 1981
17. Milani-Comparetti A, Gidoni EA: Routine developmental examination in normal and retarded children. Dev Med Child Neurol 9: 631-638, 1967
18. Trembath J: The Milani-Comparetti Motor Development Screening Test. Omaha, NE, University of Nebraska Medical Center Print Shop, 1978
19. VanderLinden D: Ability of the Milani-Comparetti Developmental Examination to predict motor outcome. Physical and Occupational Therapy in Pediatrics 5: 27 - 38, 1985
20. Stuberg WA, White PJ, Miedaner JA, Dehne PR: Item reliability of the Milani-Comparetti Motor Development Screening Test. Phys Ther 69: 328 - 335, 1989
21. Chandler L, Andrews M, Swanson M: The Movement Assessment of Infants: A Manual. Rolling Bay, WA, 1980
22. Harris SR, Haley SM, Tada WL, Swanson MW: Reliability of observational measures of the Movement Assessment of Infants. Phys Ther 64: 471-475, 1984
23. Haley SM, Harris SR, Tada WL, Swanson MW: Item reliability of the Movement Assessment of Infants. Physical and Occupational Therapy in Pediatrics 6: 21 - 39, 1986
24. Schneider JW, Lee W, Chasnoff IJ: Field Testing of the Movement Assessment of Infants. Phys Ther 68: 321 - 327, 1988
25. Darrah J, Piper MC, Byrne PJ, Warren S: The utilization of the Movement Assessment of Infants risk profile with preterm infants. Physical and Occupational Therapy in Pediatrics 11: 1 - 12, 1991
26. Bayley N: Bayley Scales of Infant Development. New York, NY, Psychological Corporation, 1969
27. Werner EE, Bayley N: The reliability of Bayley's revised scale of mental and motor development during the first year of life. Child Dev 37: 39, 1966
28. Ramey CT, Campbell FA, Nicholson JE: The predictive power of the Bayley Scales of Infant Development and the Stanford-Binet Intelligence Test in a relatively constant environment. Child Dev 44: 790, 1973
29. Coryell J, Provist B, Wilhelm IJ, Campbell SK: Stability of Bayley Motor Scale scores in the fist year of life. Phys Ther 69: 834 - 841, 1989
30. Gesell A, Halverson HM, Ilg FL, et al: The First Five Years of Life. New York, NY, Harper & Row, 1940
31. Knobloch H, Stevens F, Malone AF: Manual of Developmental Diagnosis: The Administration and Interpretation of the Revised Gesell and Amatruda Developmental and Neurologic Examination. Hagerstown, MD, Harper & Row, 1980
32. Knobloch H, Pasamanick B: Gesell and Amatruda's Developmental Diagnosis: The Evaluation and Management of Normal and Abnormal Neuropsychologic Development in Infancy and Early Childhood. Hagerstown, MD, Harper & Row, 1974
33. Knobloch H, Pasamanick B: An evaluation of the consistency and predictive value of the 40 week Gesell Developmental Schedule. Paper presented at the Regional Research Meeting of the American Psychiatric Association, Iowa City, IA, 1960
34. Folio R, Dubose RF: Peabody Developmental Motor Scales. Hingham, MA, Teaching Resources Corporation, 1983
35. Bruininks RH: Bruininks Oseretsky Test of Motor Proficiency. Examiner's Manual. Circle Pines, MN, American Guidance Service, 1978
36. Miller LJ: Miller Assessment of Preschoolers. Littleton, CO, The Foundation for Knowledge in Development, 1982
37. Berk RA, DeGangi GA: DeGangi - Berk Test of Sensory Integration: Manual. Los Angeles, CA, Western Psychological Services,1983
38. Ayres AJ: Sensory Integration and Praxis Tests. Los Angeles, CA., Western Psychological Services, 1989
39. Ayres AJ: Southern California Sensory Integration Tests (rev. ed). Los Angeles, CA., Western Psychological Services, 1980
40. Ayres AJ: Southern California Postrotary Nystagmus Test manual. Los Angeles, CA., Western Psychological Services, 1975
41. Ayres AJ: Patterns of perceptual motor dysfunctions in children: A factor analysis study. Perceptual and Motor Skills 20: 335 - 368, 1965

42. Ayres AJ: Deficits in sensory integration in educationally handicapped children. Journal of Learning Disabilities 2: 160 - 168, 1969

43. Ayres AJ: Types of sensory integrative dysfunction among disabled learners. American Journal of Occupational Therapy 26: 13 - 18, 1972

44. Ayres AJ: Cluster analyses of measures of sensory integration. American Journal of Occupational Therapy 31: 362 - 366, 1977

45. Murray EA, Cermak SA, O'Brien A: The relationship between form and space perception, constructional abilities, and clumsiness in children. American Journal of Occupational Therapy 44: 623 - 628, 1990

46. Stott D, Moyes FA, Henderson SE: Manual of Test of Motor Impairment: Henderson revision. Ontario, Canada, Brook Educational, 1984

47. McAtee S, Mack W: Relations between Design Copying and other tests of sensory integrative dysfunction: A pilot study. American Journal of Occupational Therapy 44: 596 - 601, 1990

48. Haley SM, Faas RM, Coster WJ et al : Pediatric Evaluation of Disability Inventory. Boston, MA,. New England Medical Center, 1989

49. Feldman AB, Haley SM, Coryell J: Concurrent and construct validity of the Pediatric Evaluation of Disability Inventory. Phys Ther 70: 602-610, 1990

CHAPTER 3

ORGANIZING TREATMENT SESSIONS AND ESTABLISHING BEHAVIORAL OBJECTIVES

Patricia C. Montgomery, Ph.D., PT

◆

The physical therapist who treats children is responsible for determining which treatment techniques to use, when to use them, and how long specific treatment should continue. Making the transition between didactic information and theoretical neurophysiologic frameworks to actual "hands-on" intervention can be a long, frustrating, and anxiety-producing experience for both the therapist and child. Because of the traditional academic focus on techniques, the physical therapist may not develop strategies for planning and sequencing treatment. The purpose of this chapter is to identify some of the variables that influence treatment planning. A method for selecting appropriate treatment techniques and sequence of application is suggested by working backwards from the establishment of behavioral patient objectives. Principles of motor learning that are applicable to planning and administering treatment are included.

The information presented in this chapter is intended to serve as one possible process for developing a strategy for organizing treatment. Such a framework involves a number of therapist and patient variables that will alter its applicability in different situations. In addition, many experienced clinicians have no difficulty determining the content of individual treatment sessions in relation to therapeutic goals. These clinicians, however, may not be able to describe the cognitive processes they use to make such determinations.

Therefore, a specific strategy for treatment planning and sequencing may be useful to many physical therapists, particularly the student and new graduate, who have little clinical experience. Evaluation of patient progress in relation to treatment is essential in the clinical as well as the research setting. The approach of goal setting and use of measurable behavioral objectives in relation to treatment outcome is becoming increasingly mandated by third-party payers.

VARIABLES INFLUENCING TREATMENT PLANNING AND SEQUENCING

The theoretical framework a physical therapist uses to plan intervention will be affected by both the understanding of and the degree of agreement with specific theories of motor control, motor learning, and motor development. Although physical therapy curricula contain similar content in therapeutic exercise, there will be differences in which theories are emphasized and which therapeutic techniques are taught depending on physical therapy faculty, and, in turn, their training and clinical expertise. In my opinion, this is not a negative, but a positive phenomenon as it provides physical therapists with several approaches to treatment which eventually can be validated or invalidated by clinical research. Although we may be criticized for not having one research validated treatment approach to therapeutic exercise, our profession is no different than many other health professions. For example, the oncologist may not know what causes a certain form of cancer and may not have a proven cure, but the patient is treated based on the information available at that time, while research studies are in progress which may lead to more effective treatment in the future. The analogy to the approach of the physical therapist who assesses and treats the child using current state of the art information in therapeutic exercise is clear.

A second variable affecting treatment planning and sequencing is the physical therapist's ability to integrate general assessment and treatment techniques taught in the basic curriculum with neurophysiologic techniques in the treatment of the pediatric population. For example, techniques for improving strength, endurance, and flexibility are essential in the treatment of many children. Orthopedic and cardiovascular considerations in relation to exercise, weight-bearing, various positions, and the use of adaptive devices are important, but may be neglected if the emphasis is on normalizing movement patterns and developing age appropriate motor skills through the use of specific neurophysiologic techniques.

A third variable affecting treatment is the selection of assessment tools. Norm-referenced tests are designed primarily to detect whether or not a child has a motor problem in relation to his normal peer group[1]. Criterion-referenced tests measure a child's performance against set criteria or his own previous performance, therefore providing information on the most appropriate focus of treatment. In my experience, the more physically and mentally disabled the child is, the more difficult it is to assess current abilities and potential for change and fewer standardized assessment tools are available. An in-depth discussion of assessment tools currently used in pediatrics was provided in the preceeding chapter.

Physical therapists rely on clinical observations or qualitative assessments of sensory and motor abilities to supplement the results of formal assessments or as a substitute for unavailable or inappropriate assessment tools. The applicability of clinical assessments in relation to choosing specific treatment techniques is documented in the subsequent chapters of this book.

Another variable affecting the process of treatment planning is clinical experience in determining therapeutic goals and observing change resulting in attainment of or failure to accomplish specific objectives. For example, major motor milestones, such as rolling, sitting, and crawling, may be used as functional goals. The physical therapist working with the child with severe disabilitites, however, may discover that these goals must be broken down into smaller units to effectively measure progress over specified periods of time.

DEVELOPING A STRATEGY FOR PLANNING TREATMENT

The first step in developing a strategy for planning individual treatment is not to assess the patient, but to assess your own existing framework of knowledge. What has your academic and clinical training provided which will assist you in working with children? What areas of knowledge do you need to supplement with additional information or training? A thorough understanding of normal motor development is a necessary prerequisite in assessing and treating children. If your caseload consists of children with learning disabilities who demonstrate subtle motor problems, additional study of pertinent resource material may be necessary. The physical therapist must assume the responsibility of being adequately prepared to plan appropriate treatment for specific children.

The second step is to identify the numerous variables or treatment approaches which can be used. Different theoretical frameworks emphasize different aspects. For example, mobility versus stability components of movement can be analyzed and intervention can be organized around this model. The integration of primitive postural responses along with the development of righting, equilibrium, and protective reactions also may be used as a model. Figure 1 illustrates some of the factors that can be emphasized during assessment and treatment of children. Note that sensory processing is an integral part of all other components. Each physical therapist will address the mental organization of these variables differently, but will, hopefully, create a gestalt useful in assessing and treating children in a holistic manner. The third step in planning treatment is to choose appropriate assessment tools. Most normative tests inform you as to whether the child is performing below, at, or above expectations as compared to a normal child of the same age. Few tests will tell you what to do to improve the child's performance. Normative tests, however, may reveal areas of deficits and tests are available for monitoring developmental change (refer to Chapter 2).

During the assessment process, summarize what the child can and cannot do. Make a list of the sensory tasks or motor activities he should be accomplishing. The most difficult step in the process is to determine why he cannot do the tasks or movements you have listed. The assessment procedures in Chapters 5 through 12 should assist you in delineating specific problem areas.

A decision must be made if it is reasonable to make long range goals for the child in relation to normal or

Therapeutic Exercise In Developmental Disabilities

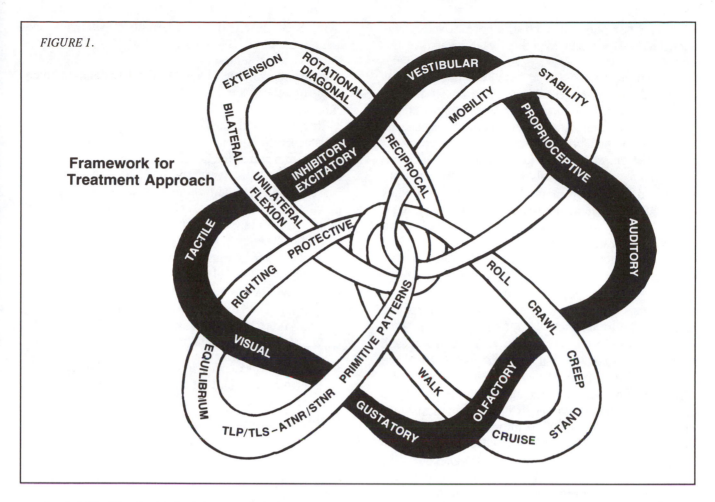

FIGURE 1.

Framework for Treatment Approach

EXTENSION · ROTATIONAL DIAGONAL · VESTIBULAR · STABILITY · BILATERAL · MOBILITY · PROPRIOCEPTIVE · INHIBITORY EXCITATORY · RECIPROCAL · UNILATERAL FLEXION · TACTILE · PROTECTIVE · AUDITORY · RIGHTING · ROLL · CRAWL · CREEP · PRIMITIVE PATTERNS · VISUAL · WALK · OLFACTORY · STAND · EQUILIBRIUM · TLP/TLS–ATNR/STNR · GUSTATORY · CRUISE

standard skills. For the high-risk preterm infant who is mildly delayed in motor skills at an adjusted age of six months, it seems appropriate to use the normal developmental model to determine long term goals, such as rolling, crawling, and walking. For the ten year old severely spastic quadriplegic child with cerebral palsy, who will probably not attain normal skill levels in motor tasks, goals which reflect improved independence or obtainment of specific functional skills are more appropriate. For example, a long term goal may be "to improve voluntary use of one upper extremity so the child is able independently to punch the keys on a computer." The issue of "quality" of movement is a sensitive one with developmental therapists. One opinion is that the best strategy is to strive for normal quality of movement. There are some children, however, who do not have the capability of normal movement and valuable time may be lost working towards unattainable goals when the major objective of the physical therapist should be to improve the child's functional abilities.

BEHAVIORAL OBJECTIVES

The physical therapist is responsible for determining therapeutic goals for the child. Although therapists know what "improving equilibrium reactions" is, various therapists may use different observational data to support the conclusion that this therapeutic goal has

been met. It is also our responsibility to describe the behavior or set of behaviors which allows other observers (therapist, physician, parent, teacher) to arrive at the same conclusion regarding the child's level of function. Precise, unambiguous specifications regarding a behavior also decrease the amount of subjectivity in the evaluation process. For example, the objective "the child will ambulate independently with a walker" does not tell us if there are any constraints on the child's abilities. If we state that "the child will ambulate independently with a reverse walker in all environments," we clarify the behavioral objective and desired functional level.

Behavioral objectives consist of a behavior which can be observed and measured. Specific criteria describing the behavior may include the conditions under which the behavior will occur. Using successful completion of a minimum number of trials or performance of a behavior during a percentage of a set time period would be examples of specified conditions.

The movement problems we identify are determined by our theoretical perspective. When we observe a child spontaneously assume an asymmetrical posture, we can hypothesize the influence of a primitive reflex pattern such as an asymmetrical tonic neck (ATNR), sensory disregard of one side of the body, or some other explanation for the motor behavior. We can be accurate in our objective descriptions of a child's posture and movement, but we only can hypothesize about underlying causes.

Physical therapy goals and functional objectives for the child also depend on the theoretical framework of the physical therapist. In hierarchial models, goals often relate to altering muscle tone, decreasing reflex patterns of movement, achieving developmental motor milestones, and improving sensory processing. In more contemporary models, goals may relate to initiation, speed, and variability of movement and to variables described in a systems approach[2]. Traditional goals of physical therapy intervention, such as those addressing strength, endurance, and flexibility also are used in pediatrics. Goals in various frameworks overlap. The essential element that ties them together is the use of functional, measurable objectives.

Therapists may have difficulty stating therapeutic goals in behavioral terms. We may agree with the goal of decreasing the influence of the ATNR in a spastic cerebral palsied child, but how do we measure the success of our treatment? One approach is to hypothesize how the ATNR interferes with the child's movement and to write behavioral objectives based on these interferences. For example, if the child cannot maintain a prone on elbows position when he turns his head (due to collapsing on the arm on the skull side), one objective would be that "the child will be able to maintain prone-on-elbows for one minute while turning his head to the left and right". By identifying a functional problem and describing motor behavior objectively, we can communicate clearly about movement parameters even though our hypotheses or assumptions about the underlying causes may be different. Several developmental problems, followed by examples of how each may interfere with function are listed below. Problems identified in hierarchial, systems, and traditional models are included. Therapeutic goals and related objectives, written in behavioral terms, are then provided to address each problem.

PROBLEM 1:
Predominance of Asymmetrical Tonic Neck (ATNR) response

Therapeutic Goal: Decrease influence of ATNR on motor skills.

Interferes with Development/Skill: In supine, when child turns head, ATNR posture assumed. Child cannot bring hands to mouth or hands together at midline.

Behavioral Objectives:

In supine, child will be able to volitionally bring either hand to his mouth. In supine, child will be able to bring his hands together at midline for hand-to-hand contact and to manipulate objects (toys).

Interferes with Development/Skill: In prone, child cannot maintain prone on elbows. As he turns his head,

shoulder girdle support decreases on the skull side and he collapses.

Behavioral Objective:

In prone, child will be able to achieve and maintain prone on elbows for one minute as he turns his head to either side.

Interferes with Development/Skill: In quadruped, child has difficulty creeping without collapsing on skull arm when he turns his head.

Behavioral Objectives:

Child can maintain a quadruped position for one minute while visually tracking a suspended ball as it swings horizontally in front of him.

Child will be able to creep a distance of ten feet and maintain upper extremity stability (does not collapse) while turning his head to either side.

Child will independently assume reverse ATNR posture in quadruped to either side (i.e. balance with left leg up and left arm on hip while looking up at ceiling).

PROBLEM 2:
Influence of Symmetrical Tonic Neck (STNR) response

Therapeutic Goal: Decrease influence of STNR in functional activities.

Interferes with Development/Skill: Child uses STNR to assume quadruped position, then "bunny-hops" (bilateral lower extremity pattern) in creeping.

Behavioral Objectives:

In hands and knees position, child can flex head and maintain hip and shoulder extension for 5 seconds.

In hands and knees position, child can extend head without sitting back on heels.

From a hands and knees position, child will be able to push up on his hands and feet and look through his legs without falling.

In a hands and knees position, child will be able to shift weight forward and backward three times without falling.

Child will creep with a reciprocal pattern 100% of the time.

Interferes with Development/Skill: Child cannot push down on water fountain button, then flex his head to drink (extended position of arms cannot be maintained).

Behavioral Objective:

Child will drink out of water fountain independently.

PROBLEM 3:
Poor head righting and head control

Therapeutic Goal: Improve head righting and control in all planes of movement.

Interferes with Development/Skill: In prone, child does not lift head off floor.

Behavioral Objectives:

In prone, child will lift head to 90 degrees, two out of three times, and maintain this position for 30 seconds to view an object.

In prone, child will lift head two of three trials to visually track a moving object across midline.

Interferes with Development/Skill: In sitting, head is extended and supported by shoulders.

Behavioral Objective:

In sitting, child will tuck chin and maintain an erect head position 50% of the time in an observation period of 5 minutes.

Interferes with Development/Skill: In rolling, child's head hits the floor.

Behavioral Objective:

Child's head does not touch floor when rolling a distance of six feet.

Interferes with Development/Skill: In sitting, child does not consistently reposition head upright when tilted.

Behavioral Objective:

Child will maintain head in midline when rocked 20 degrees in any direction from the upright in sitting.

PROBLEM 4:
Inadequate protective reactions

Therapeutic Goal: Facilitate the development of effective protective reactions in all planes of movement.

Interferes with Development/Skill: When child loses balance in sitting, he does not attempt to catch himself with his arms.

Behavioral Objectives:

When placed in sitting, child will prop on extended arms for one minute without collapsing.

In sitting, the child will successfully catch himself two of three trials when pushed off balance in a lateral direction.

Interferes with Development/Skill: Child is ambulatory, but must wear a helmet because he does not protect himself adequately when he falls.

Behavioral Objectives:

Child will be able to deliberately fall forward from a standing position and catch himself with his arms.

Child will be able to deliberately fall sideways from a standing position and catch himself with his arms.

Child will be able to deliberately fall backwards from a standing position and "sit" down with protective reactions of the arms.

In walking during the school day, child will not hit his head on the floor when he falls.

PROBLEM 5:
Vestibular processing deficits
(hypothesized from informal observation)

Therapeutic Goal: Normalize vestibular processing and response to movement-based activities.

Interferes with Development/Skill: Child does not enjoy or tolerate movement activities. He will not attempt to play on moveable equipment/toys.

Behavioral Objectives:

Child will tolerate swinging slowly on playground swing for three minutes.

Child will participate in scooter board games with his peers.

Interferes with Development/Skill: Child complains of nausea and dizziness whenever he is on moveable equipment.

Behavioral Objective:

Child can play independently on playground equipment for 10 minutes without complaining of dizziness or nausea.

Interferes with Development/Skill: Child seeks out excessive movement-based stimulation; rocks and twirls himself repeatedly as part of self-stimulatory behaviors.

Behavioral Objective:

Child will decrease rocking behavior from current level of 75% of 10 minute observation period to less than 50%.

PROBLEM 6:
Tactile processing deficit
(hypothesized from testing and observation)

Therapeutic Goal: Normalize tactile processing.

Interferes with Development/Skill: Child is tactilely defensive. He does not like to be touched, wear new clothes, or have his face or hair washed.

Behavioral Objectives:

Child will seek out hugs from adults.

Child will not cry or scream when his hair is washed.

In two of three trials, child will not demonstrate an aversive reaction to being touched by another person.

Interferes with Development/Skill: Child dislikes using his hands to explore or play in various textured mediums.

Behavioral Objectives:

Child will play independently for 5 minutes in water or sand.

Child will complete a finger painting project without assistance from adult.

PROBLEM 7:
Poor visual processing — poor focusing
and tracking abilities

Therapeutic Goal: Normalize visual processing.

Interferes with Development/Skill: Child will not look at objects placed in his visual field and does not maintain eye contact with adults or peers.

Behavioral Objectives:

Child will orient two of three trials to an object lit by a flashlight.

Child will maintain visual focus on a specific toy for 10 seconds.

Child will turn eyes and head two of three trials to follow a moving object.

Child will maintain eye contact with an adult 50% of the time during a five minute observation period.

PROBLEM 8:

Somatosensory processing deficit — child shows abnormalities in body awareness or neglects body parts

Therapeutic Goal: Normalize somatosensory processing and improve body awareness.

Interferes with Development/Skill: Child does not demonstrate good awareness of body parts and his position in space. He tends to neglect the left side in functional activities.

Behavioral Objectives:

Child actively removes sticky tape placed on right arm (must remove with left hand).

Child correctly moves body parts on verbal command (or visual imitation).

Child belly crawls using all four extremities.

PROBLEM 9:

Child has fine motor delays—demonstrates gross grasp and release only

Therapeutic Goal: Facilitate maturation of hand skills and increase independence in manipulation of objects and self-feeding.

Interferes with Development/Skill: Child cannot move object to radial side of hand or orient hand to get objects (food) to mouth.

Behavioral Objectives:

Nine out of ten times, child will grasp small objects with radial portion of hand.

Child will grasp bread stick and bring it to his mouth independently.

In two of five trials, child will use a three-finger pinch to pick up a small object (cheerio).

PROBLEM 10:

Poor control of forearm in fine motor tasks

Therapeutic Goal: Facilitate maturation of fine motor development.

Interferes with Development/Skill: Child demonstrates poor supination — uses a pronated reach for objects and is unable to orient the hand to neutral to grasp.

Behavioral Objectives:

Child will orient the forearm to neutral two of three trials to grasp a vertical dowel.

Child will supinate both arms to hold a large box.

Child will bring both forearms to neutral to grasp a large ball.

PROBLEM 11:

Poor lower extremity dissociation

Therapeutic Goal: Facilitate the ability to dissociate movement of one leg from the other during functional activities.

Interferes with Development/Skill: Child tends to use both legs together. In sitting, cannot shift weight onto one hip and put on socks or clothing.

Behavioral Objective:

In sitting on the floor, the child will shift his weight and leave one leg extended while flexing one leg to put on socks or pants.

Interferes with Development/Skill: Child "bunny-hops" in creeping.

Behavioral Objectives:

In quadruped, child will extend one leg and maintain balance for three seconds.

Child will creep with a reciprocal rather than a bilateral lower extremity pattern 100% of the time.

Interferes with Development/Skill: Child cannot shift weight in standing, but stands with legs internally rotated at hips and knees together.

Behavioral Objectives:

While holding onto a walker, the child will shift weight in standing and lift one leg for 3 seconds.

Child will independently ride a tricycle for a distance of 6 feet.

PROBLEM 12:

Difficulty initiating movement

Therapeutic Goal: Improve ability to initiate movement.

Interferes with Development/Skills: Child is slow to move in response to verbal requests. Other children and siblings assist the child, decreasing opportunities to practice motor skills and decreasing independence.

Behavioral Objectives:

In sitting, child will initiate reaching for a toy less than 3 seconds after a verbal request to "get the toy".

In prone, child will belly crawl toward a toy within 5 seconds after toy is placed on the floor.

PROBLEM 13:

Decreased frequency of voluntary movement

Therapeutic Goal: Increase frequency of attempts at independent movement.

Interferes with Development/Skill: Child does not use right upper extremity during play or when large toys requiring bilateral upper extremity use are presented to him to hold.

Behavioral Objectives:

In ring sitting, child will use his right arm, with verbal reminders, to pick up 3 of 5 puzzle pieces placed to his right.

Child will use his right hand spontaneously to clap in a game of patty-cake, imitating the therapist on five of fifteen attempts.

Child will use both hands to hold orange therapy ball, three of five trials.

PROBLEM 14:

Decreased variability of movement

Therapeutic Goal: Increase variability of movement.

Interferes with Development/Skill: Child always moves from prone to "W" sitting by pushing up on extended arms and pulling his legs underneath him.
Behavioral Objectives:

When placed on the floor in prone, child will use more than one movement pattern to get into sitting during 5 trials.

Child will assume at least two different sitting positions over a 5 minute observation period of free play.

PROBLEM 15:
Slow movement; inability to generate fast movements
Therapeutic Goal: Increase speed of movement.
Interferes with Development/Skill: In ambulation using a reverse walker, child walks too slowly to keep up with his peers in the classroom.
Behavioral Objectives:

Child will march in time (20 steps/minute) to fast music while standing with his walker.

Child will ambulate independently with his walker 20 feet in 10 seconds in the classroom.
Interferes with Development/Skill: Child moves very slowly when feeding himself and takes more than 45 minutes to finish a meal.
Behavioral Objective:

Child will feed himself and complete a meal within 30 minutes.
Interferes with Development/Skill: Child cannot pedal an adaptive tricycle fast enough to keep up with his peers as they walk.
Behavioral Objective:

Child will pedal his tricycle fast enough to keep up with his walking peers for 1 minute.

PROBLEM 16:
Poor selective attention
Therapeutic Goal: Improve selective attention during motor tasks.
Interferes with Development/Skill:

Child cannot walk independently from classroom to gym as he becomes distracted by other children.
Behavioral Objective:

Child will walk independently from classroom to gym within 10 minutes, 100% of the time.
Interferes with Development/Skill: Child does not attempt fine motor activities in classroom as he becomes distracted by other children.
Behavioral Objective:

Child will attend to a table activity for 5 minutes without being distracted by two other children working at the same table.

PROBLEM 17:
Poor abdominal strength
Therapeutic Goal: Improve abdominal strength for trunk stability and control.

Interferes with Development/Skill: Child cannot lift head in supine, but rolls to side.
Behavioral Objective:

In supine, child will independently lift up head to look at toes.
Interferes with Development/Skill: If child loses balance backwards in sitting, he attempts to right himself, but usually falls backwards.
Behavioral Objective:

In sitting with hips stabilized, child will be able to lower his trunk back 10-20 degrees and return to sitting.
Interferes with Development/Skill: Child cannot make independent transitions from sitting to hands and knees using trunk rotation, but moves forward over legs, without any trunk rotation, onto hands and knees.
Behavioral Objective:

Child will be able to rotate trunk to move from sitting to sidesitting to hands and knees and back to side-sitting on the opposite side with minimal assistance at the pelvis.

PROBLEM 18:
Child demonstrates general rigidity of movement, with poor flexibility of body parts
Therapeutic Goal: Decrease general rigidity and increase flexibility.
Interferes with Development/Skill: Child has rigid movements, especially of trunk. He does not demonstrate trunk rotation in any position and has difficulty crossing the midline of the body in upper extremity tasks.
Behavioral Objectives:

Child will roll using trunk rotation (observed separation between shoulders and pelvis), rather than log-rolling.

In tailor sitting, child will be able to rotate trunk two of three trials to view an object behind him (without moving base of support — legs and pelvis).

In two of three trials, child will cross midline of body with arm to reach for an object (rather than turning his entire body to avoid crossing the midline).

In standing, the child will be able to independently perform "windmills" — touching left foot with right hand, then right foot with left hand.

PROBLEM 19:
Poor motor planning skills
Therapeutic Goal: Improve motor planning—gross and fine motor.
Interferes with Development/Skill: Child uses an electric wheelchair but runs into objects, walls, and people.
Behavioral Objectives:

Child will successfully complete a 20 foot obstacle course two of three trials without hitting any walls or five obstacles.

When using a rear-view mirror mounted on the wheel-chair, the child will successfully back up.

The child will be able to turn the wheelchair around in a 4-foot square space in the classroom.

ESTABLISHING LONG TERM GOALS AND SHORT TERM OBJECTIVES

One example of a long term goal is that "the child will ambulate independently with a walker in the home." The therapist analyzes this task and develops short term objectives which are appropriate for eventually reaching the long term goal for the individual child. Examples of short term objectives might include:

— The child will pull to stand at furniture two of three trials when a toy is placed out of reach on the furniture.

— The child will cruise to the left or right at furniture to obtain toys.

— When placed, the child will maintain balance in upright with the walker for 5 minutes.

— The child will make forward progress with the walker for a distance of 10 feet.

— The child will demonstrate the ability to motor plan a distance of 15 feet and turn the walker to avoid two obstacles in his path.

— The child will demonstrate protective reactions each time he falls.

— The child will be able to lower himself independently from the walker to the floor or to a chair, 2 of 3 attempts.

After determining long term goals and short term objectives, the therapist then selects appropriate treatment techniques to aid the child in achieving each objective (refer to chapters 5 through 12). During treatment, the therapist continually evaluates the effectiveness of treatment techniques, adding, omitting, or revising intervention as necessary for the child's success. As the child makes progress, long term goals and short term objectives may be altered or new goals may be instated and the process begins again (Figure 2).

MOTOR LEARNING

During the past 50 years the clinical approach of physical therapists to children with neurologic disabilities has been influenced primarily by clinicians who developed a variety of neurophysiologic approaches. These neurophysiologic approaches include the theories and techniques of the Bobaths (Neurodevelopmental Treatment - NDT), Kabat, Knott, and Voss (Proprioceptive Neuromuscular Facilitation - PNF), Ayres (Sensory Integration - SI), Rood, and others and have been described in a number of publications[3,4]. Physical therapy assessment and treatment techniques, in general, have

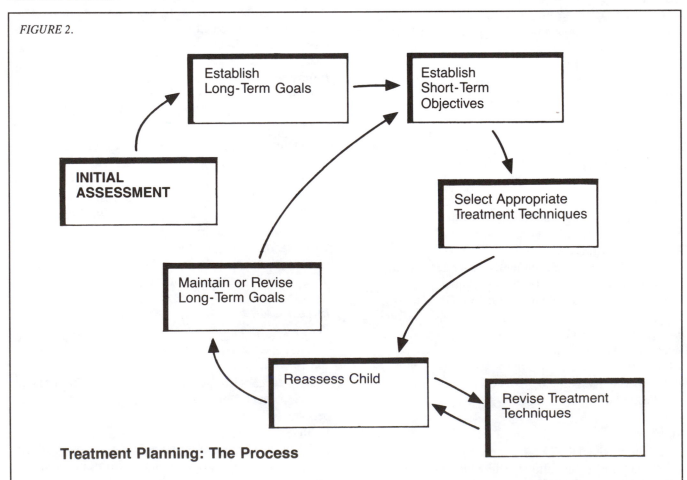

FIGURE 2.

INITIAL ASSESSMENT

Establish Long-Term Goals

Establish Short-Term Objectives

Select Appropriate Treatment Techniques

Maintain or Revise Long-Term Goals

Reassess Child

Revise Treatment Techniques

Treatment Planning: The Process

centered around issues of motor control. In recent years, physical therapists also have been influenced by research in the field of motor learning.

Movement can be described by two general classes [5]. One class of movements, such as control of our limbs and walking, appears to be determined primarily by genetic makeup and/or through growth and development and are fairly stereotyped across members of the same species. What central nervous system (CNS) structures are involved and how the CNS organizes individual and coordinated movements of the limbs and body are the basic questions in the study of motor control.

A second class of movements, such as riding a bicycle, writing, or performing a somersault, can be considered to be "learned". These movements do not appear to be genetic and require varying (usually long) periods of practice and experience to master. How movements are produced as the result of practice or experience is the major question in the study of motor learning.

Although issues of motor control and motor learning in relation to movement (genetic or practiced) may be more clearly differentiated in normal individuals, the distinction becomes blurred in children (and adults) with neurologic dysfunction. If a child has damage to CNS structures that produce a specific movement pattern, such as components of the gait cycle, he may have to practice or adapt the movements he is able to produce in order to develop ambulation. In this case, ambulation may be considered a "skill" and is perhaps a better example of motor learning than motor control.

Because most of the functional tasks we want children with neurologic deficits to perform require a combination of motor control and motor learning, understanding and applying principles of motor learning to physical therapy treatment are essential. There are few motor learning studies of children with neurologic disabilities to guide our intervention sessions, therefore we rely on information from studies of normal adults and children. We should remain cautious in application of principles of motor learning until research studies validate their use with disabled populations.

Selected motor learning issues and their application to pediatrics are described briefly. Refer to Schmidt[5,6] and Winstein[7,8] for more detailed discussions of principles of motor learning.

PERFORMANCE VS. LEARNING

Motor learning is not directly observable. It is defined as "a set of processes associated with practice or experience that leads to a relatively permanent change in skilled motor behavior" [5, p.345].

When we facilitate movement through manual guidance (handling), such as assisting the child with shoulder protraction during reaching, we are affecting the child's "performance" at that moment. We can determine his

performance directly by visually or kinesthetically observing his movements. It only would be evident that the child had "learned" a skill if he consistently and appropriately used shoulder protraction independent of intervention over a period of time. Another example of performance versus learning is the common intervention strategy of facilitating hip abduction and weight shifting during gait training through manual guidance of the pelvis of the child with spastic diplegia. If the child demonstrates this gait pattern only during treatment sessions with manual facilitation and reverts to "scissoring" when attempting movement on his own we have succeeded only in changing his performance during the treatment session. He has not acquired a skill which can be generalized to other settings. In most instances, physical therapists use handling and facilitation/inhibition techniques to assist the child initially to perform a more efficient or coordinated movement. This is an attempt to provide the child with kinesthetic information (feedback) on how this movement feels and to give him an idea of the movement(s) we want him to attempt. We decrease our handling as the child is able to produce some aspects of the movement independently. When the child is able to perform the entire movement independently and consistently, he not only has improved his performance, but also has acquired a skill. Physical therapy that has as its end result only changes in performance is not cost-effective and is of limited value to the child. The goal in physical therapy is for the child to acquire motor skills that will increase his independence in a variety of environments and decrease his dependence on the physical therapist.

TRANSFER OF LEARNING

Transfer of learning refers to a gain (or loss) in the capability for producing a movement or performing a task as the result of practice or experience of another movement or task. According to Schmidt[5], in research on transfer of learning, two major points emerge. One is that the amount of transfer between tasks appears to be quite small. The second is that the amount of transfer depends on the similarity of the tasks; the more similar the tasks, the more likely transfer will occur.

One assumption made in neurophysiologic approaches is that a motor skill learned in one position will provide positive transfer to a similar skill in another position. For example, we assume that having the child practice trunk extension in prone will assist with trunk extension in sitting and standing. Another example is the hypothesis that facilitating balance reactions while the child sits on a therapy ball will improve the child's balance while sitting on the floor.

In the first example, we need to consider that prone extension is a different task for the CNS to organize than trunk extension in sitting and standing where the biomechanical constraints and pull of gravity are quite different

(Figure 3). In the second example, responses to externally produced perturbations may be a significantly different control issue for the CNS than maintaining sitting balance through a feed-forward mechanism. The biomechanical constraints of the task also vary to the extent the sitting position on the ball differs from that on the floor.

Until research offers a clearer understanding regarding the positive transfer of practice between specific movements and skills in children with neurologic impairments, physical therapists can ensure a comprehensive approach to treatment by having the child practice the specific movements or tasks we want him to perform, in addition to those prerequisite movements or tasks we assume will provide positive transfer. This means that, in addition to practicing trunk extension in prone, we have the child practice trunk extension in sitting and standing; and, in addition to facilitating balance reactions while the child sits on a therapy ball, we provide the child with ample opportunity to practice independent floor sitting. Another technique used by physical therapists is to have the child practice components of a motor task before attempting to practice the entire task (part-whole trans-

fer). For example, we may have the child work in a standing position on balance, weight-shifting, and lower extremity control, such as kicking a ball, before having the child practice walking. According to Schmidt[5], the problem may be that practicing a part in isolation may change the motor programming of the part so it is no longer the same as in the context of the total skill.

Research suggests that the effectiveness of part-whole transfer depends on the nature of the task. When tasks are strictly serial in nature, as in an assembly line, practice of parts transfers highly to the whole task. Motor tasks are, however, seldom strictly serial in nature. For example, when reaching for an object from a standing position, milliseconds prior to lifting the arm to reach, the leg and trunk muscles must contract to provide stability and prevent a weight shift forward and possible fall. In walking there are precise temporal and spatial relationships among and between the muscles of each leg. Schmidt[5] suggested that part to whole transfer also may depend on the extent to which the movement is governed by a single motor program. Generally, if a movement is fast, it probably is governed by a single program and should be practiced as a whole. Throwing a ball is an example of a ballistic-type feed-forward movement that is better practiced as a whole. Simultaneous movements of limbs also may be governed by a single program. There is, however, little research to guide us in determining which movements and tasks may benefit from part to whole transfer. Winstein suggested that "natural breaks in the resultant velocity profile of a multisegmental movement could reflect the end of one subunit and the beginning of the next"[7, p. 74]. In summary, the assumption that breaking down a task for practice will always improve performance on the whole task can be challenged. Physical therapists should include practice on the whole task as well as practice on component parts in their approach to treatment.

VARIABLE (RANDOM) VS. CONSTANT (BLOCKED) PRACTICE

The amount of variability within a practice session may affect motor learning. Children, in particular, perform better on a novel task when earlier practice is variable as opposed to constant[5,9]. This suggests that providing variations of tasks and varying practice among tasks during treatment may be more beneficial for motor learning than having the child perform a large number of repetitions of a single movement or task. One hypothesis is that each time a component of a task or the task itself is varied, the child must concentrate anew and problem solve in relation to the required movements or task. With numerous repetitions, movement becomes automatic and the child may concentrate less and not be required to actively problem solve regarding the motor requirements. In neurophysiologic approaches, repetition is considered an essential element to improve motor control. Undoubtedly there must be a sufficient number of repetitions for the child to receive feedback about his movements and to engage in trial and error attempts at controlling movement or performing a task. The therapist must look for cues that the child is performing movement in a rote fashion with little attention to the task in order to vary the task requirements at the appropriate moments. Treatment sessions should be structured around the child's attention level and motivation. A practical example would be to have the child change positions and practice various skills several times within a 45 minute treatment session, dictated by his attention span and the difficulty of the tasks. This would be preferable to pre-determining the structure of a treatment session, for example spending 15 minutes working on prone extension, 15 minutes working on sitting balance, and 15 minutes working on gait. Schmidt stated that "blocked (constant) practice and drills are highly ineffective ways to generate learning and should almost never be used" [6, p.54]. The exception would be very early practice when the child is first acquiring a movement or basic skill. Schmidt suggested that once a movement can be performed, practice should be randomized. A related point is that practice needs to be somewhat difficult and require effort on the part of the child. The challenge for the physical therapist is to find activities that entice the child to attempt and repeat movements that require effort and concentration.

FEEDBACK/KNOWLEDGE OF RESULTS (KR)

One of the most important variables enhancing motor learning is feedback or information that is provided to the child about his performance as he attempts to move or accomplish a task. Intrinsic feedback refers to information obtained through the sensory systems (i.e., visual, proprioceptive, auditory, vestibular) as movement is attempted or produced. Extrinsic feedback refers primarily to verbal information (i.e., from a physical therapist) related to performance. Extrinsic feedback also can be provided through non-verbal means, such as a switch device that activates a musical toy each time the child's head is upright in sitting.

Knowledge of Performance vs. Knowledge of Results

Gentile[10] distinguished between knowledge of performance (KP-feedback about the movement itself) and knowledge of results (KR-feedback about the outcome of the movement). Providing the child information on how effectively the back muscles are contracting (KP) versus providing information on how effectively he is maintaining an upright sitting posture (KR) is a specific example. Most research to date has focused on information regarding movement outcome (KR). The current assumption is that the mechanisms of KR and KP are similar[6].

Traditional vs. Contemporary View

The traditional view of feedback (prior to the 1980's) was that feedback that was more frequent, more immediate, more accurate, or produced more information was the most beneficial for learning[6]. More recent research has caused a reexamination of how feedback enhances learning. It now appears that while frequent feedback may enhance motor performance, it actually may be detrimental to motor learning. This is a startling notion to physical therapists who have used feedback in the traditional manner. One hypothesis is that too frequent feedback interferes with the child's ability to learn to detect and correct errors. Less frequent feedback or fading feedback appears to be more beneficial for motor learning[6,7]. In practical terms this means the physical therapist should avoid providing feedback after every trial or attempt at movement. Schmidt[6] suggested that more guidance may be needed in complex tasks, whereas less guidance may be needed in simple motor tasks.

Various schedules of feedback have been examined experimentally and have been reviewed elsewhere[5]. One alternative to constant feedback would be to provide feedback in a summary form after several trials. Another alternative is "bandwidth KR" where feedback is given only if the movement or performance is outside a given error range. The absence of KR informs the child that his movement is acceptable. A practical example would be monitoring the child's tendency to "W-sit" during a treatment session. The physical therapist can instruct the child that kneel-sitting on his feet is acceptable, but kneel-sitting while internally rotating the hips with the feet out to the side of the body with the buttocks on the floor is unacceptable (Figures 4 and 5). The therapist decides to call the child's attention to his "W-sitting" position whenever the child sits in this unacceptable position for more than 30 seconds. The absence of feedback at other times informs the child that his sitting posture is acceptable. Another example would be calling the child's attention to foot placement only when the foot is placed outside of an area where it could serve as a base of support during a series of attempts to move from half-kneeling to standing at a sofa. Although the child may vary his foot placement from trial to trial, as long as he could shift his weight adequately to push to stand, he would receive no feedback. Bandwidth KR can be used to allow more variability of movement, prevent too frequent feedback (after every trial), and allow the child to concentrate on intrinsic feedback to monitor his movements.

Application to Pediatrics

Several principles of KR have special applicability in the treatment of children[5]. When KR is provided, it is provided during or immediately after a movement or task is completed. The interval between completion of a movement and feedback from the therapist should be "empty". In other

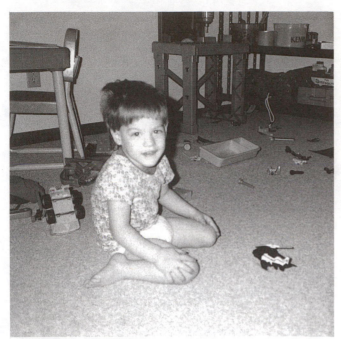

FIGURE 4. "W-sitting" with hips internally rotated and buttocks flat on floor.

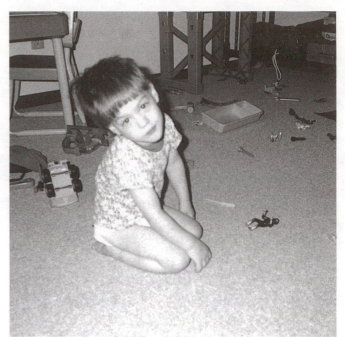

FIGURE 5. "Heel-sitting" with hips in neutral alignment and buttocks resting on feet.

words, the child should not be asked to perform other movements or be distracted by the therapist or environment. It is hypothesized that the child may be retaining in short term memory kinesthetic information regarding the movement and that this process should proceed without distractions. Therapists should be cautious about distracting the child unnecessarily by talking or calling his attention to toys or other objects in the environment.

In research with children, it has been determined that performance is disrupted when shortening the period of time following KR and when a subsequent attempt is made to repeat the movement or task.[5] The assumption is that new solutions to motor problems are being processed and a certain amount of time is necessary for this to occur. The child should be allowed to initiate repetitions of movements and tasks at his own determined speed.

GUIDANCE

Guidance refers to a number of procedures ranging from physically assisting movement (facilitation/handling) to verbally talking the child through a task[5]. In general, guidance tends to prevent the child from making errors. One hypothesis in support of facilitation and handling (guidance) is that improved quality of movement will be produced and the child will be less apt to learn incorrect movements and, therefore, will not repeat or learn these less desirable movements. In an opposite view, motor learning appears to be most effective in trial and error situations. The child must learn which internal commands lead to effective or ineffective outcomes and the only way to learn this is to make, recognize, and try to correct errors.

Although research is limited, it appears that guidance is most effective in early practice of new, unfamiliar tasks. Guidance also may be more effective for slow movements where feedback may be used for control and monitoring.

Physical guidance may be beneficial in showing the child what to do and perhaps in reducing fear when having the child attempt new motor skills. The physical therapist initially assists the child in producing a response or movement which can be improved with practice; less guidance is used as the child takes more responsibility for producing the movement.

Too much guidance, however, may act as a "crutch" preventing the child from experiencing errors and learning from his own attempts at movement. In the presence of a damaged CNS, it may be idealistic to assume that we can facilitate "normal" movement. The goal of physical therapy should be for the child to produce the most efficient and effective movement he can to accomplish independent skills. The physical therapist must decide when facilitation designed to improve "quality of movement" should be discarded and emphasis placed on alternative strategies for accomplishing a motor task. One limitation in applying motor learning principles to physical therapy is that we do not know how applicable various concepts are to infants and children with impaired cognition.

MOTOR LEARNING — SUMMARY

Feedback appears to be essential for motor learning. Providing feedback less frequently, however, may be more beneficial for learning than immediate feedback following each attempt at movement. The use of less frequent verbal feedback and less manual facilitation of

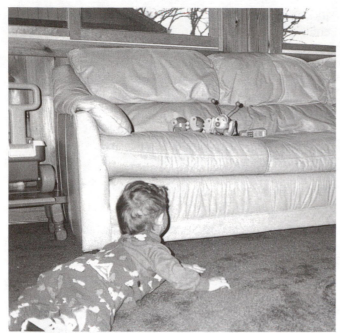

FIGURE 6. *From prone, child is unable to pull to kneeling at sofa.*

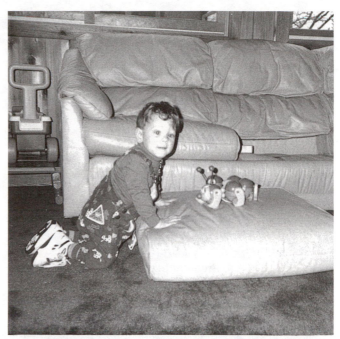

FIGURE 7. *From prone, child is able to pull to kneeling at sofa cushion.*

movement may be frustrating for the physical therapist because the child's performance may actually be worse during the treatment session. Schmidt[6] suggested that the goal of physical therapy is not necessarily to produce the best performance during therapy, but to organize practice to maximize retention (learning).

ORGANIZING TREATMENT

Context

In Gibson's[11] approach to understanding human behavior, called "ecological psychology", the child and the environment are linked. Objects in the environment are described in terms of "affordances" or what they offer the child for perceptual exploration and movement. For example, while observing a 7 month old child belly crawling on the floor, a toy is placed on an 18 inch high sofa (Figure 6). The child, who sees the toy and appears interested in it, does not attempt to reach the toy. If the sofa cushion (6 inches in height) is placed on the floor and the toy is placed on top of the cushion, the child reaches up to the sofa cushion, pulls himself up on his knees, and reaches for the toy (Figure 7). The top of the sofa was too high for the child to reach from a prone position and, therefore, did not "afford" the child a surface to pull up on. The sofa cushion, on the floor, however, was of an appropriate height and "afforded" the child the opportunity to pull up into a kneeling position to obtain the toy.

Physical therapists working with children construct affordances in the environment to elicit functional movements[12]. We also recognize the importance of practicing skills in various environments (home, school, community) related to long term functional goals. Physical

therapists want a child to perform a specific skill, such as ambulation, in a variety of environments (different contexts). Being able to walk safely in a therapy room with a tile floor and few obstacles or distractions does not ensure that the child will be able to walk safely on carpet in a cluttered, noisy, and visually distracting classroom.

To ensure use of the same skill in varied contexts, the physical therapist has the child practice the skill in each environment and makes modifications or alters training, as necessary. This often is a difficult concept for third party payers, who may prefer to reimburse therapy services that are delivered primarily on an outpatient basis in a hospital or medically related facility. Environments in which it is important for the child to function include the home, school, neighborhood, and community settings including church, shopping mall, and playground. Several physical therapy sessions spent on the neighborhood playground may appear frivolous to a third party payer. This is the best context however, for the child to learn skills that will enable him to effectively and safely move and interact with his peers in a playground setting.

The Normal Developmental Sequence

Physical therapists have used normal development as a guide for assessing and treating children with motor deficits. Normal development has been considered the "gold standard" for movement. Although the normal developmental sequence provides physical therapists with a wealth of information regarding components of movements and patterns generally used by normal children, its applicability to children with motor deficits is limited. Major developmental milestones, such as rolling, sitting, pulling to stand, and walking are important functional goals. However, how they are accomplished does not need to mirror "normal". Consider the child with arthrogryposis. He will be limited in how he moves because of lack of specific muscles and certain joint limitations. This child will not be able to produce "normal" movement using the same muscles and joint range of motion of normal peers. Yet, by using the muscles and joint range available to him, the child with arthrogryposis may be able to accomplish the motor skills necessary to function independently. Do we conclude that the "quality" of his movements is poor because they do not "look like" the movements produced by a normal peer?

Perhaps movements should be judged primarily by their effectiveness in accomplishing a task. For example, rather than considering gait in terms of heel-strike, stance, toe-off, etc., or the specific muscles involved in each phase, gait should be assessed in terms of its major functional components, namely support and propulsion in stance, clearance of the foot, and a transfer of momentum in swing[13]. If children with arthrogryposis, cerebral palsy, or spina bifida are able to accomplish the functional components of ambulation perhaps the "quality" of their movements should be considered good, regardless of how closely they approximate normal movement.

Another important issue in evaluating the quality of movement is to determine the potential for the development of secondary problems. Postures such as "W-sitting" when used excessively may produce decreased range of motion in hip external rotation, knee instability, and contribute to ankle eversion and a poor base of support in standing. Continued use of a pronated reach will limit active forearm supination and muscle tightness may result. The child and family must be informed about the risk of secondary problems and, together with the developmental therapist, make decisions about which patterns of movements are acceptable.

The developmental sequence of skill acquisition has been demonstrated to be variable[14,15]. This is a compelling argument for not using the developmental sequence as a rigid, prescriptive model for treatment. In a developmental, hierarchal model, the child would practice skills in a specific sequence (i.e., rolling, then sitting, then crawling) and may not practice a "higher" skill before a "lower" skill is mastered (i.e., delaying practice of ambulation until sitting balance is accomplished). Arguments for and against using the developmental sequence as a model in the treatment of children and adults were discussed at the II STEP conference[16-18].

An alternative approach to using a developmental sequence would be to have the child practice a variety of age-appropriate functional tasks that he might reasonably be expected to accomplish. A two year old child with spastic diplegia, for example, may have difficulty maintaining floor sitting due to increased muscle activity or tightness of the hamstrings, yet he may be able to control his balance in upright using a walker. This child may never master the task of independent floor sitting and if we follow the developmental sequence prescriptively, we would not allow him to practice ambulation skills. The alternative approach is to work on a variety of skills simultaneously, allowing the child to progress with the acquisition of skills at varying rates as allowed by neurologic, biomechanical, cognitive, and other factors (systems approach).

Sequencing Treatment

Usually many deficits occur simultaneously in the child with a developmental disability. For example, a child with spastic diplegia may demonstrate deficits in sensory processing, motor control, strength, and attention. In organizing treatment and attempting to address various problems simultaneously, there are two general treatment sequences to consider. The first is the overall sequence of treatment over an extended period of time, for example, a three month period or a school year. Careful formulation of long term goals and short term objectives will aid the therapist in obtaining a mental overview of the necessary emphasis in treatment. The second consideration is sequencing treatment within an individual treatment session which may vary from a half-hour to an hour or longer.

Considerations in determining the content of an individual treatment session are the mental abilities of the child, his motivation, age, and endurance. A "play" versus a "work" approach can be varied depending on the age, personality, and interests of the child. Toys can be used quite effectively to motivate the young child and infant and to maintain interest during therapy. If a child resists or fatigues during certain activities, such as abdominal strengthening, three or four treatment techniques designed to strengthen the abdominal muscles can be interspersed during an individual session.

Techniques for behavior management can be employed to assist in specific sensory or motor tasks and also as a way to modify negative behavior during therapy. Checklists of exercises, which when completed yield a reward, are often helpful to motivate the child and to help the child be more organized during therapy. A small kitchen timer can be used to designate specific "work" (15 minutes) versus "play" (3 minutes) sessions, or specific rewards can be given for each 15 minute "crying-free" session.

A final, but perhaps the most crucial, consideration is the availability of caregivers for carryover of treatment. Whenever possible, the physical therapist should involve the family, school personnel, and other caregivers in the child's therapy program. Clearly defined behavioral objectives will assist in this process and the therapist can facilitate the child's progress by training others in the child's environment in related therapeutic activities, and, when necessary, the use of adaptive equipment.

DOCUMENTING PROGRESS

Physical therapists are responsible not only for determining functional objectives for the child, but also for determining whether the objectives have been met. Various methods for charting progress have been described[19]. An important component is to differentiate motor performance from motor learning. One method to determine whether functional objectives have been learned is to observe the child at the beginning of the treatment session to document his performance before treatment begins. Another method is to have the parent or teacher chart specific movements or tasks (i.e., number of times the child assumes all fours independently) between treatment sessions.

SUMMARY

Developing a strategy for planning and sequencing treatment requires the therapist to impose organization on the variables affecting this process. Although individual therapists will have differing theoretical frameworks, the use of well-defined, long term goals and short term objectives will improve communication among professionals, parents, and third-party payers about the child's current functioning, physical therapy intervention, and progress. ❏

SUGGESTED READINGS

1. Ilmer S, Drews J: Differential analysis of selected prompts and neurological variables in motor assessment of moderately mentally retarded children. Am J Ment Defic 5:508-517, 1980
2. Mager RF: Preparing instructional objectives. ed 2. Belmont, CA, Pitman Learning, 1975
3. O'Neill DL, Harris SR: Developing goals and objectives for handicapped children. Phys Ther 62: 295-298, 1982
4. Popovich D: A prescriptive behavioral checklist for the severely and profoundsoderately and Severely Handicapped. ed 3. Columbus, OH, Charles E. Merrill Publishing Co, 1987, pp 110-149
5. Turnball HR, et al: Developing and Implementing IEP's. Columbus, OH, Charles E. Merrill Publishing Co., 1978
6. Zimmerman J. Goals and Objectives for Developing Normal Movement Patterns. Rockville, MD, Aspen Publishing, 1988

REFERENCES

1. Montgomery P, Connolly B. Norm-referenced and criterion-referenced tests: Use in pediatrics and application to task analysis of motor skill. Phys Ther 67:1873-1876, 1987
2. Horak FB: Chapter 4. Assumptions underlying motor control for neurologic rehabilitation. In Contemporary Management of Motor Control Problems:Proceedings of the II Step Conference, Foundation for Physical Therapy. Fredericksburg, VA, 1991, pp 85-87
3. Northwestern University Special Therapeutic Exercise Project (NUSTEP). Am J Phys Med 46:1967
4. Connolly B, Montgomery P: Chapter 1. Framework for assessment and treatment. In Montgomery P, Connolly B (eds): Motor Control and Physical Therapy. Chattanooga Group, Hixson, TN, 1991, pp 1-11
5. Schmidt RA: Motor Control and Learning: A Behavioral Emphasis. ed 2. Champaign, Ill: Human Kinetics Publisher Inc., 1988
6. Schmidt RA: Chapter 7. Motor learning principles for physical therapy. In Contemporary Management of Motor Control Problems:Proceedings of II Step Conference, Foundation for Physical Therapy. Fredericksburg, VA, 1991, pp 49-64
7. Winstein CJ. Chapter 8. Designing practice for motor learning: Clinical implications. In Contemporary Management of Motor Control Problems: Proceedings of II Step Conference, Foundation for Physical Therapy, Fredericksburg, VA, 1991, pp 65-76
8. Winstein CJ: Knowledge of results and motor learning-Implications for physical therapy. Phys Ther 71:140-149, 1991
9. Shapiro DC, Schmidt RA. The schema theory: Recent evidence and developmental implications. In Kelso JAS, Clark JE (eds): The Development of Movement Control and Coordination. New York: Wiley, 1981
10. Gentile AM: A working model of skill acquisition with application to teaching. Quest 17:3-23,1972
11. Gibson JJ: The Ecological Approach to Visual Perception. Boston, MA: Houghton Mifflin Co, 1979
12. Fetters L: Chapter 22. Cerebral Palsy: Contemporary treatment concepts. In Contemporary Management of Motor Control Problems: Proceedings of II STEP Conference. Foundation for Physical Therapy, Fredericksburg, VA, 1991, pp 219-224
13. Oatis CA: Chapter 11. Perspectives on the evaluation and treatment of gait disorders. In Motor Control and Physical Therapy. Chattanooga Group, Hixson, TN, 1991, pp 141-155
14. Cintas H: Cross cultural variation in motor development. Physical & Occupational Therapy in Pediatrics 8:1-20, 1988
15. VanSant A. Chapter 2. Motor control, motor learning, and motor development. In Montgomery P, Connolly B (eds): Motor Control and Physical Therapy. Chattanooga Group, Hixson, TN, 1991, pp 13-28
16. Attermeier S: Chapter 10. Should the normal motor developmental sequence be used as a theoretical model in patient treatment? In Contemporary Management of Motor Control Problems: Proceedings of the II STEP Conference. Foundation for Physical Therapy, Fredericksburg, VA, 1991, pp 85-87
17. Atwater SW: Chapter 11. Should the normal developmental sequence be used as a theoretical model in pediatric physical therapy? In Contemporary Management of Motor Control Problems: Proceedings of the II STEP Conference. Foundation for Physical Therapy, Fredericksburg, VA,1991, pp 89-93
18. VanSant AF: Chapter 12. Should the normal developmental sequence be used as a theoretical model to progress adult patients? In Contemporary Management of Motor Control Problems: Foundation for Physical Therapy, Fredericksburg, VA, 1991, pp 95-97
19. Effgen S: Systematic delivery and recording of intervention assistance. Pediatric Physical Therapy 3:63-68, 1991

CHAPTER 4

THE CHILDREN

Barbara H. Connolly, Ed.D., PT
Patricia C. Montgomery, Ph.D., PT

◆

One of the major problems experienced by the student, new graduate, or clinician inexperienced in pediatric developmental therapy is integrating theory with practice. A problem solving approach can be helpful for developing skill in the practical application of assessment and treatment techniques. To facilitate a problem solving approach, we have selected four case studies that represent common problems encountered by the clinician. Contributing authors were asked to address the developmental problems observed in each of these children and to develop goals and objectives for an "ideal" treatment program. A composite clinical picture of each child is presented in this chapter and should be reviewed briefly before proceeding to the subsequent chapters.

CASE NO. 1 — JASON
Cerebral Palsy, Right Hemiparesis, 18 Months

General Description: Estimated to have normal IQ; delayed speech development; no surgeries; typical hemiplegic posture with less weight bearing on the right side, upper extremity retracted and flexed, pelvis retracted; has just begun ambulation.

NICU: First born of non-identical twins; birthweight of 1660 grams; APGARs 7 at one minute, 9 at five minutes; no mechanical ventilation; discharged after 40 days on caffeine-citrate due to bradycardia with feedings; follow-up at 2 months gestational age non-remarkable; follow-up at 6 months definitely asymmetrical; referred for services.

Sensory: Neglect of right side, more in upper extremity; tactile defensive behaviors noted; hypersensitive palmar and plantar grasp.

Head and Trunk: Asymmetrical posture with slight anterior tilt of pelvis; shoulder retraction on right; tightened hip and lateral trunk flexors on right; trunk tone increases with activity; poor dissociation of pelvis and shoulder; limited trunk rotation.

Righting and Equilibrium Reactions: Rights head in all planes; lacks complete trunk rotation to diagonal movement; in sitting, demonstrates protective reactions on left, right arm initiates movement forward and sidewards but without full extension and weight bearing; equilibrium reactions in sitting are adequate to the left but inadequate to the right; in standing, no staggering reactions present, prefers to use left sided protective reactions in response to displacement, cannot stand on the tilt board.

Respiratory/Oral Motor: Subtle asymmetries in oral

structures, does not lateralize well to right with tongue, chews solid food only on left; drools when stressed; relies more on gestures for communication, consonants limited in quantity/quality; gasps for breath after drinking.

Ambulation: Increased tone in right lower extremity, distal greater than proximal; short swing phase on right; short stride length with backward rotation of pelvis, minimal knee and ankle flexion at midswing; short stance phase on right with genu recurvatum, foot in valgus at midstance; initiates walking with left side, turns and changes direction from left side only.

Hand Function: Sensory disregard; inactivity of right shoulder girdle; humeral extension, adduction, internal rotation; weakness in elbow extension; lack of isolated forearm and wrist movement; hypersensitive palmar grasp, hand function limited to gross grasp.

Educational Setting: Home based program; private physical therapy and speech therapy.

CASE NO. 2 — JILL
Cerebral Palsy, Spastic Quadriparesis, Mental Retardation, 7 Years

General Description: IQ estimated at 60 (mild retardation); easily motivated; multiple surgeries (heelcord and adductor releases); poor respiratory patterns; few words; feeding problems; postural asymmetry; mild scoliosis; non-ambulatory with poor potential for ambulation.

NICU: Full term; normal pregnancy; APGARs 5 at one minute and 8 at five minutes; neonatal seizures; EEG abnormal; on mechanical ventilation several days; feeding difficulties initially; discharged on anticonvulsants and bottle feeding; follow-up at 4 months, decreased head growth, normal eye exam and BAER.

Sensory: Movement through space results in autonomic distress, tonic reflexes evident; hypersensitive in oral area with increased lip retraction and head extension.

Head and Trunk: Kyphotic posture in upper back with head and neck hyperextension; poor head control; no ability to sit without support; tightness in capital extensors, pectorals, shoulder girdle, hip flexors, lumbar extensors; indented sternum.

Righting and Equilibrium: Maintains head in neutral when held vertical, cannot right head when tilted; raises head momentarily in prone, but not supine; protective and equilibrium reactions absent.

Respiratory/Oral Motor: Rib cage generally immobile; asynchronous respiratory pattern; respiratory coordination during feeding poor with much coughing and choking; attempts to say few words; severe cheek/lip retraction and jaw thrusting with retraction; tongue thick in contour and retracted.

Ambulation: Non-ambulatory with poor potential for assisted ambulation.

Hand Function: Poor ocular control, lacks downward gaze; shoulder girdle immobility, reach limited to 60 degrees of humeral abduction; attempts to grasp, but hand closes involuntarily prior to obtaining object; no release or manipulation.

Educational Setting: Full day special education classroom with occupational therapy, physical therapy, and speech therapy services.

CASE NO. 3 — TAYLOR
Myelomeningocele, Repaired L 1-2, 4 Years

General Description: Normal IQ; as infant, shunted for hydrocephalus; equinovarus deformities, surgery for bilateral hip dislocation; currently exhibits minimal hip flexor and hip adductor tightness bilaterally; visual perceptual problems; has been using a free standing orthosis (parapodium), but is ready for long leg braces and crutches; self propels in wheelchair.

NICU: Full term, born by cesarean section due to fetal distress and breech presentation; primary closure of myelomeningocele; V-P shunt on day 5; increased apnea and use of respirator; questionable seizures but normal EEG, suspected Arnold Chiari malformation with surgical release of posterior fossa; serial casting for foot deformities; following 4 month hospital stay, discharged home on cardiorespiratory monitor due to continued apnea; referred for physical therapy services.

Sensory: Loss of cutaneous and proprioceptive sensation below T-12; visual acuity problems, wears glasses; difficulty with figure-ground discrimination; bending head to look at floor disturbs balance.

Head and Trunk: Weak abdominal muscles; holds breath during use of upper extremities, blocks ability to rotate trunk; poor active trunk extension; at rest hangs on ligaments; rolling completed with poor leg dissociation; in four point, lordotic posture, hangs on shoulder girdle.

Righting and Equilibrium: Has normal head righting and protective reactions in sitting; in sitting, trunk righting reactions are inadequate; standing without external support not possible.

Respiratory/Oral Motor: Oral motor activity within normal limits; mean sentence length of 3-4 words; sounds produced are within normal limits; needs complete evaluation of language functioning; inadequate abdominal strength to support sustained exhalation.

Ambulation: Limited voluntary control of lower extremities; standing posture dependent upon external support; swing-to gait with walker and parapodium, limited speed, poor endurance; balance in standing with new orthosis poor.

Hand Function: Normal grasp, manipulation, and release; visual motor integration delays; cannot accomplish lower body dressing independently; lacks upper extremity strength for efficient use of ambulation aids.

Educational Setting: Special education preschool;

considering placement in a regular kindergarten; PT to identify potential problems and solutions for regular school placement.

CASE NO. 4 — ASHLEY
Down Syndrome, 15 Months

General Description: IQ estimated to be 75, generalized hypotonia; poor shoulder and hip stability in quadruped; pulls to stand, wide base of support, knee hyperextension, not attempting to cruise; trunk is kyphotic in sitting but lordotic in quadruped; uses several words; feeding problems.

NICU: Full term, 26 year old primipara mother, uncomplicated pregnancy; esophageal atresia, primary repair not possible, gastrostomy present for first 6 months; ventricular septal defect, surgically repaired at 8 months; chronic otitis media, mild conductive hearing loss, PE tubes at 12 months; prolonged hospitalization; family refused physical therapy for child for 10 months.

Sensory: Responds to tactile, proprioceptive, and vestibular input with increased tone and stability.

Head and Trunk: Shoulders elevated, shortened capital extensor muscles; poor tolerance for handling particularly around the neck and shoulders; poor grading of trunk extension and flexion, minimal rotation; generally apprehensive about movement.

Righting and Equilibrium: Head righting reactions present; inadequate protective and equilibrium reactions in sitting, quadruped, and standing.

Respiratory/Oral Motor: Low muscle tone provides poor base for oral motor, respiratory-phonatory functioning; suckle pattern used in feeding, tongue thick in contour, protrudes from mouth; mouth breather; drinks from cup only at snack time; solids inconsistently presented.

Ambulation: Pulls to stand; in standing, spine lordotic, knees hyperextended, feet pronated; uses straight plane movement; needs assistance to take steps.

Hand Function: Grasps but cannot release with control; flings objects to dispose of them, no goal directed play; cannot pick up pellet sized objects; in movement transitions, locks elbows into extension and externally rotates humerus.

Educational Setting: Mother-infant early intervention program twice weekly with physical therapy, occupational therapy, and speech therapy consultation.

CONCLUSION

The preceding descriptions can be used to guide you through the information in chapters 6-13. Each of these chapters presents a specific perspective for assessing and treating children with developmental disabilities. Chapter 14 will provide an integrated approach to the assessment and treatment of each of the four children used in the case studies. ❏

CHAPTER 5

PHYSICAL THERAPY IN THE NICU

Carolyn Fiterman, M.S., PT
Meredith Hinds Harris, Ed.D., PT

◆

The neonatal intensive care unit (NICU) is certainly a window into the twenty-first century (Figure 1). It is advanced technology in the highest degree. When entering the NICU we are initially aware of the brightness, the constant noise level, and the scurrying around of a variety of intense looking people.[1] On closer examination we are attracted to babies attached to an incredible number of monitors, electrodes, machines, and tubes. A different language is spoken here: terms like "spells", ABG, TCM, CPAP, and BPD often are heard in addition to the medical terminology with which the physical therapist is more familiar.[2-5]

Personnel in the NICU include the neonatologist (a pediatrician who has two years of additional training in how to deal with the preterm or critically ill full term newborn) and the perinatologist (an obstetrician who specializes in high risk pregnancies). Many units also have a variety of medical residents from several different specialties, such as pediatrics, obstetrics, and family practice. Nurses in the NICU have training which requires additional hours of supervised practice and inservice experience. Some units have nurses with specialty training and expertise, called neonatal nurse clinicians or practitioners. Their roles differ from unit to unit. In some units they provide transport services to

bring critically ill babies from distant places to the center; in others they provide primary care and function like resident physicians.

When we think of the babies admitted to a NICU the typical image is that of very tiny, preterm infants. This may be due to the massive amounts of publicity in the popular press regarding these babies. Another reason the small baby comes to mind is because the length of hospital stay is long and the cost enormous. Technological advances are making it possible for many babies born three months early and weighing less than two pounds to survive. These babies are at risk for potential damage to many organ systems. Possible problems include retinopathy of prematurity (ROP), intracranial hemorrhage (ICH), necrotizing enterocolitis (NEC), hyaline membrane disease (HMD), bronchopulmonary dysplasia (BPD), apnea, bradycardia, sepsis, and meningitis.[3-6] Long term hospitalization often disrupts normal parent-child relationships. The need for continual medical intervention, often including the use of heart and respiratory rate monitors after discharge, makes it difficult for the parents of these children to believe that these babies are "normal".

Although the long term prognosis for many of these infants is good, the cost, both financially and emotion-

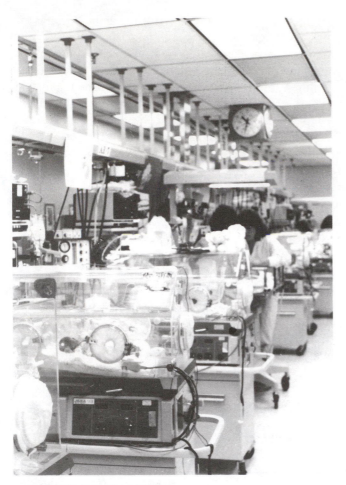

FIGURE 1. Typical NICU.

ally, may result in irreparable damage to the structure of the family. Many mothers of preterm infants are both young and unmarried and have received little if any prenatal care.[7] The number of infants admitted to the NICU because of maternal drug and multiple substance abuse is on the increase. Each type of substance carries with it a unique and not necessarily well understood risk to any of the disorders already addressed for the infant in need of the special care of the NICU. With maternal substance abuse and sporadic or absent prenatal care, there is increased risk of prematurity, intrauterine growth retardation, gastrourinary malformations, low birth weight, infections, cardiac and limb malformations, and increased risk to infection from Human Immunodeficiency Virus (HIV). Infants affected by substance abuse also may have to cope with narcotic abstinence syndrome (NAS) characterized by neurobehavioral sequelae.[8-12] Because of the perinatal drug abuse problem, HIV infection, and an economically deprived family situation, the newborn infants and their health care providers face problems about which long term outcome is still undetermined.[13]

The best predictor of long term outcome for preterm infants is not birth weight or medical complications, but the socio-economic status of the family.[14-19] While smaller and earlier babies are surviving, it is important to note that in many units half of the admissions are for babies weighing 2500 grams (approximately 5 1/2 pounds) or more. Many of these babies are at significant risk for developmental disabilities, and therapists also should concentrate time and effort on these infants, as well as the small preterm infants.

Examples of babies other than preterm infants who may be admitted to the NICU are those with neonatal sepsis or infection. Infants who are full term or preterm have few capabilities to combat infection. Infants may contract infections in-utero, while passing through the birth canal, or after birth. Certain types of infections that may be virtually harmless to adults are potentially fatal to infants. Although there have been great advances in antibiotic therapy, infant infections often become systemic via the blood system and eventually may result in meningitis because of immaturity in the blood/brain barrier.[6] Even with advanced technology, infants may die as a result of "neonatal sepsis syndrome". Surviving infants may be neurologically impaired and certainly should be closely monitored by the neonatal physical therapist. Infants at risk for HIV infection because of maternal HIV infection are at increased risk for frequent periodic opportunistic infections and sexually transmitted diseases. Infants who are in this high risk category should be assessed carefully and closely monitored over time for potential neurologic impairment or developmental delay.[20-23]

At first glance, the fat, rosy-cheeked infants of diabetic mothers (IDM) look healthy, and we assume that these are very healthy children. However, these babies are generally large for gestational age (LGA) and are at risk for congenital anomalies and difficulty with glucose metabolism. Unless they are managed medically immediately, hypoglycemic seizures may result. Another typical finding in IDM is feeding difficulties. The infants often are initially lethargic, and feeding patterns may be even less mature than gestational age would indicate.[3-4] Keeping gestational age in mind, the therapist can be of great assistance to both the nursing staff and the parents by offering techniques to increase alertness, as well as suggestions for positioning and oral motor facilitation.[24-26]

The differentiation between preterm, appropriate for gestational age (AGA), and small for dates or small for gestational age (SGA), or intrauterine growth retarded (IUGR) babies is important. Causes of poor intrauterine growth include: maternal smoking, drugs, or alcohol; intrauterine infections; and placental insufficiency. Because brain growth is so critical prior to birth and during the first year of life, anything that compromises this growth may decrease both the number and size of neurons.[5] Little or no evidence has been documented for regeneration of neurons following this critical period. In studies where SGA children were followed on a long term basis, two outcomes were documented. These children generally did not catch up with their growth parameters, and remained smaller than their age peers and other family members. Additionally, they often had difficulty in school, particularly with attending skills, even if they were intellectually normal. [27-29] If possible, the etiology of growth retardation should be ascertained, because certain types of intrauterine infections are particularly devastating to the central nervous system (CNS). TORCH infections (see glossary) may result in significant microcephaly and in some cases visual or auditory defects. [3-4]

Children with perinatal asphyxia have received inadequate oxygen prior to, during, or shortly after birth. Apgar scores [30] or blood pH may give an indication of the severity of oxygen deprivation, but some babies appear normal on follow-up even when early indicators seem predictive of significant impairment. Other infants sustain severe brain damage with minimal indication of asphyxia. Full term babies seem to be at a greater risk for brain damage due to asphyxia. This may be because their central nervous systems are relatively more mature, just as an adult has less capacity to demonstrate neural plasticity than a child. It may also be related to the relative oxygen needs of a full term nervous system as compared to an immature nervous system. Certain drugs such as cocaine when ingested during pregnancy put the infant at risk for hypoxia, decreased cardiac output, uterine arterial vasoconstriction, impaired oxygen transport, intracranial hemorrhages, or infarct. Clinical symptoms may or may not be present immediately nor detectable. [31] The severity of the neurological insult may be evaluated partially by the presence or absence of secondary complications, including seizures, the need for ventilator support, and kidney damage. All of these factors are indicators of significant neurological damage. If none of these indicators are present, but the child demonstrates feeding difficulties, long term problems are still a possibility. [32]

A variety of syndromes and congenital anomalies are observed in infants in the NICU. Included in this category are chromosomal abnormalities, such as Down syndrome (trisomy 21), other lethal trisomies (13 and 18), birth defects including myelomeningocele and cleft palate, congenital cardiac and limb defects secondary to maternal drug use, and problems related to lack of intrauterine space (e.g. arthrogryposis and club foot). All of these problems indicate the necessity for therapeutic intervention in the NICU, parent counseling regarding long term implications, and a variety of therapy services following discharge. This group of infants is probably the easiest to identify regarding the need for services. However, some of these infants never are admitted to intensive care and others remain in the NICU for only a very short period of time. Because of the need for a variety of other specialty consultations, physical therapy may be forgotten or ignored. Depending on the setting, it may be appropriate for the acute hospital to provide long term intervention for these babies and families, or, in many cases, referral to local community agencies as outpatients might better meet their needs. Children referred to social service agencies for foster care need to be carefully tracked to ensure that their health, therapeutic services, and developmental progress are carefully monitored and not lost during per-iods of family disruption or a placement process. [21-23]

THE ROLE OF THE PHYSICAL THERAPIST IN THE NICU

Physical therapists constantly are looking for new frontiers in providing therapy. Any physical therapist involved in pediatric therapy probably has considered that if only they had begun treatment earlier, with a specific child, the results of intervention would be improved. Logically, then, we look to the NICU as the earliest type of "hands on" treatment. Fetal ultrasound films even have been used to assess movement abnormalities. [33] How we might intervene if abnormalities are noted, we can only guess. Enthusiastic, energetic physical therapists may descend on the unsuspecting neonatal unit certain that they will be able to right the wrongs of years of delayed referrals, and that they will be able to improve the developmental outcome of any baby with whom they interact. The staff of most neonatal units are very protective of the needs of the babies, and are, perhaps justifiably, suspicious of new personnel and new techniques. It is important to display competence, yet, be patient to gain the confidence of the nursing personnel, as well as the physicians, in order to gain acceptance as an important member of the NICU team.

Understanding fetal development is a prerequisite for beginning intervention programs in the NICU. It would be as foolish to try bottle feeding with a baby of 30 weeks gestation as it would be to begin self feeding with a two month old normal child. The last trimester of fetal development should be studied intensely so inappropriate activities or inaccurate predictions regarding abnormalities of movement or muscle tone based on previous experience with full term or older infants can be modified. [34-35] For example, the full term child is generally flexed, while the more preterm the baby is, the more relative extension is noted (Figure 2). [36] Although non-nutritive sucking may begin as early as 17 weeks post conception, nutritive sucking and therefore bottle or breast feeding rarely is accomplished prior to 34 weeks. [34] Sick and preterm babies have difficulty maintaining homeostasis, i.e. temperature, blood pressure, heart, and respiratory control. Their sleep cycles are brief and often disturbed. [37-38] Organization of sensory stimuli and state control often are disrupted or impaired in infants exposed to drugs or alcohol in utero. Activities that the therapist thinks may provide positive input to these fragile babies may be potentially life threaten-

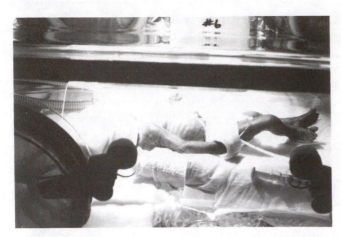

FIGURE 2. Typical extension of the preterm with supine positioning. Note lack of subcutaneous fat.

ing. The terminology "infant stimulation" is probably one of the most inappropriate concepts in treating any child, and particularly those in the NICU. These babies are already over-stimulated both visually and auditorily. The tactile, vestibular, and proprioceptive input they are receiving is not comparable to the intrauterine environment, nor is it similar to that a full term baby would receive in the first few days of life. [1,39]

If therapists can have any impact on the neonatal environment it is hoped that they might help parents and staff members understand the sensory and motor needs of these babies and to help normalize sensory experiences whenever possible. [40-42] Very few therapists are willing or able to be available seven days a week, or 24 hours a day. As noted previously, the awake and alert times of the ill neonate are brief at best. Optimally, therapists should be available in the unit for several long blocks of time during the day, rather than setting a specific schedule for when to provide therapy. Generally speaking, it is contraindicated to evaluate or treat a baby just after a feeding or stressful medical procedure. Because a baby's optimal time for intervention might occur when the therapist is not available, it is essential to train both parents and nursing staff in specific intervention techniques, as well as the principles of therapeutic intervention. Some therapists think that they alone are capable of providing these services. The most successful treatment strategies are those that are integrated into the total lifestyle of the baby and carried out throughout the waking hours. Inservice education, as well as role modeling of useful techniques, will enhance normalization of the baby's sensory-motor and behavioral environment.

Physical therapy in the NICU is a relatively new entity. There have been many studies showing both positive and negative outcomes related to short term intervention techniques. [40,43-48] There have been very few studies on whether early intervention techniques have long term positive outcomes for children and families. [5,49-51] The guiding therapeutic principle should be to

"do no harm" and if benefit results, so much the better. Long term effects are difficult to assess, because the older the child, the more difficult it is to differentiate whether the outcome is related to the primary insult, the intervention, the genetic complement, or the environment.

ASSESSMENT TECHNIQUES

The assessment of the newborn begins long before he is admitted to the NICU. Although the physical therapist is not directly involved with these assessments, it is important to become familiar with the terminology and to understand what has been done previously to enhance quality of life. Early in the pregnancy, the obstetrician monitors weight gain and fundiscopic height of the mother. Ultrasound examination also may be done to evaluate fetal growth. Ultrasound is capable of evaluating the status of the heart and kidneys and can determine whether intrauterine hydrocephalus is present. Amniocentesis may be done to determine whether the fetus has certain genetic abnormalities such as Down syndrome, and is used late in the pregnancy to determine lung maturity. Mothers are taught to monitor fetal movements and to inform their physicians of any change in these patterns.

Once labor begins, both external heart rate monitors and internal probes can be used to determine if the baby is well oxygenated. Immediately after birth, at one and five minutes of age, Apgar scores [30] are obtained. The following five measures are assessed: heart rate, respiratory effort, muscle tone, reflex irritability, and color. Each item is scored 0, 1, or 2, with the best possible score being 2 and the lowest score being 0. The Apgar is an evaluation of neonatal well being and is not meant to determine long term neurologic outcome. Rather, it is an indication for the delivery room personnel to act immediately, if the score is low, to resuscitate the infant. Low five minute Apgar scores may be indicative of long term neurologic sequelae, and these infants should be monitored carefully.

Another early evaluation is the gestational age assessment originally described by Dubowitz, (Figure 3). [36] This assessment includes two broad categories: external signs (edema, skin texture, skin color, lanugo, plantar creases, nipple formation, breast size, ear form and firmness, and genitals) and neurological signs related to muscle tone, positioning, and response to handling. Physical therapists may be involved in the neurologic part of this assessment, and it may be useful later as a determiner of neurologic maturation of muscle tone.

A number of authors have described evaluations for newborn and preterm infants (Figure 4). [52-57] These evaluations stress assessment of positioning at rest, excursion of passive motion, and reflexes and are therefore quite passive in nature. Although there are differences in these evaluations, there also are similarities. Both Amiel-

Therapeutic Exercise In Developmental Disabilities

FIGURE 3. Dubowitz (front).
—Reprinted with permission.

CLINICAL ESTIMATION OF GESTATIONAL AGE

AN APPROXIMATION BASED ON PUBLISHED DATA

EXAMINATION FIRST HOURS

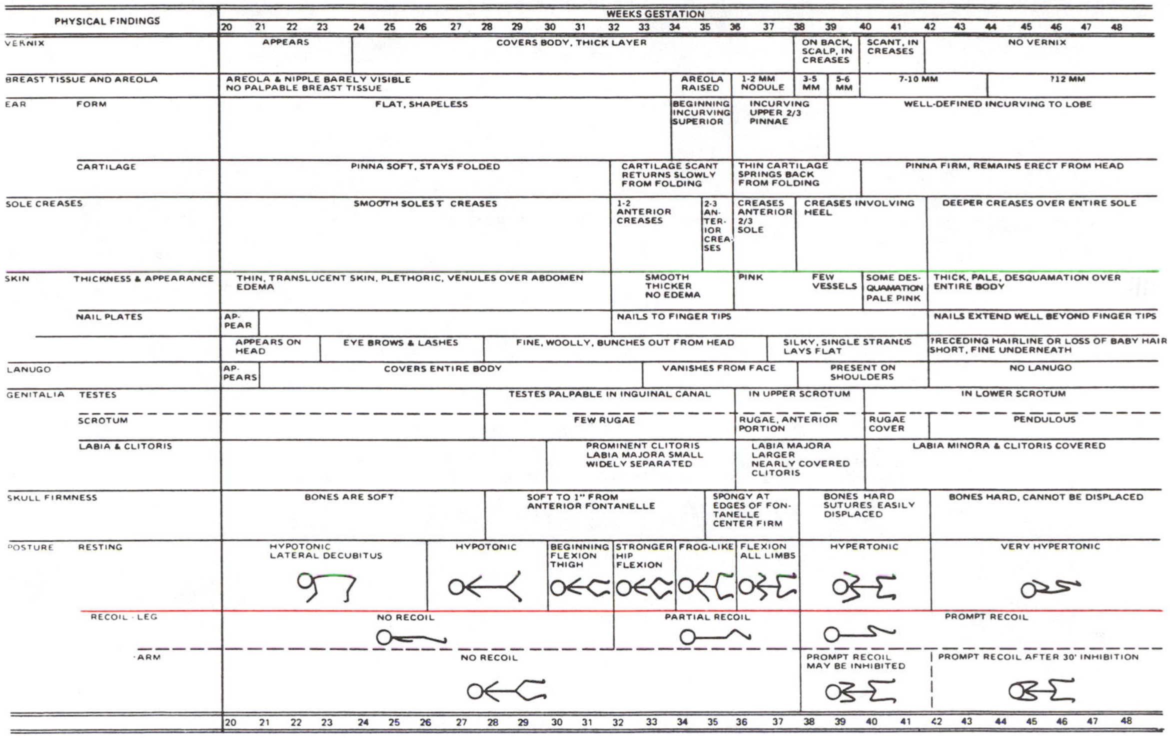

WEEKS GESTATION — 20 21 22 23 24 25 26 27 28 29 30 31 32 33 34 35 36 37 38 39 40 41 42 43 44 45 46 47 48

PHYSICAL FINDINGS		Descriptions across weeks gestation
VERNIX		APPEARS / COVERS BODY, THICK LAYER / ON BACK, SCALP, IN CREASES / SCANT, IN CREASES / NO VERNIX
BREAST TISSUE AND AREOLA		AREOLA & NIPPLE BARELY VISIBLE, NO PALPABLE BREAST TISSUE / AREOLA RAISED / 1-2 MM NODULE / 3-5 MM / 5-6 MM / 7-10 MM / ?12 MM
EAR	FORM	FLAT, SHAPELESS / BEGINNING INCURVING SUPERIOR / INCURVING UPPER 2/3 PINNAE / WELL-DEFINED INCURVING TO LOBE
	CARTILAGE	PINNA SOFT, STAYS FOLDED / CARTILAGE SCANT RETURNS SLOWLY FROM FOLDING / THIN CARTILAGE SPRINGS BACK FROM FOLDING / PINNA FIRM, REMAINS ERECT FROM HEAD
SOLE CREASES		SMOOTH SOLES ? CREASES / 1-2 ANTERIOR CREASES / 2-3 ANTERIOR CREASES / CREASES ANTERIOR 2/3 SOLE / CREASES INVOLVING HEEL / DEEPER CREASES OVER ENTIRE SOLE
SKIN	THICKNESS & APPEARANCE	THIN, TRANSLUCENT SKIN, PLETHORIC, VENULES OVER ABDOMEN EDEMA / SMOOTH THICKER NO EDEMA / PINK / FEW VESSELS / SOME DESQUAMATION PALE PINK / THICK, PALE, DESQUAMATION OVER ENTIRE BODY
	NAIL PLATES	AP-PEAR / NAILS TO FINGER TIPS / NAILS EXTEND WELL BEYOND FINGER TIPS
	(hair)	APPEARS ON HEAD / EYE BROWS & LASHES / FINE, WOOLLY, BUNCHES OUT FROM HEAD / SILKY, SINGLE STRANDS LAYS FLAT / ?RECEDING HAIRLINE OR LOSS OF BABY HAIR SHORT, FINE UNDERNEATH
LANUGO		AP-PEARS / COVERS ENTIRE BODY / VANISHES FROM FACE / PRESENT ON SHOULDERS / NO LANUGO
GENITALIA	TESTES	TESTES PALPABLE IN INGUINAL CANAL / IN UPPER SCROTUM / IN LOWER SCROTUM
	SCROTUM	FEW RUGAE / RUGAE, ANTERIOR PORTION / RUGAE COVER / PENDULOUS
	LABIA & CLITORIS	PROMINENT CLITORIS LABIA MAJORA SMALL WIDELY SEPARATED / LABIA MAJORA LARGER NEARLY COVERED CLITORIS / LABIA MINORA & CLITORIS COVERED
SKULL FIRMNESS		BONES ARE SOFT / SOFT TO 1" FROM ANTERIOR FONTANELLE / SPONGY AT EDGES OF FONTANELLE CENTER FIRM / BONES HARD SUTURES EASILY DISPLACED / BONES HARD, CANNOT BE DISPLACED
POSTURE	RESTING	HYPOTONIC LATERAL DECUBITUS / HYPOTONIC / BEGINNING FLEXION THIGH / STRONGER HIP FLEXION / FROG-LIKE / FLEXION ALL LIMBS / HYPERTONIC / VERY HYPERTONIC
	RECOIL – LEG	NO RECOIL / PARTIAL RECOIL / PROMPT RECOIL
	– ARM	NO RECOIL / PROMPT RECOIL MAY BE INHIBITED / PROMPT RECOIL AFTER 30' INHIBITION

FIGURE 3. Dubowitz (back).

CLINICAL ESTIMATION OF GESTATIONAL AGE

AN APPROXIMATION BASED ON PUBLISHED DATA

CONFIRMATORY NEUROLOGIC EXAMINATION TO BE DONE AFTER 24 HOURS

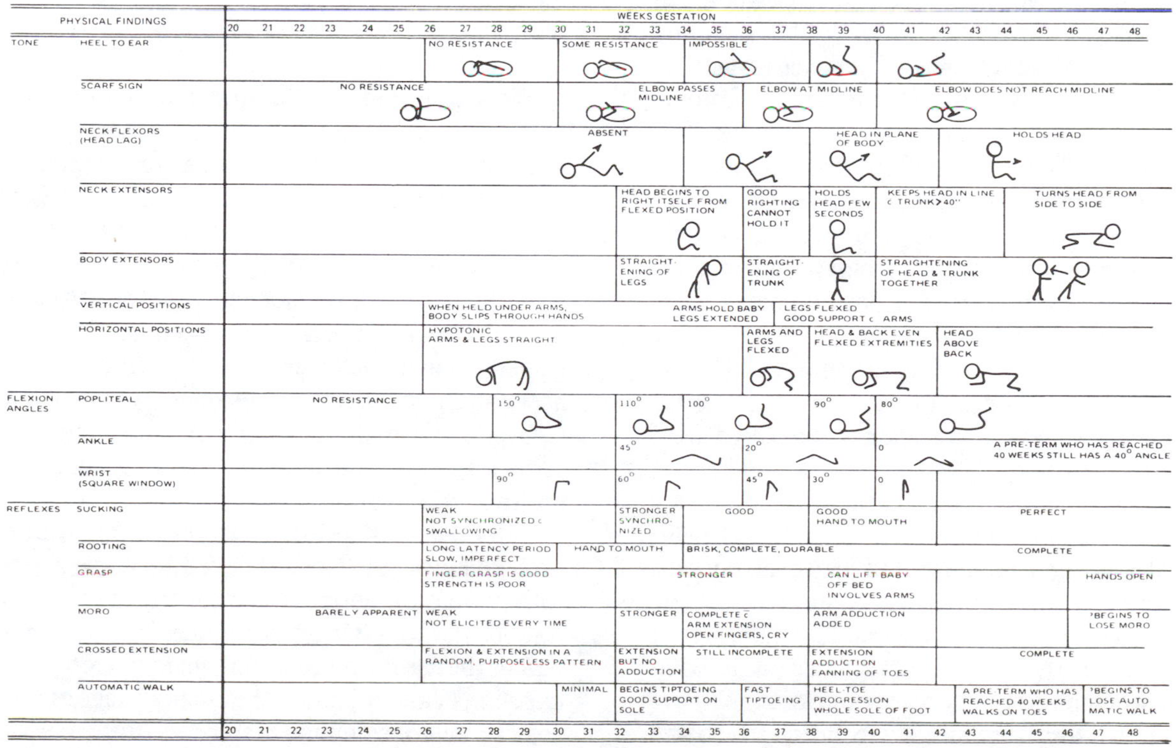

WEEKS GESTATION — 20 21 22 23 24 25 26 27 28 29 30 31 32 33 34 35 36 37 38 39 40 41 42 43 44 45 46 47 48

PHYSICAL FINDINGS		Descriptions across weeks gestation
TONE	HEEL TO EAR	NO RESISTANCE / SOME RESISTANCE / IMPOSSIBLE
	SCARF SIGN	NO RESISTANCE / ELBOW PASSES MIDLINE / ELBOW AT MIDLINE / ELBOW DOES NOT REACH MIDLINE
	NECK FLEXORS (HEAD LAG)	ABSENT / HEAD IN PLANE OF BODY / HOLDS HEAD
	NECK EXTENSORS	HEAD BEGINS TO RIGHT ITSELF FROM FLEXED POSITION / GOOD RIGHTING CANNOT HOLD IT / HOLDS HEAD FEW SECONDS / KEEPS HEAD IN LINE c TRUNK >40" / TURNS HEAD FROM SIDE TO SIDE
	BODY EXTENSORS	STRAIGHTENING OF LEGS / STRAIGHTENING OF TRUNK / STRAIGHTENING OF HEAD & TRUNK TOGETHER
	VERTICAL POSITIONS	WHEN HELD UNDER ARMS, BODY SLIPS THROUGH HANDS / ARMS HOLD BABY LEGS EXTENDED / LEGS FLEXED GOOD SUPPORT c ARMS
	HORIZONTAL POSITIONS	HYPOTONIC ARMS & LEGS STRAIGHT / ARMS AND LEGS FLEXED / HEAD & BACK EVEN FLEXED EXTREMITIES / HEAD ABOVE BACK
FLEXION ANGLES	POPLITEAL	NO RESISTANCE / 150° / 110° / 100° / 90° / 80°
	ANKLE	45° / 20° / 0° / A PRE-TERM WHO HAS REACHED 40 WEEKS STILL HAS A 40° ANGLE
	WRIST (SQUARE WINDOW)	90° / 60° / 45° / 30° / 0°
REFLEXES	SUCKING	WEAK NOT SYNCHRONIZED c SWALLOWING / STRONGER SYNCHRONIZED / GOOD / GOOD HAND TO MOUTH / PERFECT
	ROOTING	LONG LATENCY PERIOD SLOW, IMPERFECT / HAND TO MOUTH / BRISK, COMPLETE, DURABLE / COMPLETE
	GRASP	FINGER GRASP IS GOOD STRENGTH IS POOR / STRONGER / CAN LIFT BABY OFF BED INVOLVES ARMS / HANDS OPEN
	MORO	BARELY APPARENT / WEAK NOT ELICITED EVERY TIME / STRONGER / COMPLETE c ARM EXTENSION OPEN FINGERS, CRY / ARM ADDUCTION ADDED / ?BEGINS TO LOSE MORO
	CROSSED EXTENSION	FLEXION & EXTENSION IN A RANDOM, PURPOSELESS PATTERN / EXTENSION BUT NO ADDUCTION / STILL INCOMPLETE / EXTENSION ADDUCTION FANNING OF TOES / COMPLETE
	AUTOMATIC WALK	MINIMAL / BEGINS TIPTOEING GOOD SUPPORT ON SOLE / FAST TIPTOEING / HEEL-TOE PROGRESSION WHOLE SOLE OF FOOT / A PRE-TERM WHO HAS REACHED 40 WEEKS WALKS ON TOES / ?BEGINS TO LOSE AUTOMATIC WALK

Neonatal Evaluation Form*

Name: _____ Testing Date: _____
D.O.B.: _____ Gestational Age: _____ Day of Life: _____
Birth Weight: _____ Present Weight: _____
Type of Birth: _____
Apgar: _____ 1 min. _____ 5 min. _____ Diagnosis: _____
Parental History: _____ Perinatal History: _____ Neonatal History:

		Primary Walking:	
Predominant State:	_____	response	N/absent
Posture:	N/Ext/Fl/other	scissors	no/plantigrade/
scissors	no/yes		tiptoe
lateral preference	no/R/L	symmetry	equal/↓R L/ab R L
strong ATNR	no/R/L	Placing:	
Motor Activity:		response	N/poor
amount	N/↑/↓	symmetry	equal/R↓/L↓
symmetry	equal /R ⟩L/L ⟩ R	Eyes:	
focal twitching	no/R/L	visual focus	yes/no
jittery/clonic	no/R/L	visual tracking-smooth/jerky/___°	
tremulous	no/yes	doll eye/nystagmus	
Oral Motor:			yes/↓R L
head shape	symmetrical/R/L	Auditory:	
rooting	N/↓R L/ab R L	response (loud)	yes/no/startle
sucking	N/↓/ab/Asym/uncoord	symmetry (soft)	N/↓R L/ab R L
palate	N/nar/high/cleft	Moro:	
gag	N/↑/↓	threshold	N/low/high
respiration	N/reverse/shal/	symmetry	equal/↓R L/ab R L
	labored/stridor	Cry:	
Pull to Sit:	N/sl.↓/sev.↓/↑tone	amount	N/↑/↓/ab
Palmar Grasp:		high pitch	no/yes
response	N/↑/↓	monotonous	no/yes
symmetry	equal/R /L	Primitive Crawl:	N/↓/absent
cortical thumb	occasional/oblig.	Tactile:	
Hip Abduc. Resist.:	N/↑R L/↓R L	touch	N/hypo/hyper
Planter Grasp:	N/↓R L/↑R L	pain	N/hypo/hyper
Toe Signs:	↑R L/↓R L	Tone:	
Ventral Suspension:	N/floppy/↑	amount	N/↑/↓
Gallant:	equal/↓R L/ab R L	symmetry	equal/↑R L/↓R L
Upright suspension:	N/slips/flops/R↓/L↓	distribution	generalized/
			UE ⟩ LE/LE ⟩ UE
		State Change:	N/irrit./depr.

Feeding Problems:

Summary:

* Adapted from Neurodevelopmental Problems in Early Childhood; CM Drillien & MB Drummond, editors

FIGURE 4.
Neonatal Evaluation Form

Tison[53] and Korner[55] considered gestational age in the development of their exams. The Prechtl examination[57] is designed for the full term newborn, but it must be noted that a preterm infant, at term, is not precisely like a baby born at term because of differences in the environment. It is possible for a baby to have significant neurologic abnormalities including structural deficits (hydrocephalus, porencephaly, or intra-cranial hemorrhage) and still look "normal" on these initial evaluations. For this reason, we must consider carefully the medical history, including prenatal risk factors, and perform serial evaluations over a period of time to predict accurately long term outcomes.

Prechtl[57] incorporated states of alertness of the newborn in the total assessment of neurologic status. He noted that even the reflex character of the baby varied depending on whether he was in deep or light sleep, awake, drowsy, alert, or crying. Korner[55], in an attempt to standardize her evaluation, noted state for each item.

Brazelton[54] refined the concept of state of alertness in his newborn behavioral assessment scale (NBAS). Although neurologic reflex items are included, this is not the focus of the NBAS. Care is taken to assess the baby at his optimal time in the wake-sleep cycle. In addition, a variety of sensory modalities are presented to the sleeping infant to assess his initial responses, as well as his ability to accommodate sensory input. The NBAS is the only newborn assessment that recognizes individual differences and responses to environmental input. This assessment has been continually revised[5,58] (see Chapter 2).

We need to consider the state of the infant in any type of evaluation. Although it may be possible to wake an infant to perform an evaluation, a more optimal picture of the infant's abilities will be obtained by waiting until the baby arouses naturally. In studies where babies were not awakened either for medical care or for other invasive procedures, medical personnel did not need to wait more than ten minutes to perform a procedure.[37,38] Babies also gained weight faster and were discharged from the hospital sooner when they were not wakened unnecessarily. From a financial perspective, anything that can be done to shorten hospital stay will be regarded as a positive intervention.

Individual variability occurs in infants with no two babies being exactly alike, even identical twins. The baby's state of alertness, the time of day, the general activity in the NICU, other procedures that have preceded the examination, medical concerns such as infection or anemia, and the gestational age of the infant need to be considered. In addition, the cultural background of the infant should be considered.[59] Studies

Therapeutic Exercise In Developmental Disabilities

have indicated some basic differences. Black babies generally have higher muscle tone than caucasian babies, and Asian babies generally have lower muscle tone. We must be cautious not to discount abnormal muscle tone just because of cultural variability. We do not want to ignore a black baby with increased muscle tone just because of ethnicity, or over alarm a parent of a child with high "normal" tone.

THERAPEUTIC TECHNIQUES

Before beginning a therapeutic program in the NICU, neuromuscular facilitation techniques should be reviewed because the principles apply to the immature neonate. Particular emphasis should be placed on the techniques of Bobath (NDT)[24,60,61] and Rood.[62] A good understanding of the general principles of facilitation and especially inhibition is vital in establishing credibility with other professionals working with these babies. Any handling technique can be inhibitory or facilitatory depending on how it is administered. Slow, rhythmic movement tends to be calming, while rapid irregular movement is alerting. Changing the position of the infant, even when using the same sensory input, may result in a different response. Unless the physical therapist understands the neuromuscular implications of handling and positioning, it is not possible to explain to other medical personnel why certain techniques are useful. Ludington-Hoe[39,63] advocates "stimulation" (increased sensory input), however, "inhibition" may be the essential element. Two basic principles must be adhered to when dealing with the fragile population in the NICU. WHEN IN DOUBT, DO NOTHING! ! !, and DO NO HARM! ! !

Many articles describe specific techniques of rocking, stroking, swaddling, positioning, talking, and providing certain types of tactile and visual input, and report improved scores on infant intelligence scales.[40,45,47,64-72] Other studies demonstrate little or no change in outcome.[73,74] These widely divergent results may be due to the fact that many of these intervention strategies do not address the total baby in the context of his environment, but instead attempt to manipulate isolated variables. The physical therapist must consider all the sensory and motor avenues available to the neonate: visual, auditory, tactile, olfactory, gustatory, kinesthetic, proprioceptive, and vestibular. When observing motor responses to sensory input, changes in heart and respiratory rates, sweating, and color change should be considered. Als[52] described various avoidance techniques observed in preterm infants in response to over-stimulation. These included sneezing, coughing, eye closing, and, in extreme circumstances, apnea, bradycardia, vomiting, and defecating. This is not to imply that whenever we observe these responses the infant is being overstimulated, but to consider sensory overload when we are not observing the desired motor output. When treating adults or older children, if the desired response

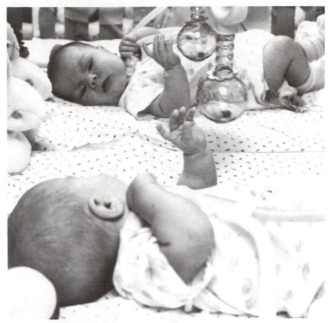

FIGURE 5. Use of a mirror in the crib.

is not elicited, the therapist may increase sensory input. This strategy may not be useful with the neonate, and is potentially harmful.

When developing a treatment plan it is helpful to compare the environments of the fetus, the NICU, and the home. The intrauterine environment is one of constant tactile input, decreased visual input, constant noise (maternal heart beat, digestion), and both active movement generated by the baby and passive movement generated by the mother. The NICU has constant bright lights, loud mechanical noises, and provides little movement for the infant.[1,75] The home environment might include dim lights, children and animal noises, cooking smells, music, and varying amounts of movement. Parents and NICU staff can be encouraged to make the NICU environment either more like the intrauterine or the home environment by placing a diaper over the top of the isolette to decrease the glare of bright lights and closing isolette doors carefully to decrease loud noises. Tactile input to the infant's body with the whole hand, rather than with the fingertips to the extremities, will help to calm him. Mirrors, pictures of faces, and toys with faces can be placed inside the isolette when parents cannot be present (Figure 5). Water beds can be used to encourage active movement and for increased vestibular input.[44] The preterm infant has little body fat and therefore has difficulty retaining body heat. Also, the temperature control mechanism is not fully mature. Care must be taken to avoid chilling which will increase caloric needs and energy requirements in these babies.[3,4]

Babies who have been in the NICU may not be able to adjust to the relative dark and quiet of home when discharged. If this is the case, the parents should be encouraged to use a night light and a radio until the baby is able to tolerate the decreased sensory input.

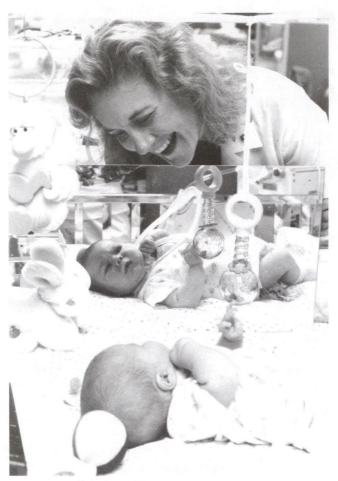

FIGURE 6. Infants prefer faces to objects.

Theories of child development continually change. At one time it was believed that infants were without skills or preferences at birth. We now know that infants are born with certain preferences and capabilities.[54,76,77] In the visual area, they prefer the human face. Even when the elements of a face are rearranged in a visual presentation, they are not as interesting to the baby as a face (Figure 6). In the area of color, the preference is for red and yellow, probably because these colors can be diffused through the mother's abdomen, and can be seen before birth. Sharp contrasts in color and lines, such as stripes or checkerboard patterns also are attractive. In the auditory area, babies prefer voices to other sounds, and the female voice to the male.[76] Researchers now are trying to determine what types of music are most appealing to the newborn and some authors are advocating the development of rhythm.[76] Neonates prefer sweet to salty and bitter tastes.[77] A breastfeeding baby can differentiate his own mother from another breastfeeding mother by the smell of the breast pad.[76,77] Certain speeds of rocking are preferred, probably those most similar to the human heart rate. We now appreciate that the newborn comes into the world with certain specific sensory and motor systems for interacting with the environment. Less research has been done regarding the sensory capabilities of the preterm infant because of his fragile

medical status. We will assume that the sensory preferences identified in full term babies are similar to those of the preterm, and provide an enriching environment, being careful not to produce sensory overload. Research alerts us to specific caution on sensory stimulation for infants exposed to drugs as these infants may be hyperirritable and disorganized by visual, auditory, tactile, and vestibular input unless it is carefully modulated and monitored.

Before administering intervention techniques, observe the infant at rest, and how he responds when nursing care or other procedures are done. Is the baby able to maintain his heart and respiratory rate? Does he startle whenever he is touched? Are his movements smooth or jerky? Is he usually positioned on his back, or facing only one direction? When are his eyes open? These and other questions should be asked before beginning to handle the baby. Do not begin physical therapy immediately following feeding. The baby will not be able to respond optimally, and the nursing staff will not welcome your services if the baby vomits.

Whenever possible encourage sidelying positioning which allows the baby to bring his hands together and toward his mouth for self calming (Figure 7). Sidelying promotes a balance between flexion and extension. Generally, skin to skin contact is a positive experience for infants, and bringing the hands together or to the mouth will provide more normal sensory input than putting a pacifier or your finger in the infant's mouth. Skin to skin contact can be both calming and alerting. When the baby is no longer on a respirator, or is medically stable, visual responses can be enhanced by positioning him upright. Sweeney[78,79] suggested the use of hydrotherapy for the very irritable infant, to provide neutral warmth while allowing active movement. Extreme care must be used when attempting these

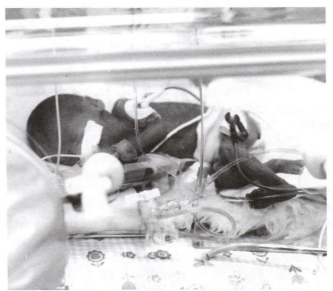

FIGURE 7. Use of sidelying to enhance hands together and hand to mouth behavior.

techniques. As mentioned previously, use of the whole hand rather than the finger tips is preferable, and less irritating to the baby. Physiologic flexion develops in the last trimester, partially in response to decreased space and partially as an active process in neurological development.[34-35] Infants who are born before they have a chance to develop physiologic flexion, or who demonstrate extensor overactivity and are then placed supine for long periods of time, may have difficulty developing flexor patterns because the supine position facilitate extension, and because it is difficult for these babies to flex against gravity. To help the infant develop normal movement patterns prone positioning should be attempted if it is not medically contradicted (Figure 8). Sidelying with tactile input on the anterior surface of the infant's body also will facilitate flexion. Another method useful in encouraging flexor responses is the use of non-nutritive sucking. Swaddling can be used to provide tactile input and to encourage flexion.

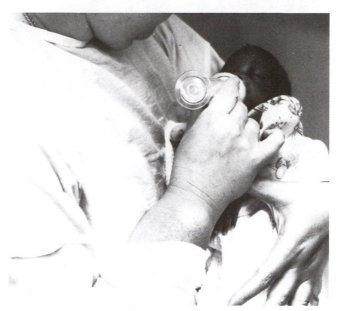

FIGURE 9. *Positioning to encourage sucking.*

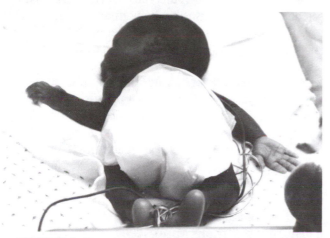

FIGURE 8. *Use of prone position to facilitate flexion.*

The physical therapist often is asked to evaluate a baby because of difficulty with feeding. Therefore, being well versed on normal oral motor reflexes,[25,26] as well as potential pathological patterns that may occur, is important. Although non-nutritive sucking may begin as early as 17-18 weeks post-conception, nutritive sucking (the skills necessary for successful feeding) do not emerge until approximately 34 weeks gestation, or six weeks before full term delivery.[35] The sucking response can be strengthened by encouraging non-nutritive sucking prior to the time that bottle feeding is initiated.[80,81] In addition to waiting to begin feeding until the infant is gestationally ready, it is important to evaluate the strength and rhythm of sucking. Does the infant use coordinated "stripping" or back and forth movements of his tongue, seal the lips adequately to prevent loss of fluid around the nipple, and remember to breathe when feeding?

Before feeding an infant, assess muscle tone and state of alertness. A floppy, sleeping baby or an agitated, screaming baby are not in optimal states for successful feeding. Facilitatory or inhibitory input, such as fast or slow rocking, can be used to prepare the baby and also to facilitate sucking. Mechanical problems might contribute to feeding difficulties. Certainly, cleft lip or palate presents unique problems and special nipples and bottles have been devised for these babies. Many babies with cleft palates also have small jaws which contribute to further difficulties because of airway obstruction by the tongue. Sidelying or even prone positioning might be necessary for such infants. Occasionally the airway obstruction becomes life threatening and surgical intervention becomes necessary to correct this problem.

The preterm infant who has required mechanical ventilation for a prolonged period of time often has a very high palate because of distortion from the endotracheal tube. If this baby is weak, bringing the tongue up to the palate in order to begin sucking may be difficult. Gentle pressure with the nipple either up against the palate or down on the tongue may assist this infant to initiate feeding.

Generally, the principles for feeding any child or adult with feeding difficulties apply to the neonate as well. Avoid neck extension as it opens the airway and can result in aspiration. Jaw control might be necessary for the infant having difficulty with lip closure. Slight traction to elongate the neck may facilitate swallowing. Swaddling or other positioning to encourage flexion will facilitate sucking, which is a flexion activity (Figure 9). Rocking can be used to encourage sucking. In a preterm infant who has difficulty remaining awake for an entire feeding, it might be useful to unwrap the baby, hold him slightly away from your body, and use short bursts of periodic moderately fast rocking to increase alertness.

Babies should be watched carefully during the process of feeding (Figure 10). It is not uncommon for them to have periods of apnea or bradycardia during feeding.

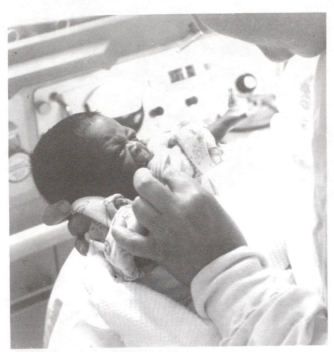

FIGURE 10. Evaluation of sucking, which produced a gag reflex and bradycardia.

Subtle changes in color, particularly perioral cyanosis, or just a pale appearance should be noted. There are many causes of these "spells" during feeding, including neurological immaturity and inability to coordinate sucking, swallowing, and breathing. Another cause of feeding bradycardia might be vagal hypersensitivity which may result when feeding tubes are passed down the throat. It is important to inform the medical staff if abnormal feeding patterns persist, because they may be indicative of more complex medical problems such as anemia or generalized infection.

There are many different kinds of feeding nipples used in the NICU. Our first inclination is to use the softest nipple with very small babies. Experience has shown that this may not always be the best strategy. Encouraging a stronger sucking pattern with a harder nipple may encourage a more mature pattern to develop and enhance muscle strength in the neck and oral motor areas. The formula may flow rapidly through the softer nipple, making it more difficult for the baby to handle a larger amount of fluid in his mouth, causing choking. Each infant should be evaluated carefully as to the type of nipple which will optimally suit his stage of development and his unique feeding problems.

Why is it important for the physical therapist to look at feeding problems? The most obvious reason is to address the whole child. Babies in the NICU generally feed every four hours. If it takes an hour or more to feed a baby each time, this is comparable to a full time job for the parent. Difficulty with feeding may interfere with parent-child interaction and may diminish the mother's feelings of self esteem if she feels that she is unable to

successfully nourish her child.[7] In addition to these issues, babies with unexplained feeding difficulties not related to immaturity are at risk for additional neurologic abnormalities. Because so much of the newborn neurological examination is not predictive of long term outcome, feeding is a very important factor in assessing neuromotor functioning. Infants with significant feeding difficulties, even when they do not develop major motor handicaps, are at risk for speech and language abnormalities because the same muscles necessary for successful feeding are used in speech production.[82]

Physical therapists in the NICU should view themselves as teachers and role models for both the staff and the parents. It is imperative to establish inservice education programs for parents and nursing staff, and to provide orientation for resident physicians, which includes both practical examples of intervention strategies, as well as the theoretical basis for treatment. In addition, role modeling with proper positioning and handling techniques is essential. If inservice and orientation programs are successful, there will be an increase in referrals as staff members come to recognize the value of, and become comfortable in, requesting physical therapy consultation.

Parents often ask what kinds of toys to purchase for their infants. In the NICU, seeing the baby in the crib or isolette may be difficult because of the stuffed toys, music boxes, and pictures. If parents and NICU staff understand the general sensory capabilities of the child, they will do a better job of selecting appropriate toys. For example, encourage the use of brightly colored toys with faces.[83] A tape recording of the family when at home, or some special music can be used when the parents are not visiting. Mirrors provide a face to look at whenever the baby is awake. Try to see objects as the baby sees them. A baby sees objects best if they are 7-10 inches from his face.[34,35] Pictures should be lying down if the baby is lying down when looking at them. Do not put toys at the baby's feet, unless you are merely trying to decorate the room. Encourage flexion by placing objects slightly below eye level.

There is nothing magical about any particular toy that will make babies happier or smarter. Although some toys may help to alert a certain baby, the best thing to use is the human touch, voice, and face. Toys are useful when there are not any caretakers to interact with the baby, but they do not take the place of people. The most expensive toys are not necessarily better than cheaper toys that are well made, safe, and provide interesting sensory experiences.

It is not always possible to identify children with neuromuscular abnormalities in the NICU. For this reason, a systematic method of providing periodic follow-up for those children who are at high risk for long term disabilities should be established. In reviewing criteria for follow-up in numerous NICUs,[84,85] it becomes apparent that similar categories are used. It is not necessary to follow every infant that briefly has been admitted to the NICU. Typical follow-up criteria include:

1) Low birth weight. (This can mean anything from below 2000 to below 1250 grams.)
2) Perinatal asphyxia, often determined by Apgar scores.
3) Infants requiring mechanical ventilation. (The length of time on a respirator varies.)
4) Intrauterine growth retardation.
5) Neurological abnormality. (Seizures, abnormal muscle tone, intra-cranial hemorrhage, congenital or acquired hydrocephalus.)
6) Documented sepsis or meningitis.
7) Congenital anomalies, birth defects, and chromosome abnormalities.
8) Vision and hearing defects.
9) Neonatal Abstinence Syndrome (NAS) or narcotic withdrawal.
10) Gastrointestinal abnormalities or prolonged feeding difficulties which may lead to failure to thrive.
11) High risk indicators of potential HIV infection.

These criteria generally encompass 40-50% of those children admitted to the NICU. Most clinics adjust for prematurity, using the child's due date as an estimation of birthdate. There is some variation in how long clinics use this adjustment. If a child is not showing "catch up" by two years of age, long term delays are suspected. Preterm infants, if they are appropriate for gestational age, are not destined to be small. Their ultimate growth is more determined by the genetic complement rather than the size at birth. Growth patterns of preterm infants are different from full term babies. Often they show very rapid catch up growth with the head growing fastest. The weight catches up next, and finally, height. It is important to reassure parents that this rapid head growth is normal for their child. If the child is properly nourished, growth often reaches the normal growth parameters within the first year of life.

Most major neurologic handicaps can be identified within the first year of life with careful attention to quality of movement, as well as to quantity of motor development.[86-89] Long term language and cognitive development generally take longer to determine.

Approximately 5% of live births are transferred to tertiary centers for medical management. Of those infants who require such services, approximately 15% have major developmental abnormalities.[90] Although smaller babies are surviving, there have not been significant changes in the percentage of children with developmental disabilities.[91-93] Therapists working in schools, hospitals, and other clinics mistakenly believe that few infants in NICU settings develop normally. It is

difficult to accurately assess whether NICU graduates are at greater risk for problems such as dyslexia and other learning disabilities. Because environmental factors become more significant with increasing age, it is difficult to assess how much of the problem is related to prematurity and how much to other factors.[94]

The NICU is an exciting place for the physical therapist to work. Medical professionals and families work as a team to optimize the outcome of high risk infants. The information presented in this chapter is only a brief introduction for the therapist interested in working in this setting. Previous pediatric experience as well as supervised clinical practice in the NICU are strongly recommended. The physical therapist must exhibit professionalism as well as expertise in order to become an integral member of the NICU team.

CASE STUDIES

CASE NO. 1 — JASON
Cerebral Palsy, Right Hemiparesis, 18 Months

Jason was the first born of non-identical twins delivered by cesarean birth eight weeks prematurely. His Apgar scores were 7 at one minute and 9 at five minutes. His birth weight (1660 grams, or 3 pounds, 4½ ounces), head circumference, and length were appropriate for gestational age. He did not require any mechanical ventilation at birth. A cranial ultrasound at three days of age showed a left sided germinal matrix hemorrhage with normal sized ventricles. A follow-up ultrasound one week later, however, revealed complete reabsorption of the clot and normal ventricular size bilaterally. A Brazelton Neonatal Behavior Assessment Scale initially was performed when Jason was three weeks old (35 weeks post-conceptional age). At that time, Jason demonstrated few self-calming strategies, such as non-nutritive sucking or hand to mouth activities, and his tendon reflexes were generally brisk. Trunk incurvation was diminished slightly on the right. There was significant ankle clonus bilaterally and he was jittery. He was on caffeine citrate which was being used to control apnea and bradycardia spells which occurred particularly during feeding. This medication has been noted to result in some generalized jitteriness and increased muscle tone in infants.

Jason was re-evaluated by the physical therapist at seven weeks of age (39 weeks post-conception). At that time the asymmetry was no longer apparent, but he continued to be difficult to calm and was jittery. Jason and his twin were discharged at 40 days of age on caffeine-citrate. Jason did not receive P.T. services in the NICU, nor were any recommended at discharge, even though there were early, subtle, transient findings of asymmetry and jitteriness. The use of theophylline or caffeine citrate to control apnea and bradycardia spells can result in jitteriness, as well as increased muscle tone, thereby making it difficult to accurately assess the neurological status of these babies. The majority of children who present with a history like Jason's develop normally. There have not been comprehensive long term studies done to evaluate the outcome of therapeutic doses of caffeine.

The twins were seen in follow-up clinic at four months of age (two months corrected gestational age). Jason continued to be irritable and preferred to hold his head to the right, but his examination was otherwise "normal".

The next visit was scheduled at Jason's six months adjusted chronological age (eight months true chronological age). At this time his mother remarked that Jason was "left handed". The neurological evaluation was markedly asymmetrical, with a persistent asymmetrical tonic neck reflex to the right, fisting of the right hand with the thumb flexed in the palm, and 5-7 beats of ankle clonus on the right. The Bayley Scales of Infant Development were administered by the physical therapist at this visit, and Jason was age appropriate when adjusted for prematurity.

The abnormal neurologic findings were discussed with his parents, and a more complete neurologic examination was recommended. Jason was referred for physical therapy intervention in their local community. Neurologic abnormalities in children like Jason may not become obvious before 6-9 months of age. It is becoming increasingly difficult to locate therapy services for "at risk" infants without documented diagnostic criteria. For this reason, it is important for NICU follow-up clinics to monitor closely such infants and refer them for services as soon as abnormalities become apparent.

CASE NO. 2 — JILL
Cerebral Palsy, Spastic Quadriparesis, Mental Retardation, 7 Years

Jill was the product of a full term, uncomplicated pregnancy. She was the first child for her 30 year old mother. The delivery was very rapid and Apgar scores were 5 at one minute and 8 at five minutes. There were no initial problems and Jill was placed in the normal newborn nursery. The nurses in the nursery noted some unusual eye movements and occasional stiffening of Jill's extremities when she was four hours old, and called the staff from the neonatal intensive care nursery. Jill was immediately transferred to the NICU and given a loading dose of phenobarbital. Her seizures continued, and several other anti-convulsants were added, following an examination by the pediatric neurologist. The increase in medication resulted in respiratory depression and Jill was placed on a respirator at 12 hours of age (Figure 11). The EEG was markedly abnormal at this time. Over the next several days the seizures gradually

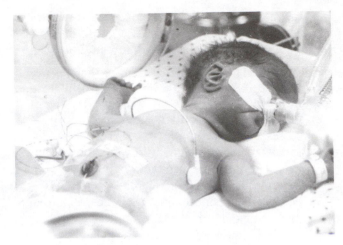

FIGURE 11. *Jill on respirator.*

subsided, medications were decreased, and Jill was weaned from the respirator.

Initial physical therapy evaluation at five days of age, using the Brazelton and Dubowitz Scales, revealed a sleepy child with generalized hypotonicity, absent suck, and diminished gag response. Over the next week, the feeding pattern improved and Jill was sent home bottle feeding. Feeding techniques recommended by the physical therapist to the parents and nursing staff included rapid rocking prior to and during feeding for vestibular input, perioral stroking, positioning in midline with slight neck flexion, using a pacifier between feedings to strengthen the suck, and positioning upright as possible to improve alertness.

The physical therapist met with the parents, the pediatric neurologist, and the neonatologist to discuss long term prognosis and program planning. A brain stem auditory evoked (BAER) test was administered because of neonatal seizures, and the response time was slightly delayed. An eye exam was recommended at two months of age because she required assisted ventilation.

Prior to discharge, the parents were instructed in positioning and handling techniques. Jill initially presented as a child with low muscle tone, but with potential for increased tone with time, which mandated close monitoring of her home program. The parents were given a handout discussing the use of toys to enhance visual and auditory skills. Jill's stay in the NICU was short, but she will need long term programming. It is extremely important for the physical therapist working in the NICU to maintain good communication with community agencies providing therapy services. Because of her history of prolonged seizures and early feeding problems, Jill was referred for homebound physical therapy services when she was discharged from the hospital.

When seen initially in follow-up clinic at four months of age, Jill was a very irritable child, with generalized

Therapeutic Exercise In Developmental Disabilities

increased muscle tone. At this visit, a decrease in her head growth was noted because of the significant neonatal insult. The eye exam and a repeat of the BAER were normal. The need for continued therapy services as well as future educational needs were discussed, and the parents were referred to the local agency for family support services.

CASE NO. 3 — TAYLOR
Myelomeningocele, Repaired L 1-2, 4 Years

Taylor was a child born at full term who was delivered by cesarean section because of fetal distress and breech presentation. A large lumbar myelomeningocele was noted immediately at birth and he was transferred to the neonatal intensive care unit. The neurosurgeon, after examining the infant, explained to the parents the long term implications of myelomeningocele, including paralysis, potential mental retardation, hydrocephalus, bowel and bladder dysfunction, and the need for long term care and many surgical procedures. They were given the option of an immediate operation, and they chose to have primary closure of the myelomeningocele.

Taylor was examined by the physical therapist prior to the surgery. It was noted that he had 90° hip flexion contractures, and knee flexion was limited to 60°. He also had severe equinovarus deformities of both feet. There was no response to sensory input of touch, pressure, or pin prick on either lower extremity.

Following primary closure of the myelomeningocele, the physical therapist met with the parents to discuss the long term rehabilitation goals for Taylor, including the good potential for assisted ambulation. The parents were instructed in range of motion techniques, and advised regarding skin precautions because of the sensory loss. Emphasis was placed on developing good head and trunk control, upper extremity skills, maintaining lower extremity mobility, and cognitive skills. They were given a list of books on normal development which were available in the hospital parent library. They were encouraged to be aware of the positive aspects of Taylor's development and not only his disability. Referral was made, with their permission, to the local spina bifida association, which has an excellent parent to parent support network. Referral also was made to state services for crippled children, to assist with some of the financial burden associated with having a child with a long term disability requiring continuing medical and surgical intervention, as well as orthotic and transport equipment.

Three days following primary closure of the myelomeningocele, a bulging fontanelle was noted. Cranial ultrasound revealed enlarged ventricles, and a ventricular-peritoneal shunting was performed on day five. Taylor continued to have severe apnea spells and was placed on a respirator. The neurosurgeon recommended an EEG to rule out seizures, and fortunately the EEG essentially was normal. An Arnold-Chiari malformation was suspected as causing compression of the brain stem and the resultant apnea spells. At two weeks of age, a surgical decompression of the posterior fossa was performed. The apnea improved and the respirator was discontinued, but Taylor continued to have apnea several times a day requiring stimulation to resume breathing.

Because of the medical concerns, little attention was paid to rehabilitation services. However, the foot deformities were being treated with serial casting by the orthopedic surgeon. During this time the physical therapist performed passive range of motion to the lower extremities of the child, and instructed both parents and the nursing staff on range of motion and prone positioning to reduce hip flexion contractures. Suggestions for toys were given to the family to encourage them to look at Taylor's need for normal sensory input in the relatively abnormal hospital environment.

The apnea spells continued and Taylor remained in the NICU for four months. Every attempt was made to provide a variety of sensory-motor experiences appropriate for his age that would not compromise his medical status (Figure 12). Discharge plans were eventually made, with a cardio-respiratory monitor for home use. He was referred to a physical therapist for homebound treatment once a week and to the myelomeningocele clinic at the local children's orthopedic hospital outpatient department. Because so many community services were available to this family, Taylor was not scheduled to return to the NICU follow-up clinic.

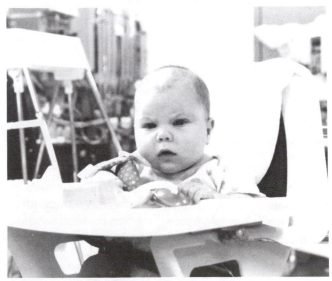

FIGURE 12. Four-month-old child in NICU experiences normal upright positioning.

CASE NO. 4 — ASHLEY
Down Syndrome, 15 Months

Ashley was the first child born to a 26 year old woman. The pregnancy was uncomplicated, and Ashley was born at full term. Characteristics of Down syndrome were noted in the baby at the time of delivery. She was transferred to the NICU because of a heart murmur. Cardiac echogram revealed a rather large ventricular septal defect. On further examination, an esophageal atresia was noted. Primary repair of the esophageal atresia was not possible, and a gastrostomy was performed. No oral feedings were permitted. However, Ashley had a fair suck on a nuk pacifier, and this was encouraged.

Activities suggested to Ashley's parents included positioning in various ways: upright with as little support as necessary to enhance head and trunk control, prone to encourage head control and upper extremity weight bearing, and sidelying to encourage hands together and hand to mouth activities (Figure 13). There is no contraindication to prone positioning in a child with a gastrostomy. After the first week post-operatively, these children can be positioned safely in prone. Most children do not require any special devices for prone positioning, but for those that do, a small cut-out in a foam rubber block or wedge to accommodate the tube is sufficient. The earlier these children are placed in prone positions, the easier it is for them, their parents, and the nursing staff. Other suggestions given to Ashley's parents included wrist rattles and bells on her hands and feet to encourage movement, water toys to encourage movement against the resistance of water, holding her while in a rocking chair, use of a baby swing for vestibular input, and olfactory input with pleasant odors (cinnamon, cherry) during non-nutritive sucking.

Ashley was discharged from the hospital at six weeks of age. Because of concerns regarding medical complications the family refused to become involved with an infant therapy program. They were unwilling to follow a program of activities suggested to enhance motor development. They had many toys for Ashley, but these were used generally to provide visual and auditory stimulation and not movement.

At six months of age the esophageal atresia was repaired. At eight months of age the heart defect was surgically corrected. At ten months of age the family finally consented to become involved in an infant therapy program. When initially seen by the physical therapist at ten months of age Ashley was very hypotonic even for a child with Down syndrome. She was prop-sitting momentarily, had moderate head lag when pulled to sit, and would bear minimal weight on her legs. Ashley had many ear infections and finally received PE (pressure equalizing) tubes at 12 months of age. She has a mild conductive hearing loss.

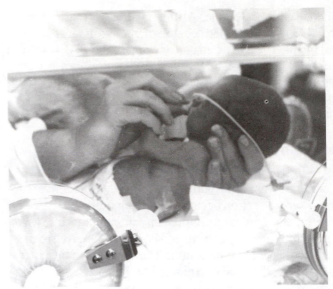

FIGURE 13. *Facilitating hand to mouth.*

In children like Ashley, with complex medical problems, the family may not be willing or able to participate even in non-stressful therapeutic activities. All of their energy is concentrated on the child's acute medical needs. Experience has shown that such families will eventually recognize the need for physical therapy services, as the child's delay become more apparent, and the child grows larger and more difficult to handle. It is important to continue to reinforce the need for such services. Often the best way to do this is for the primary physician or a specialist (cardiologist) to suggest programming to the family, because they will continue to see these children on a regular basis. The physical therapist in the NICU as well as those in the community must constantly work to keep physicians informed regarding the need for developmental physical therapy services and their availability. ❏

GLOSSARY

A and B SPELLS:
Apnea—absence of respiration for 20 seconds;
Bradycardia—heart rate less than 90 per minute,
accompanied by cyanosis.

AGA: Appropriately grown for gestational age.

ANOXIA: Absence of oxygen.

ASPHYXIA: A condition in which there is a deficiency of
oxygen and an increase in carbon dioxide in the blood
and tissues. Perinatal asphyxia is lack of oxygen just
prior to, during, or shortly after birth.

ASPIRATION: Breathing a foreign substance such as
meconium, formula, or stomach contents into the lungs;
may cause aspiration pneumonia.

ATELECTASIS: Collapse of the air sacks in the lungs.

BETAMETHASONE: A steroid given to a mother before a
threatened preterm birth to help the baby's lungs mature.

BILIRUBIN: A yellowish substance produced when red blood
cells break down; may cause jaundice, and in large
amounts, kernicterus, with resultant basal ganglia
damage and possible athetoid type cerebral palsy.

BLOOD GAS: A sample of blood which measures how much
oxygen, carbon dioxide, and acid it contains; ABG—
arterial blood gas; VBC—venous blood gas.

**BRAIN STEM AUDITORY EVOKED RESPONSE TEST
(BAER):** A method for early detection of hearing loss in
neonates in which brain wave response to a variety of
sound levels is assessed.

BRONCHOPULMONARY DYSPLASIA (BPD): Iatrogenic
condition, characterized by changes and alterations of
the normal development of the air passages of the lungs
and lung tissues generally following prolonged treatment
with a respirator.

CHALASIA: Relaxation or immaturity of the sphincter between
the esophagus and the stomach resulting in vomiting;
also may be referred to as gastroesophageal reflux
(GER).

CONTINUOUS POSITIVE AIRWAY PRESSURE (CPAP): The
constant flow of air being blown into the lungs by a
respirator.

DISSEMINATED INTRAVASCULAR COAGULATION (DIC):
A condition in which the platelets and other clotting
factors of the blood are consumed because of infection,
hypoxia, acidosis or other diseases or injuries; this
results in excessive bleeding and often requires
transfusions.

DUCTUS ARTERIOSUS: A fetal blood vessel extending from
the pulmonary artery to the aorta; PDA—patent ductus
arteriosus; a condition in which this vessel fails to close
after birth which results in poor oxygenation and
generally requires either medical or surgical intervention
for closure.

ECLAMPSIA: Toxemia of pregnancy accompanied by high
blood pressure, albuminuria, oliguria, tonic and clonic
convulsions and coma; may occur before, during, or after
childbirth.

ENDOTRACHEAL INTUBATION: Passage of a small plastic
tube through the trachea, past the vocal cords, and into
the bronchial tree for assisted ventilation.

ERYTHROBLASTOSIS FETALIS: Blood type incompatibility
between the mother and baby, causing maternal
antibodies to attack neonatal blood cells, and causing
severe anemia and jaundice in the newborn.

GAVAGE FEEDING: Feedings given through a tube passed
through the nose or mouth and into the stomach in
babies who are too immature to bottle feed, or who are
otherwise unable to feed orally.

HUMAN IMMUNODEFICIENCY VIRUS (HIV) INFECTION:
Systemic fatal infection which severely compromises the
immune system, and causes neurological and
developmental deficits; presents a widely variant clinical
picture

HYALINE MEMBRANE DISEASE (HMD): Respiratory
disease that affects preterm babies; it is caused by a
lack of surfactant, a substance that prevents collapse of
the alveoli.

HYPERALIMENTATION: Intervenous administration of
glucose, protein, minerals, and vitamins; used when oral
feedings cannot be initiated; this is also called total
parenteral nutrition (TPN).

INDOMETHACIN: A drug used to close the patent ductus
arteriosus.

INFANT OF A DIABETIC MOTHER (IDM): These babies are
often LGA (large for gestational age) and are at high risk
for both prenatal and postnatal complications.

LOADING DOSE: Sufficient amount of medication to obtain a
therapeutic blood level.

L/S RATIO: A ratio between two factors in surfactant (lecithin
and sphingomyelin) in the amniotic fluid: this ratio is used
as an indicator of lung maturity in the fetus.

MATERNAL SUBSTANCE ABUSE: Use of potentially
teratogenic substances during pregnancy which may
have adverse effect on the fetus; includes drugs such as
heroin, cocaine, alcohol, and cigarettes.

MECONIUM: A greenish-black tarry material present in the
fetal intestine before birth, and usually passed in the first
few days after birth; this may be passed in utero if the
baby is in distress before birth; aspiration of meconium
results in asphyxia and severe respiratory complications.

NECROTIZING ENTEROCOLITIS (NEC): A condition in
which there is diffuse or patchy necrosis of the mucosa or
submucosa of the small or large bowel, probably due to
ischemia and prematurity.

NEONATE: A baby less than four weeks of age.

NEONATAL ABSTINENCE SYNDROME: neurobehavioral
sequelae identified in infants prenatally exposed to
narcotic drugs.

NON-NUTRITIVE SUCKING: Sucking on finger or pacifier,
purpose is not for oral intake.

OCCIPITAL FRONTAL CIRCUMFERENCE (OFC): Head size
measurement.

OLIGOHYDRAMNIOS: A greatly reduced amount of amniotic
fluid.

PaCO$_2$: Partial pressure of carbon dioxide in arterial blood.

PaO$_2$: Partial pressure of oxygen in arterial blood.

PAVULON: A drug which acts on the myoneural junction and
produces temporary paralysis; often used to prevent a
baby from "fighting" the respirator.

PERIODIC BREATHING: Breathing interrupted by pauses of
10 or more seconds; common in preterm babies.

PERSISTENT FETAL CIRCULATION (PFC): A condition in
which the blood continues to flow through the ductus
arteriosus and bypass the lungs; this usually occurs in
term and post-term infants following hypoxia.

PLACENTA ABRUPTIO: Premature separation of the
placenta from the uterus with resultant bleeding and
neonatal asphyxia.

PLACENTA PREVIA: A condition in which the placenta is
abnormally positioned over the cervix, thereby preventing
a normal vaginal delivery.

PNEUMOGRAM: Monitoring a baby's heart rate and
respiratory patterns for several hours to detect any
abnormalities either during waking or sleeping.

POLYCYTHEMIA: Abnormally high number of red blood cells, causing "sluggish" circulation; this is also called hyperviscosity.

POLYHYDRAMNIOS: Excessive amount of amniotic fluid.

POSITIVE END EXPIRATORY PRESSURE (PEEP): A constant amount of pressure exerted by the respirator to keep the lungs expanded.

PREMATURE RUPTURE OF MEMBRANES (PROM): The breaking of the membrane surrounding the fetus before the beginning of labor; this results in an increased possibility of infection.

RESPIRATORY DISTRESS SYNDROME (RDS): Terminology used interchangeably with hyaline membrane disease.

RETINOPATHY OF PREMATURITY (ROP): A condition of the eyes related to prematurity, oxygen concentration, and possibly other factors, affecting the blood vessels of the eyes that can result in blindness; previously called retrolental fibroplasia (RLF).

SEPSIS: Generalized infection characterized by proliferation of bacteria in the bloodstream, due to the fact the newborn has little capacity to localize or encapsulate infections.

SEPTAL DEFECTS: Congenital defects in the heart muscle; VSD—ventricular septal defect is an opening between the right and left ventricles; ASD—atrial septal defect is between the right and left atria; these defects generally require surgical repair.

SEXUALLY TRANSMITTED DISEASES: Infection passed prenatally or perinatally to the infant whose mother is infected; examples include syphilis, herpes, gonorrhea.

SMALL FOR GESTATIONAL AGE (SGA): Newborn whose growth parameters (weight, length, and head circumference) are less than the fifth percentile for gestational age; also called intrauterine growth retardation (IUGR).

SURFACTANT: A substance manufactured by the lungs to prevent alveolar collapse.

THEOPHYLLINE: A stimulant drug used in the treatment of apnea; caffeine citrate is also used for this purpose.

TOCOLYTIC DRUGS: Drugs used to stop premature labor (e.g. ritodrine).

TORCH TITERS: A blood test to determine the presence of certain viral agents including toxoplasmosis, rubella, cytomegalovirus (CMV), and herpes.

TRANSCUTANEOUS MONITOR (TCM): A device to monitor oxygen concentration in the blood by means of a skin electrode.

TRANSIENT TACHYPNEA NEONATORUM (TTN): Rapid respiratory rate generally seen in term infants born by cesarean or with precipitous deliveries, related to poorly absorbed lung fluid; also called wet lung.

VERNIX: White, fatty substance that protects the fetus skin in utero.

READING LIST FOR PARENTS

1. Barker, LW, Williams, H: Your Babies First 30 Months. New York, NY, HP Books: Fisher Publishing Company, 1981
2. Brazelton, TB: Doctor and Child. New York, NY, Dell Publishing Company, Inc., 1970
3. Brazelton, TB: Infants and Toddlers. New York, NY, Dell Publishing Company, Inc.,1969
4. Brazelton, TB: Toddlers and Parents. New York, NY, Dell Publishing Company, Inc.,1974
5. Caplan, F, Caplan, T: The Early Childhood Years (The 2 - 6 year old). New York, NY. Putnam Publishing, 1983
6. Chase, PA, Rubin, RR (eds): The First Wondrous Year. New York, NY, Johnson and Johnson Child Development Publications, Collier Books, 1978
7. Dorris, M: The Broken Cord. New York, NY, Harper Collins Publishers, 1989
8. Gordon, IJ: Baby Learning Through Baby Play. New York, NY, St. Martin's Press, 1970
9. Gordon, IJ: Child Learning Through Child Play. New York, NY, St. Martin's Press, 1972
10. Kelly. P (ed): First Year Baby Care. Wayzata, MN, Meadowbrook Press, 1983
11. Leach, P: The Child Care Encyclopedia. New York, NY, Alfred A. Knoff Publishing,1983
12. Leach, P: Your Baby and Child from Birth to Age Five. New York, NY, Alfred A. Knoff Publishing, 1977
13. Rubin, RR, Fisher, JJ, Doering: Your Toddler. New York, NY, Johnson and Johnson Child Development Publications, Collier Books, 1980
14. Smith, HW: Survival Handbook for Preschool Mothers. Chicago, IL, Folley Publications, 1977

REFERENCES

1. Lawson K, Daum C, Turkewitz G: Environmental characteristics of a neonatal intensive care unit. Child Dev 48:1633-1639, 1977
2. Harrison H: The Premature Baby Book. New York, NY, St. Martin's Press, 1983
3. Klaus MH, Fanaroff AA: Care of the High Risk Neonate. Philadelphia, PA, WB Saunders Company, 1973
4. Korones SB: High Risk Newborn Infants, ed. 2. St. Louis, MO, CV Mosby Company, 1976
5. Lubchenco LO: The High Risk Infant, Philadelphia, PA, WB Saunders, 1976
6. Philip AGS: Neonate Sepsis and Meningitis. Boston, MA, GK Hall Company, 1985
7. Johnson SH: High Risk Parenting: Nursing Assessment and Strategies for the Family at Risk. Philadelphia, PA, JB Lippincott Company, 1979
8. Plant ML, Plant MA: Maternal use of alcohol and other drugs during pregnancy and birth abnormalities: Further results from a prospective study: Alcohol and Alcoholism 23: 229 - 233, 1988
9. Neuspiel DR, Hamel SC: Cocaine and infant behavior. Developmental and Behavioral Pediatrics 12:55 - 64, 1991
10. Cherukuri R, Minkoff H, Feldman J, Parekh A, Glass L: A Cohort Study of Alkaloidal Cocaine ("Crack") in Pregnancy. Obstretrics and Gynecology 72: 147- 151, 1988
11. Chasnoff I, Bussey ME, Savich R, Stack CM: Perinatal cerebral infarction and maternal cocaine use. J Pediatr 108:456-459, 1986
12. Chasnoff I, Burns WJ, Schnoll SH, Burns KA: Cocaine Use in Pregnancy. New England Journal of Medicine 313:666-669, 1985
13. Bryson YJ: Perinatal acquired immunodeficiency disease. Report of the 100th Ross Conference in Pediatric Research. Ross Laboratories, Columbus, OH, 1991
14. Dyer J: High Risk Infants: Does Government Care? (presented at Contemporary Issues in High Risk Infant Follow-Up). Madison, WI, Oct 1982
15. Gorsh PA, Davison MF, Brazelton TB: Stages of behavioral organization in the high risk neonate: theoretical and clinical considerations. Seminars in Perinatology 3:61-72, 1979
16. Harper PA, Fisher LK, Rider RV: Neurological and intellectual status of prematures at 3-5 years of age. J Pediatr 55:679-690, 1959
17. Lewis M, Wilson, CD: Infant development in lower class American families. Hum Dev 15:112-127, 1972
18. Newberger CM: The cognitive structure of parenthood: designing a descriptive measure. New Directions for Child Dev 7:45-67, 1980
19. Wiener G, Rider RV, Oppel W, et al: Correlates of low birth weight: Psychological status at 6-7 years of age. Pediatr Res 2:110-118, 1968
20. Belman AL: AIDS and Pediatric Neurology. Neurologic Clinics, 8:571-603, 1990
21. Grosz J and Hopkins K: Family Circumstances Affecting Caregivers and Brothers and Sisters in Crocker AC, Cohen HJ and Kastner TA (eds): HIV Infection and Developmental Disabilities. Paul H Brookes, Baltimore, 1992, pp. 43-52
22. Cohen HJ and Diamond GW: Developmental Assessment of Children with HIV Infection in Crocker AC, Cohen HJ and Kastner TA (eds): HIV Infection and Developmental Disabilities. Paul H Brookes, Baltimore, 1992, pp. 53-62
23. Harris MH: Habilitative and Rehabilitative Needs of Children with HIV Infection in Crocker AC, Cohen HJ and Kastner TA (eds): HIV Infection and Developmental Disabilities. Paul H Brookes, Baltimore, 1992, pp. 85 - 94
24. Bly L: NDT Baby Course, Minneapolis, MN, Nov 1984
25. Morris SE: The Normal Acquisition of Oral Feeding Skills: Implications for assessment and treatment. New York, NY, Therapeutic Media Inc, 1982
26. Mueller HA: Facilitating Feeding and Prespeech. In PH Pearson and C Williams (eds): Physical Therapy Services in Developmental Disabilities. Springfield, IL, Charles C. Thomas, 1972
27. Babson S, Kongos, J: Preschool intelligence of undersized term infants. Am J Dis Child 117:553-169, 1969
28. Fitzhardinge PM, Steven EM: Small for date infants: Neurological and intellectual sequelae. Pediatr 50:50, 1972
29. Markarin M: SGA infant term and preterm. Presented at Tomorrow: A follow-up on prenatal care. San Diego, CA, Nov 1980
30. Apgar V, Beck J: Is My Baby All Right. New York, NY, Trident Press, 1973
31. Zuckerman B, Frank DA, Hingson R, et al: Effects of maternal marijuana and cocaine use on fetal growth. New England Journal of Medicine 320:762-768, 1989
32. Gluck L: Intrauterine Asphyxia and the Developing Fetal Brain. Chicago, IL, Year Book Medical Publishers, Inc., 1977
33. Milani-Comparetti, A: The Prenatal Development of Movement: Implications for Developmental Diagnosis (seminar presented). St. Paul, MN, Oct 1980
34. Moore KL: The Developing Human. ed.2, Philadelphia, PA, WB Saunders, 1977
35. Nilsson L: A Child is Born. New York, NY, Dell Publishing Co, 1966
36. Dubowitz LM, Dubowitz V: Clinical assessment of gestational age in the newborn infant J Pediatr 77:1-10, 1970
37. Barnard KE: The effect of stimulation on the sleep behavior of the premature infant. Commun News Res 6:12-40, 1973
38. Dreyfus-Brisac C: Organization of Sleep in Prematures: Implications for Caregiving. In Lewis M, Rosenblum LA (eds): The Effect of the Infant on its Caregivers. New York, NY, John Wiley, 1974
39. Ludington-Hoe S: Parents Guide to Infant Stimulation. Los Angeles, CA, Infant Stimulation Education Assoc, 1983
40. Blackburn S: Fostering behavioral development of high risk infants. J Obstr Gyn Nurs (supplement), 1983
41. Long JG, Lucey JR, Philip AG: Noise and hypoxia in the ICU. Pediatr 65:143-145,1981
42. Martin RJ, et al: Effect of supine and prone position on arterial oxygen tension in the preterm infant. Pediatr 63:528, 1979
43. Crook CK, Lipsin LP: Neonatal nutrition sucking: effects of toxic stimulation upon sucking rhythm and heart rate. Child Dev 47:518-522, 1976
44. Korner AF, Kraemer HC, Haffner ME, Cosper LM: Effects of waterbed floatation on premature infants: A pilot study. Pediatr 56:361-367, 1975
45. Korner AF, Schneider P, Forrest T: Effects of vestibular-proprioceptive stimulation on the neurobehavioral development of preterm infants: A pilot study. Neuropediatr 14:170-175, 1983
46. Orgill AA, et al: Early development of infants 1000 grams or less at birth. Arch Dis Child 57:823-827, 1982
47. Scarr-Salapatek S, Williams ML: The effects of early stimulation on low birth weight infants. Child Dev 44:94-101, 1973
48. VandenBerg K: Revising the traditional model: An individualized approach to developmental interventions in the intensive care nursery neonatal network. J of Neonatal Nurs 3, 1985

---

49. Clark D, Ensher G, LeFever J: From newborn nursery to public school: Comprehensive services for high risk infants (presented at Contemporary Issues in High Risk Infant Follow-Up). Madison, WI, Oct 1982

50. Kitchen W, et al: A longitudinal study of very low birth weight infants: An overview of performance at 8 years of age. Dev Med and Child Neurol 22:172-198, 1980

51. Weiner G: The relationship of birth weight and length of gestation to intellectual development at ages 8-10. J Pediatr 76:694, 1970

52. Als H, Lester BM, Brazelton TB: Dynamics of the Behavioral Organization of the Premature Infant: A theoretical perspective. In Field T (ed): Infants Born at risk. New York, NY, Spectrum, 1979

53. Amiel-Tison C, Grenier A: Neurological evaluation of the newborn and the infant. New York, NY, Mason Publications, Inc., 1983

54. Brazelton TB: Neonatal Behavioral Assessment Scale. Clinics in Developmental Medicine 50, Philadelphia, JB Lippincott Co., 1973

55. Korner AF, Thom A, Forrest T: Neurobehavioral Maturity Assessment for Preterm Infants (NB-MAP) (presented at Sensori-Motor Integration seminar). San Diego, CA, July 1985

56. O'Doherty N: Neurological Examination of the Newborn. In Drillion CM, Drummond MB (eds): Neurodevelopmental Problems in Early Childhood. Oxford, England, Blackwell Scientific Publications, 1977

57. Prechtl H, Beintema D: The Neurological Examination of the Full Term Newborn Infant. Clinics in Developmental Medicine 12, Philadelphia, PA, JB Lippincott, 1964

58. Horowitz FD, Brown CC (eds): Toward a Model of Early Infant Development. In Infants at Risk Assessment and Intervention. Johnson and Johnson Baby Products Co, Pediatric Round Table 5, 1981

59. Freedman DG: Ethnic Differences in Babies. Hum Nature, Jan 1979

60. Bobath B: Abnormal Postural Reflex Activity Caused by Brain Lesions. London, UK, Wm Heineman Med Books Ltd., 1971

61. Semens S: The Bobath concept in treatment of neurological disorders. Am J Phys Med 46:732-788, 1967

62. Stockmeyer SA: An interpretation of the approach of Rood to the treatment of neuromuscular dysfunction. Am J Phys Med 46:900-972, 1967

63. Ludington-Hoe S: How to Have a Smarter Baby. New York, NY, Scribner and Sons, 1985

64. Caldwell BM: The rationale for early intervention. Exceptional Children 717-726, 1970

65. Field TM, et al: Tactile/Kinesthetic stimulation effects on preterm neonates. Pediatr 77:654-658, 1986

66. Goodman M, et al: Effect of early neurodevelopmental therapy in normal and at-risk survivors of neonatal intensive care. Lancet 1327-1330, 1985

67. Leib SA, Bensfield G, Guidubaldi J: Effects of early intervention and stimulation on the preterm infant. Pediatr 66:83-89, 1980

68. Powell LF: The effect of extra stimulation on the development of low birth weight infants and on natural behavior. Child Dev 45:106, 1974

69. Widmayer SM, Field TM: Effects of Brazelton demonstrations for mothers on the development of preterm infants. Pediatr 67:711-714, 1981

70. Ferry PC: On growing new neurons: Are early intervention programs effective? Pediatr 67:38-41, 1981

71. Hayes JS: Premature infant development: The relationship of neonatal stimulation, birth condition, and home environment. Pediatric Nursing: 33-36, 1980

72. Kromer M, Chomorro I, Green D, Knudtson F: Extra tactile stimulation of the premature infant. Nursing Research: 324-332, 1975

73. Murphy TF, Nichter CA, Liden CB: Developmental outcome of the high-risk infant: A review of methodological issues. Seminars in Perinatology 6:353-364,1982

74. Masland RL: Unproven methods of treatment. Pediatr 57:713, 1976

75. Blackburn S: The neonatal ICU: A high risk environment. Am J Nurs 82:1708-1712, 1982

76. Bower TGR: A Primer of Infant Development. San Francisco, CA, WH Freeman and Co., 1977

77. McCall R: Infants: The New Knowledge. Cambridge, MA, Harvard University Press, 1979

78. Sweeney JK: Neonatal hydrotherapy: An adjunct to developmental intervention in an intensive care nursery setting. Phys Occup Ther Pediatr 3:20, 1983

79. Sweeney JK: Neonates at developmental risk. In Neurological Rehabilitation, Umphred, DA (ed): St. Louis, MO, CV Mosby Company, 1985

80. Field T, et al: Effects of non-nutritive sucking during tube feedings of ICU Preterm Neonates. Pediatr 70:381-84, 1982

81. Measil CP, Anderson GC: Nonnutritive sucking during tube feedings: Effect upon clinical course in premature infants. J Obst Gynec and Neonatal Nurs 8:265-272, 1979

82. Illingworth R: Sucking and swallowing difficulties in infancy: diagnostic problems of dysphagia. Arch Dis Child 44:238, 1969

83. Goren C, Sarty M, Wu PYK: Visual following and pattern discrimination of face-like stimuli by newborn infants. Pediatr 56:544-548, 1975

84. Wisconsin Association for Perinatal Care: Contemporary Issues in High Risk Infant Follow-up. Madison, WI, Oct 1985

85. Division of Neonatal/Perinatal Medicine and the Office of Continuing Education—School of Medicine, University of California, San Diego: Tomorrow: A Follow-up on Perinatal Care. San Diego, CA, Nov 1980

86. Ellison P: Evaluation of Abnormal Tone (presented at Contemporary Issues in High Risk Infant Follow-up). Madison, WI (Wisconsin Assoc. for Perinatal Care), Oct 1982

87. Ellison PH, et al: A scoring system for the Milani Comparetti and Gidoni method of neurologic assessment in infancy. Phys Ther 63:1414-1423, 1983

88. Ellison PH: Neurological development of the high risk infant. Clinics in Perinatology 11:1, 1984

89. Ellison PH, Hom JL, Browning CA: Construction of an Infant Neurological International Battery (INFANIB) for the assessment of neurological integrity in infancy. Phys Ther 65:1326-1331, 1985

90. Cohen SE, et al: Perinatal risk and developmental outcome in preterm infants. Seminars in Perinatology 6:334-339, 1982

91. Kitchen WH, et al: Changing outcome over 13 years of very low birthweight infants. Seminars in Perinatology 6:373-388, 1982

92. Williams JF, Davies PA: Very low birthweight and later intelligence. Dev Med Child Neurol 16:709-728, 1974

93. Yu VYH, Hollingsworth E: Improving prognosis for infants weighing 1000 grams or less at birth. Arch Dis Child 55:422-426, 1979

94. Hunt JV, Tooley WH, Harvin D: Learning disabilities in children with birthweights 1500 grams or less. Seminars in Perinatology 6:280-287, 1982

ADDITIONAL RECOMMENDED READINGS

1. Banus BS: The Developmental Therapist, New York, NY. Charles Slack Pub., Inc., 1971
2. Bly L: The Components of Normal Movement During the First Year of Life and Abnormal Development, Chicago. IL. Neuro Dev Treatment Assoc. 1983
3. Bobath B: The Very Early Treatment of Cerebral Palsy. Develop Med Child Neurol 9:171-190, 1967
4. Brown CC: Infants at Risk: Assessment and Intervention: An Update for Health Care Professional and Parents. Pediatric Round Table Series, No. 5, Johnson and Johnson Baby Products Co., 1981
5. Connor FP, Williamson GG, Siepp JM: Program Guide for Infants with Neuromotor and Other Developmental Disabilities. New York, NY. Teachers' College Press, 1978
6. Crocker AC, Cohen HJ, Kastner A: HIV Infection and Developmental Disabilities. Baltimore, MD. Paul H Brookes Publishing, 1991
7. Dickson JM: A Model for Physical Therapy in the Neonatal Intensive Care Nursery. Phys Ther 61:45-48, 1981
8. Drillien CM, Drummond MB (eds): Neurodevelopmental Problems in Early Childhood: Assessment and Management. Oxford, England, Blackwell Scientific Publications, 1977
9. Egan DF, Illingworth RS, MacKeith RC: Developmental Screening 0-5 years. Philadelphia, PA, Clinics in Developmental Medicine 30, J.B. Lippincott, 1969
10. Erickson M: Assessment and Management of Developmental Changes in Children. St. Louis, MO, C.V. Mosby Co., 1976
11. Espenschade AS, Eckert HM: Motor Development. Columbus, OH, Charles E. Merrill Pub. Co., 1967
12. Finnie NR: Handling the Young Cerebral Palsy Child at Home, ed 2. New York, NY. E.P. Dutton, 1975
13. Gabel S, Erickson MT: Child Development and Developmental Disabilities. Boston, MA, Little Brown Co., 1980
14. Holle B: Motor Development in Children. New York, NY. J.B. Lippincott, 1977
15. Holt K (ed): Movement and Child Development: Clinics in Developmental Medicine 55, Wm Heineman Medical Books Ltd., 1975
16. Illingworth RS: The Development of the Infant and Young Child: Normal and Abnormal, ed 4. Edinburgh, E.S. Livingstone, 1971
17. Illingworth RS: The Normal Child: Some Problems of the Early Years and their Treatment. Edinburgh, Churchill Livingstone, 1983
18. Kaback MM: Genetic Issues in Pediatric and Obstetric Practice. Chicago, IL. Yearbook Medical Publications, Inc., 1981
19. Klaus MH, Kennell JH: Parent-Infant Bonding. St. Louis. MO. C.V. Mosby, 1983
20. Lewis M, Taft LT: Developmental Disabilities—Theory Assessment and Intervention. New York, NY. SP Medical and Scientific Books, 1982
21. Lowrey GH: Growth and Development of Children. Chicago, IL. Medical Pub., 1978
22. Paine RS, Oppe TE: Neurological Examination of Children. London, Wm Heineman Medical Books Ltd., 1966
23. Papile L, et al: Incidence and Evaluation of Subependymal and Intraventricular Hemorrhage: A Study of Infants with Birth Weight less than 1500 Grams. J Pediatr 92:529, 1978
24. Ramey, CT, Trohanis, PL: Finding and Educating High Risk Handicapped Infants. Baltimore, MD. University Park Press, 1982
25. Van Blankenstein M. Welberger UR, LeHaas JA: The Development of the Infant. London, Wm Heineman Medical Books Ltd., 1978
26. Volpe JJ: Perinatal Hypoxic Ischemic Brain Injury. Pediatr Clin North Am 23:383, 1976
27. Wilhelm JJ: The Neurologically Suspect Neonate. In Campbell SK (ed): Pediatric Neurologic Physical Therapy. New York, NY. Churchill Livingstone, 1984
28. Wright JM: Fetal Alcohol Syndrome: The Social Work Connection. Health and Soc Work 6:5-10, 1981

CHAPTER 6

SENSORY CONSIDERATION IN THERAPEUTIC INTERVENTIONS

Rebecca Porter, Ph.D., PT

◆

While experimental studies suggest that learned movements can continue to be performed in the absence of sensory input [1,2], many children with developmental disabilities face the task of both learning and performing movements with diminished or discrepant sensory information. The multitude of neuroanatomical pathways communicating afferent information to the motor control centers of the central nervous system (CNS) supports the critical nature of sensory input.

The sensory systems provide a primary media through which a therapist influences the motor behavior of a child with a developmental disability. Our touch, voice, and way of moving the child provide his CNS with a multitude of sensory data to be received, processed, and acted on. The effectiveness of our handling techniques depends, in part, on our orchestration of the sensory information reaching the child's CNS. Our intervention techniques are based on manipulation of sensory input through one or more sensory systems.

The information in this chapter deals with the broad general category of developmental disabilities. An assumption has been made that the movement problems of children are of a central origin and affect mechanisms of processing and responding to sensory information. Children with a peripheral nerve lesion or lower motor neuron dysfunction would require different approaches.

SENSORY INFORMATION

Within the normal process of motor learning, the ability to use sensory information appropriately is a critical component. The CNS must differentiate between movement related and non-movement related information. As we consider the processing of sensory information, keep in mind that the CNS is analyzing sensory input available prior to the movement as well as the data generated as the result of the movement (feedback). Figure 1 diagrams the categorization of sensory information. As discussed in Chapter 3, intrinsic and extrinsic feedback in the form of both knowledge of results and knowledge of performance are critical variables in the process of motor learning.

Peripheral feedback provides the CNS with information on the results of movement. Was the movement of the arm successful in positioning the hand to grasp the cup? Was the speed of movement of the protective extension reaction sufficient to stop the displacement of the child's center of gravity? The child gains knowledge of the results of his movement from both internal and external sources. Internal sources of feedback include information from the sensory receptors, such as muscle

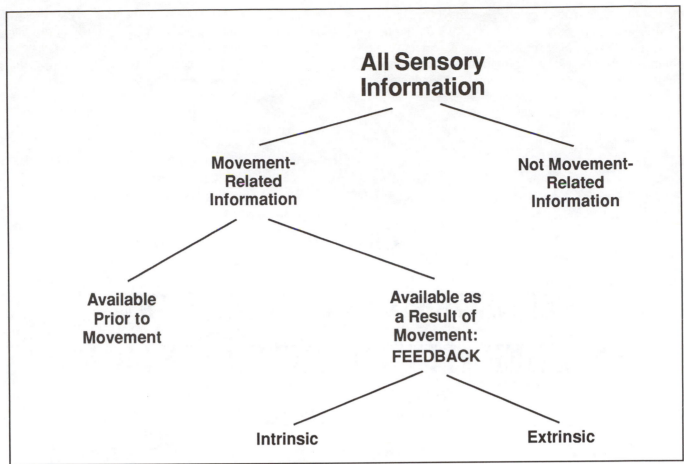

FIGURE 1. Utilization of sensory information in the process of motor control.
Adapted from Schmidt, Motor Control and Learning[2]

spindles, golgi tendon organs (which contribute to our "feel" of the movement), and vestibular receptors (which contribute to our sense of position in space). External sources of information include visual and auditory input. Depending on the characteristics of the visual and auditory input, the information may be used as intrinsic feedback in which the information is compared to a learned reference of correctness which provides an error-detection mechanism or as extrinsic feedback which supplements or augments the intrinsic feedback. [2]

In the clinical setting, the therapist can act to augment intrinsic or extrinsic feedback or both. If the therapist provides a guiding resistance to the movement pattern, intrinsic proprioceptive information is increased. Extrinsic feedback can be increased by the therapist providing verbal commentary on the quality of the movement task — "Good hold!" (knowledge of performance) or commentary on the outcome of the movement — "Good step!" (knowledge of results).

While peripheral feedback plays a role in learning movement, once movements are learned, central monitoring of the movement increases in importance. As you first learn a motor pattern such as playing a piano, multiple sources of peripheral feedback inform you of the results of your finger movements. You attend to the feel of the movement, the sound produced by the move-

ment, and the scowl of your teacher as you hit the wrong key. Once the movement is learned, the movements flow into each other without the need for delayed internal and external verifications of correctness of one movement before the next movement is made. Therapeutic handling techniques are designed to lead to this progression of motor learning and control.

Before a child can develop balance within a posture, he must have the sensory experience of being in the posture. Proprioceptive, vestibular, tactile, and visual information received by the CNS are unique to each particular posture. No amount of practice of head control in prone on elbows can provide an equivalent sensory picture of the responses necessary for head control in sitting or standing. (See discussion of Transfer of Learning in Chapter 3). As the therapist handles the child within and moving between various postures, the handling techniques should not interfere with the experience of being in the posture. The therapist's role is to assist the child in producing a normal movement response. Incorrect sensory feedback due to overcontrol or undercontrol of the child by the therapist or due to the child's central processing difficulties can result in altered or inappropriate postural alignment and movement. In either case, the therapist must correct or compensate for the problem to assist the child in learning to produce

Therapeutic Exercise In Developmental Disabilities

the most efficient and effective movements possible.

Multiple mechanisms are available within the normally functioning CNS to protect the higher centers from bombardment of sensory information. Some receptors, particularly the exteroceptors, demonstrate adaptation to a maintained stimulus. Awareness of a bandaid on your finger fades quickly after it is placed on the skin, as the cutaneous receptors adapt to the continuous stimulation. With other receptors, it is crucially important that adaptation does not occur. Imagine the difficulties we would have moving if the vestibular macula did not inform us continuously of our position in relation to gravity.

With the magnitude of divergence of sensory information, a system of inhibition is necessary to assure that the cortex receives a clear representation of sensory input. The systems of feedforward, feedback, and local inhibition assure that a clear sensory message ascends through the long ascending pathways and synaptic connections to the cortex and other motor control centers. If these inhibitory mechanisms are not functioning appropriately, the cortex may receive a confused sensory picture, resulting in an inappropriate movement.

Sensory pathways not only have ascending, but also descending connections with the higher centers. The descending connections allow the higher centers to suppress or shut down ascending information from receptors. The CNS can attend selectively to or enhance a particular set of sensory information while ignoring or suppressing another set. It allows the student to concentrate on the teacher's instructions despite the noise of other children in the hallway. Deficits with the complex mechanism of selectively attending to particular avenues of sensory information present major problems for a child attempting to learn in an unstructured school environment.

CHARACTERISTICS OF SENSORY SYSTEMS

No sensory system should be classified as inherently facilitory or inhibitory. Each system has the potential for increasing or decreasing the level of activity of the CNS depending on the manner in which the sensory stimulus is delivered. Rood formulated general guidelines which assist in predicting the types of motor response which will be elicited based on the characteristics of the delivery of the sensory input. A quick brief stimulus results in a burst of motor activity. One can predict that a light stroke to the arm of a child may elicit a phasic burst to withdraw from the stimulus. Rapid, repetitive stimulation results in a more maintained response. Repetitive tapping or mechanical vibration of a muscle are techniques which have been used to induce a sustained contraction of the muscle.

Slow, rhythmical, repetitive stimuli decrease the level of responsiveness of the individual. Parents instinctively rock fussy infants to calm them. Monotone, droning instructors have deactivated the minds of students for

centuries. A maintained stimulus, such as gravity, should elicit a maintained response. The influence of gravity should elicit continuously the automatic responses necessary to maintain a posture. When considering the response to a maintained stimulus, we must evaluate the potential adaptation of the receptor to the stimulus. A maintained cutaneous input should result in accommodation of the receptors and therefore a decreased rate of firing of these sensory pathways.

The therapist should consider additional influences on a child's response to sensory input. The set point of the autonomic nervous system (ANS) is a critical determinant. A child who is tense and sympathetically dominated may respond to a friendly pat with a startle and withdrawal. Variations in the sympathetic or parasympathetic set of the child result in variations in the response to a particular handling technique. The technique which was effective yesterday may produce less optimal responses today because the child's ANS is activating sympathetic responses.

Past experiences also influence the interpretation of sensory data. A particular cologne or aftershave may elicit parasympathetic responses if associated by the child with the scent of a loving parent. The same scent could elicit sympathetic responses if it were associated with the scent of an abusive parent.

The therapist must evaluate the number of sensory channels being stimulated by a particular handling technique. Depending on the functional and maturational level of the CNS, the child may not be able to respond appropriately to techniques or environments which provide multimodal stimulation. The child may be able to attend to controlling the position of his head when he is sitting with the therapist controlling the position of his pelvis, only if there are no other distractions, including the therapist talking. Gradually, and in a controlled manner, the therapist should introduce additional sources of input so that the child can function within a more typical environment. Responsibility to control the amount and types of sensory input requires the therapist constantly to analyze the stimuli the child is receiving to avoid inappropriate stimulation.

Our motor responses are specific to the environmental context of the moment. It is the sensory system information which provides the CNS with the internal and external information to assess the constraints under which the movement is to be performed. Gentile's Taxonomy of Motor Tasks provides therapists with a system for analyzing the complexity of different movement tasks.[3] Inherent in understanding the complexity of the movement is an analysis of the spatial and temporal attributes of the environment and the body's movement. From the perspective of the child's nervous system, the larger the quantity and diversity of sensory information which must be received and processed, the more difficult the process becomes. Walking and chewing gum at the same time is a more complex task than either alone. The addition of an object to carry or manipulate further complicates the task. As you plan your treatment progression for a particular child, remember to consider the load of sensory information which must be analyzed in order to produce the appropriate movement pattern under a given set of environmental constraints.

SELECTION OF SENSORY INPUT

Each intervention technique should be selected to assist the child in producing an adaptive response. A response is considered to be adaptive if it indicates a higher level of function than the previous behavior of the child. Farber defines an adaptive response to sensory stimuli as a "behavior of a more advanced, organized, flexible, or productive nature than that which occurred before stimulation."[4] We attempt to assist the child to produce higher level, more appropriate, and more functional movement. This is the measurement tool we can use to determine if we selected correctly the appropriate intervention techniques.

Chapter 3 introduced the concept of using sensory input to provide guidance as a teaching technique to assist the individual in learning to perform a specific movement pattern. Remember that the strongest effect of guidance is to alter the performance of the movement pattern during a specific trial. When the child is unable to execute a movement pattern which is effective and efficient, the physical therapist is responsible for selecting the treatment technique which will enable the child to make a better response. Guidance in the form of therapist enhanced sensory input is reduced as the child takes more responsibility for producing an adaptive response and moving independently.

The process of selecting an appropriate technique can seem overwhelming to the inexperienced clinician. The following general guidelines may assist in the process of selecting sensory techniques to be used in a particular program.

The therapist should select sensory stimuli which are more naturally occurring in preference to those which are artificial. An electric vibrator may elicit the contraction of a muscle, but is not the type of stimulus to which the child will respond in a typical movement situation. Preferentially, the activation of muscles can be achieved by weight bearing, vestibular input, or cutaneous facilitation. These are the types of sensory information which the child will be required to respond to outside of the therapeutic setting.

Interventions should be developmentally appropriate for the child. Appropriateness must be considered in terms of physical, mental, and social development. Working on locomotion in all fours may be perceived as demeaning by a teenager with a developmental delay.

Although quadruped may be therapeutically appropriate for the movement problems, the therapist must either convince the teenager to accept the rationale or select another posture.

The type of sensory stimulation should be appropriate to the activity. The postural neck musculature respond to vestibular input and to proprioceptive information such as approximation through the cervical spine. Rapid, quick stretch is not a stimulus to which these muscles routinely are subjected. Intervention techniques based on approximation or vestibular input would be more appropriate to activate these muscles than quick stretch.

The quality of the adaptive response frequently is enhanced if the child can respond to sensory cues other than cortically processed verbal commands. In our daily activities, many postural movements are made in response to intrinsic sensory cues. We hold our heads erect in response to vestibular, proprioceptive, and visual information, not in response to being told to pick up our heads and tuck our chins. Therapy should attempt to elicit automatic postural adjustments in response to the demands of the situation or the desire to accomplish the task. The more automatic movement becomes, the more likely it will be incorporated in the child's repertoire of movements outside of the therapy setting.

The therapist should use the least amount of control or the least amount of sensory input necessary to elicit an adaptive response. Throughout the intervention process, the therapist must remember that a primary goal is to remove the intervention. The therapist must assess constantly if components of the intervention strategy can be withdrawn. If the child is working on head control in sitting with the therapist controlling the position of the pelvis in all planes, the therapist could challenge the child by gradually relinquishing control in movements requiring flexion. As this control is beginning to be mastered by the child, control of extension is gradually relinquished by the therapist. As long as the therapist retains total control, the child will not have the opportunity to learn the appropriate movements in response to incoming sensory messages.

ASSESSMENT

In assessing the status of sensory systems in children with developmental disabilities, the therapist basically is evaluating the perception of sensation. We are looking for indications that the information is being received and processed, thus producing appropriate motor responses or providing correct feedback for internally produced movement. This intent is different from the purpose of sensory testing in children with peripheral nerve or spinal cord lesions. In these cases, the therapist is more concerned with the presence of sensation rather than the interpretation of sensory information.

The goal of the assessment is to determine which

sensory systems functionally are intact. The therapist then can design intervention strategies based on these systems. For example, if the child does not respond to vestibular input or responds inappropriately, then techniques which use other sensory systems should be the primary focus in the initial interventions.

Guard against overtesting of the sensory systems. A complete neurological sensory examination can be time consuming, fatiguing, and tedious for the child. Before beginning a comprehensive evaluation, try to target specific sensory systems on which your assessment should focus. If the physician's neurologic examination is available, review the results to identify areas which should be explored further. Interviews of parents, teachers, or caregivers may provide indications of sensory dysfunction. Does the child seem to attend to visual or auditory input consistently? Does the child explore or attempt to tactilely explore objects with his mouth or with both hands equally? Does the child withdraw from touch, which could indicate tactile defensiveness? How does the child react to being moved through space? Does he appear to enjoy movement or is he fearful? How accurate is the child in reaching for objects? Answers to questions such as these will provide the therapist with insight on the functioning of the various sensory systems.

Therapists can gather similar information from movement assessments of the child. Does the child orient appropriately to gravity? Does the child seem to perceive correctly the relation of his body parts? Can he accurately place the extremities for support or for reaching? From this process, the therapist should be able to target specific sensory systems for further evaluation. For information on the specifics of a detailed neurological examination, refer to the recommended readings at the end of the chapter. Examples of assessing each sensory system within a therapeutic framework will be discussed in combination with treatment techniques.

The sensory assessment should not only establish the level of integrity of a particular sensory system, but also must attempt to determine the child's sensory preferences. A child might enjoy vestibular input while being less comfortable with cutaneous/proprioceptive input. The therapist must investigate if this indicates a like/dislike or represents dysfunction within a system. Although the determination may be difficult to make, the therapist should attend to behavioral cues. For example, consistent increases in activity level and aversion responses to tactile input may indicate tactile defensiveness.

Assessment of function of sensory systems should encompass more than looking at each system in isolation. The child may attend preferentially to a particular input or to input on one half of the body when presented with multiple inputs. In the presence of auditory distractors, the child may be unable to process visual input. The child with hemiplegia may be able to attend to cutaneous input on the involved side if it is presented in isolation. If the child is touched on both sides simultaneously, he may report only the touch on the uninvolved side (cortical inattention or bilateral extinction). Preferential attending to certain sensory modalities may account for the difficulties some children have in making the transition from a controlled therapeutic environment to a more typical environment with its multitude of simultaneous competing information.

Postural control or balance requires the integration of sensory input to construct an awareness of the location of the body's center of gravity as well as the ability to perform an appropriate musculoskeletal response. Visual, vestibular, and somatosensory information are combined into the perception of one's orientation in relationship to gravity, the support surface, and surrounding objects.[5] Deficits in any of these systems will affect balance control particularly in situations when the remaining alternative sensory inputs are not available or are in conflict. A child with reduced vestibular function may increase the reliance on visual references to maintain postural control. For this child, the performance of balance tasks will be increasingly difficult as the level of illumination decreases or the eyes are closed. The therapist must monitor the child's responses throughout the assessment process for indications of difficulties with intersensory integration in relationship to postural control.

INTERTWINING ASSESSMENT AND TREATMENT TECHNIQUES

This section will present examples of treatment techniques based on input via the major sensory systems. Methods of assessing the child's response to the sensory input will be discussed. Treatment and assessment are integrated in this section since therapists frequently are conducting both simultaneously. The therapist may use the child's responses to intervention techniques to evaluate the function of one or more sensory systems.

Cutaneous Input

Receptors located in the skin are responsible for touch and temperature information. Therapists can stimulate touch receptors to either inhibit or facilitate motor activity. Static, maintained contact of a surface with the child's skin should result in adaptation of touch receptors and inhibition of the muscles underlying the skin.[6] Therapists use this technique by resting their hands on the skin overlying spastic muscles to inhibit the muscles. Care must be taken to maintain a constant, even pressure on the child's skin. Changing pressures could result in an increase in the activity of the underlying muscle. This concept is used in the construction of splints.[4] The static surface should be in contact with the surface overlying the spastic muscle. Straps are placed preferentially over the antagonists to the spastic muscles. The therapist assesses the success of the use of inhibitory, maintained touch by the response of the child. Has the level of spasticity decreased? Is the child able to make a more functional movement?

When the therapist attempts to facilitate the response of a muscle, manual contacts should be placed over the muscle belly. A changing, non-static pressure is used. Cutaneous receptors make spinal cord level synaptic connections with gamma motoneurons.[7] Cutaneous input may enhance the sensitivity of the muscle spindle and, therefore, positively influence the response of the muscle. Just as with inhibitory touch, the effectiveness of the technique is assessed by evaluating changes in the child's response.

Temperature receptors increase their rate of firing as the skin temperature changes. The concept of neutral warmth can be used when the therapist attempts to decrease the overall level of the child's activity or spasticity in a limb. The therapist attempts to create an environment in which neither the temperature nor cutaneous receptors are being stimulated to fire above the base firing rate. This environment is created by wrapping the child or the body part in lightweight toweling or a sheet blanket (Figure 2). The neutral environment is maintained until the desired response occurs. If the child is wrapped for too long, the increase in skin temperature may result in an increase in activity rather than a decrease. This is analogous to the restlessness created when you become too warm while sleeping and attempt to kick off the covers.

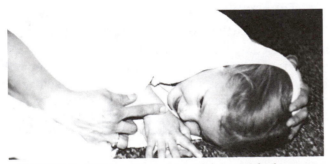

FIGURE 2. Child positioned in sidelying with sheet blanket for neutral warmth to decrease overall level of activity. Note therapist's control of the hand position of the child and use of approximation to control head position.

— Photos by William D. Porter

Therapists should attend to the temperature of the room in which they are working with a child. In the optimal setting, the temperature would be adjusted to meet the needs of each child. A child with hypotonia would be treated in a slightly cooler room and a child with hypertonia in a warmer room. In selecting the appropriate room temperature, the therapist should consider the baseline skin temperature of the child. The baseline skin temperature will vary with the child's

health and the temperature of the child's previous environment. Remember that the temperature receptors are reporting deviations from baseline. It is important, therefore, to consider whether the child has been in a warm, muggy environment or a windy, cold environment before arriving for therapy. This may affect the baseline of muscle activity and the type of temperature input the therapist chooses to use.

When considering the effects of temperature changes on the child, remember to consider your hand temperature. Therapist-child rapport can quickly be disturbed by a cold hand placed on a warm abdomen.

In general, sensory inputs which evoke a withdrawal response or which are interpreted by the child as noxious or painful are counterproductive to the goal of learning to make adaptive movements. A child with a developmental disability may demonstrate an aversive response to light touch which may be described as tactile defensiveness. The therapist can help the child prepare for the therapy session by allowing him to desensitize the skin by vigorous rubbing with various textures and media. The child may tolerate the process better if he is allowed to control the input. When the therapist uses cutaneous input to guide the child through a movement pattern, a firm touch should be employed.

Vestibular Input

Vestibular input can either arouse or depress the level of activity of the postural extensors and the level of alertness of the child, depending on the characteristics of the stimuli. Slow, rhythmical repetitive rocking, rolling, or swinging typically relax and calm the child. Parents combine the concepts of neutral warmth and repetitive vestibular input by wrapping a fussy baby in a blanket and slowly rocking the child to sleep. Rapid, nonrhythmical stimulation with stops, starts, and changes in direction of movement is arousing and increases postural tone. Encouraging a child to move prone on a scooter board requires him to use the postural extensors, while allowing vestibular input to reinforce the activity of the postural muscles (Figure 3).

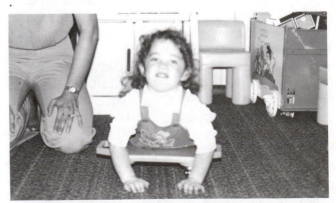

FIGURE 3. Use of a scooter to facilitate postural extension. The child can control the amount of vestibular stimulation being provided.

Inversion is a technique used by therapists to stimulate the vestibular receptors to elicit a response similar to the Landau response or pivot prone posture. According to McGraw, the child progresses through four developmental stages in response to inversion.[8] Initially, the infant responds to inversion with increased flexion and emotional arousal. The next stage is the extension response, which is the response sought when inversion is used as a therapeutic intervention. Crying is seldom heard during this phase. Later, inversion of the infant results in attempts to appropriately right the head to the horizon. Crying is frequent since these attempts are not successful. In the final stage, the child seems to recognize the futility of reversing the inverted position and hangs relaxed. Therapists should be aware of these developmental stages. If a child responds to inversion with a flexion response rather than the expected extension response, inversion may not be a developmentally appropriate technique. The therapist may need to use other forms of sensory stimulation to activate extension and introduce inversion later.

Some therapists use the post-rotatory nystagmus test developed by Ayres as an indicator of the integrity of the vestibular system.[9] The duration of nystagmus is measured following ten rotations of the child in a 20 second period. The head of the child must remain flexed at 30 degrees during the duration of the rotation. Other sensory stimuli, particularly visual, should be controlled during the rotations since they may influence the results. The test indicates the integrity of the vestibulo-ocular connections, but does not necessarily provide information concerning the multiple diverse connections between the vestibular system and other parts of the CNS.

Proprioceptive Input

Proprioceptive, or more generally, somatosensory input is provided by almost every handling technique used by therapists. Many techniques have used the concept of reciprocal innervation to affect spasticity. The antagonist of the spastic muscle is activated to achieve inhibition of the spastic muscle. A therapist might use a quick stretch to the triceps brachii followed by resistance to inhibit a spastic biceps brachii (Figures 4-6). The quick stretch elongates the equatorial region of the muscle spindle, increasing the discharge rate of the Ia fiber. The Ia fiber monosynaptically connects with an alpha motoneuron innervating a motor unit in the triceps resulting in a contraction of those fibers. Resistance helps maintain the contraction response of the muscle, so that the phasic burst following the quick stretch becomes a maintained or tonic response. Activation of the triceps

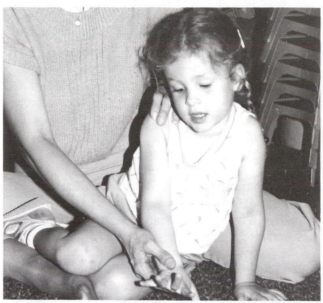

FIGURE 5.

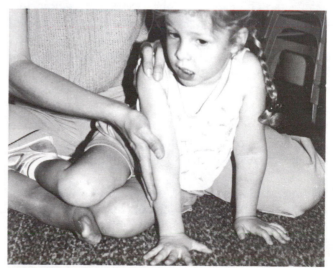

FIGURE 6.

In Figure 4, the therapist applies a quick stretch to the triceps brachii followed by resistance to extension to augment the contraction of the triceps brachii as seen in Figure 5. Figure 6 demonstrates the target posture with the activated triceps being used in a support response.

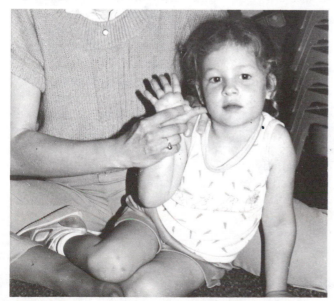

FIGURE 4.

reciprocally should inhibit the spastic biceps. If the therapeutic goal is to facilitate a particular muscle, a quick stretch followed by resistance can be used to attempt to activate the hyporesponsive muscle.

A mechanical vibrator with the proper characteristics will produce a muscle contraction. The vibrator should have an amplitude 1-2 mm[10] with a frequency of 100-125 Hz (cycles per second).[6] The vibration increases the discharge rate of the Ia fiber from the muscle spindle resulting in a contraction of the muscle being vibrated. Although the technique may be effective in producing a contraction, it is difficult to use a vibrator within the context of producing functional, adaptive behaviors. Since vibration is not a stimulus which evokes movement responses in a normal framework of movement patterns, it should be reserved for occasions when other techniques are not effective.

Joint receptors appear to influence the type of contraction produced by muscles crossing the joint. Approximation, or compression of the joint space, seems to elicit a holding contraction, particularly in the joint alignment typical for weight bearing (Figure 6). Traction or separation of the joint spaces assists with movement. As the therapist assists the child with movement between postures, traction can be added to an extremity to facilitate the transition. Once the child has assumed a posture, approximation can be added through the extremities in weight bearing positions or through the vertebral column to reinforce the holding contraction necessary to maintain the position.

The therapist may alter the child's proprioceptive (and to some extent, other system input) by using guidance assistance/resistance to facilitate movement. The purpose of the guidance assistance/resistance is to enable the child to experience movement within the environmental context in which the response should occur. This technique is employed when the child has been unable to use trial and error learning to refine a movement pattern.

Tests for proprioception frequently are not appropriate for the child with developmental disabilities. The young child or a child with marked limitations cannot reproduce the postures with one extremity that a therapist has created with the opposite extremity (position sense). The child may not understand or be able to communicate when the therapist moves a toe or finger up or down (kinesthesis or movement sense). In these cases, the therapist must evaluate how the child moves and uses his extremities to gain an assessment of the ability to act on proprioceptive information. A child may allow an extremity to lag behind when moving between postures or fail to appropriately position the extremity when assuming a resting position despite his ability to move the extremity. In this case, the therapist would suspect that the child lacks proprioceptive input or is unable to process the input in order to know the location of the extremity. The therapist's observational skills will be the primary tool to assess proprioception in the majority of children with developmental disabilities.

Visual Input

As discussed previously, visual information is one of the critical elements for maintaining postural control, particularly in individuals with vestibular system deficits. Assessment of static and dynamic balance tasks with and without vision will provide clues to the child's reliance on visual input.

Woollacott reported that young infants commit more errors in their responses to perturbations when visual information also is being processed.[11] Apparently infants learn to use the visual input in conjunction with other sensory information over time as motor control is mastered in various postures.

When children have difficulty in maintaining appropriate vertical alignment in sitting or standing, some therapists use positioning in front of a mirror. This tactic encourages the substitution of visual information for attention to internal cues (somatosensory and vestibular input) indicating appropriate alignment. Attention to internal cues is necessary to remain aligned when the mirror is removed. The reversal of movements that occurs when viewing actions in a mirror may cause some children initially to hesitate in moving, resulting in errors in moving toward a target. Therapists should consider the effects of substituting visual information for proprioceptive/vestibular cues when deciding to use mirrors in teaching maintenance of vertical alignment postures or movements within those postures with various children.

Auditory Input

If a child has difficulty processing multiple sensory inputs selectively, extraneous sounds from the environment often are distracting. With this child, the therapist should select a treatment environment which eliminates extraneous auditory inputs. As the child masters a particular task, background noises should be added. The goal should be eventually to progress the child to performing the task within a non-isolated environment.

The therapist's voice is an important therapeutic tool. Tone, volume, rate, and rhythm of speech must be modulated to meet the needs of the child. A child with spasticity, who is easily upset, should respond best to a soothing, slow paced, repetitive speech pattern. The child with hypotonia, who is lethargic, may need more authoritative, brisk verbal cues. Therapists should not confuse the need to be authoritative with being loud. Therapists can apply the general rules of sensory input discussed previously to the therapeutic use of their voices.

SUMMARY

The most effective therapists engage in a constant analysis of the child's response to their handling. This analysis includes consideration of all the sensory input the child is receiving. The therapist should note the conditions under which appropriate and inappropriate responses are made. Evaluation of these observations can lead the therapist to the construction of more effective intervention programs. Suggested readings to explore these topics further are included at the end of this chapter.

As assessment and treatment techniques are discussed in other chapters of this text, consider the type and quality of sensory input which underlies the technique. For example, in Chapter 8, the type of sensory stimulus which elicits each of the postural reactions is presented. If the child can not appropriately process that type (or types) of sensory input, the response may not be demonstrated or the response may be degraded. This represents a very different problem from the child who can not demonstrate the appropriate response due to muscle weakness. Just as the CNS must integrate input from multiple sensory systems, the reader is encouraged to integrate the information from this chapter with the concepts throughout this text.

Conclusion

Therapists working with children with developmental disabilities use manipulation of sensory input as a primary means of improving movement abilities. While some handling techniques obviously are designed to alter sensory input (inversion, quick stretch), other techniques evoke subtle changes in postural alignment altering the proprioceptive inflow and changing the motor response. While this chapter has surveyed sensory considerations in handling children, information from other chapters can be included within the scope of this topic. The challenge offered to us by children is to observe skillfully, analyze objectively, and manipulate creatively their movements until the highest and most functional level of independency is achieved.

Case Studies

Case No. 1 — Jason
Cerebral Palsy, Right Hemiparesis, 18 Months

In observing Jason's play, the therapist notes that Jason does not spontaneously use his right upper extremity to assist in manipulating objects. This observation plus others made during the intervention session leads the therapist to conclude that Jason is demonstrating sensory neglect of the involved extremities, particularly the right upper extremity. Jason will turn his head to look at an object that touches him on the right. However, if the therapist touches both the right and left sides simultaneously, Jason seems to notice only the contact on the left. This observation reinforces the therapist's conclusion that Jason demonstrates sensory neglect. Jason's mother reports that he does not like to snuggle on her lap.

He cries or fidgets when she tries to kiss his neck. Jason grimaces, fusses, or pulls away when the therapist lightly touches him on the right side. The therapist concludes that Jason is tactilely defensive on the right side. When objects are placed in Jason's right hand, he grasps them tightly and cannot control release. Contact of the ball of the foot with the floor results in a plantar grasp response. The therapist notes that Jason's standing posture improves when the therapist controls the position of the pelvis and approximates through the right lower extremity to reinforce weight bearing through the heel. The results of testing for righting and equilibrium reactions suggest that the vestibular system information is being interpreted appropriately, however, motor control dysfunction interferes with a complete response on the right side.

General treatment goals would include the following: increase awareness of the right extremities, particularly the upper extremity; decrease tactile defensiveness; decrease influence of palmar grasp reflex, (increase voluntary release) and decrease influence of plantar grasp reflex (increase full foot contact in stance).

To assess the progress being made toward meeting the general treatment goals, the therapist establishes several measurable functional objectives for Jason. Jason's ability to perform the tasks will be evaluated at the conclusion of the intervention session. Following treatment, Jason will be able to perform the following tasks:

1. In sitting, lift an 8 inch diameter ball 5 inches from the table top using both upper extremities (with the therapist assisting the right extremity). Jason must be seated in an appropriate chair to permit his feet to rest on the floor. The table height should be adjusted to provide a comfortable working surface. The therapist can use approximation through the right lower leg to reinforce a flat position of the foot.

2. In sitting, with his right hand placed on an 8 inch diameter ball placed 12 inches in front of him, he will roll the ball from side to side 5 times without losing contact with the ball.

3. Tolerate the contact of the handler (his therapist or one of his parents) on his right upper extremity for 1 minute without signs of emotional distress.

4. In spontaneous play, attempt to use the right upper extremity in an appropriate manner 5 times during a 3 minute observation period.

5. In standing at a table, maintain a neutral foot flat position of the right lower extremity for 1 minute while playing with a toy.

To progress Jason toward meeting these objectives, the therapist could include the following activities as part of the intervention program. The session should begin with Jason, one of the parents, or the therapist rubbing different textures or materials over the left and right sides of Jason's body. The contact with Jason's skin should be steady and continuous. Materials with rougher textures such as toweling or cotton sheet blankets should be used initially (Figure 7). The handlers also should use their hands to rub Jason's skin so that Jason is comfortable with the touching that will follow during the session. The therapist can assist Jason in rubbing shaving cream over his extremities as a reward for tolerating the contact (Figure 8).

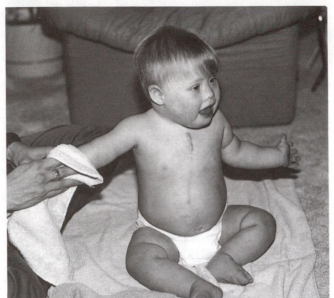

FIGURE 7. Use of toweling to increase the child's tolerance for the therapist's manual contacts with the extremity during the treatment session.

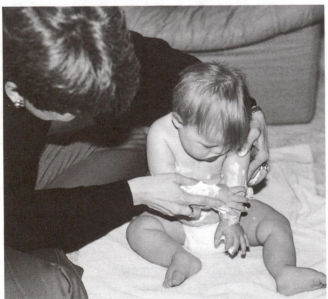

FIGURE 8. Participation of the child in activities such as spreading foam over the trunk and extremities may increase the child's tolerance for these types of interventions.

Appropriately seated at a table, the therapist should position Jason's right arm so that he is weight bearing through the elbow with his hand flat on the table. Jason is allowed to play in this position for a few minutes. Then he is encouraged to participate in activities such as

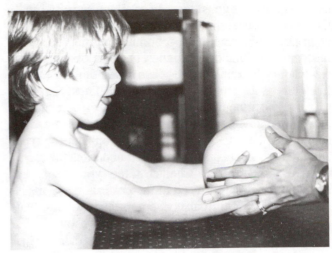

FIGURE 9.

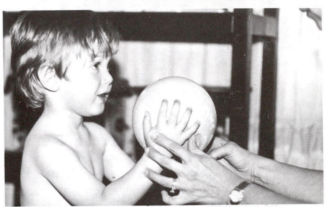

FIGURE 10.

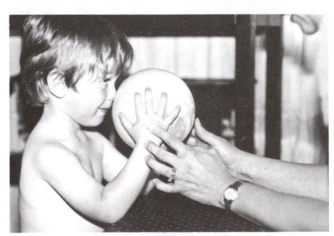

FIGURE 11.

As shown in Figures 9, 10 and 11, ball activities to promote inhibition of inappropriate overflow in the right upper extremity and to promote two handed activities.

washing or finger painting his right arm. These activities are designed to increase his awareness of his right arm and to decrease tactile defensiveness.

Following inhibition of inappropriate upper extremity posturing as discussed in Chapter 11, Jason should

Therapeutic Exercise In Developmental Disabilities

engage in two-handed activities with an 8 inch diameter ball. With the therapist controlling the position of the right extremity and the weight of the ball, Jason should push the ball away from his chest and pull it back. After several repetitions, Jason should be guided to lift the ball from the support surface and return it (Figures 9-11). The therapist should attempt to reduce the amount of external control required to keep Jason's right hand in contact with the ball. The therapist also should assist Jason in pronation and supination movements (Figure 12). This activity will require more control by the therapist since this is a developmentally advanced activity. It is included to work toward appropriate range of motion and to promote inhibition of inappropriate movements.

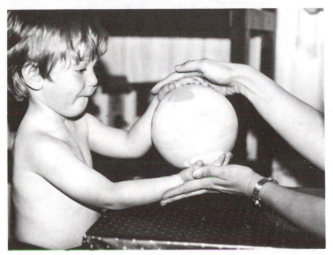

FIGURE 12. *Use of ball to promote supination range of motion of right forearm and inhibition of inappropriate posturing.*

Chapter 10 addresses developing ambulation skills. The weight bearing activities presented in the treatment sequence are effective activities in inhibiting the influence of the plantar grasp reflex. When an appropriate weight bearing posture is achieved, approximation through the pelvis reinforces maintenance of the position. Activities such as weight shifting and bending and straightening the knees assist Jason in learning the appropriate motor control in this posture.

CASE No. 2 — JILL
Cerebral Palsy, Spastic Quadriparesis, Mental Retardation, 7 Years

Jill's parents report that she does not like to be moved between positions. Her therapist notes that movement through space results in signs of autonomic distress, such as increased respiration and heart rate, increased perspiration, crying, and increased spasticity. Tonic reflexes are evident in her attempts to move. Righting reactions are not present beyond her ability to maintain her head in neutral when she is held vertical; however, the assessment of her ability to respond to vestibular input is complicated by the pattern of muscle tightness. She typically postures with her head extended and her mouth open with her lips and tongue retracted. Any touch to the lips or skin overlying the oral musculature results in increased lip retraction and increased head extension.

General treatment goals include increasing tolerance of movement, increasing attempts at voluntary movements, improving jaw closure, and improving lip closure.

Following treatment, Jill be able to perform the following tasks:

1. Positioned in a hammock, tolerate slow anteroposterior swinging for 3 minutes with an increase in the baseline pulse of 20 beats per minute or less.

2. Positioned in her adapted wheelchair, maintain jaw closure for one minute with no more than one assist from the handler.

3. Positioned in her adapted wheelchair, maintain lip closure for one minute with no more than one assist from the handler.

4. Positioned in her adapted wheelchair, appropriately close lips and jaw on the rim of a drinking glass with no assistance from the handler.

5. Positioned in her vertical stander, hold her head erect for 3-5 minutes.

Jill's intervention program must include a systematic introduction of activities to stimulate the vestibular system to increase her tolerance for movement. Positioned securely in supine in a hammock, she can be rocked gently in an anteroposterior direction. The initial excursion of the swing would be small. The amplitude and frequency of swings gradually will increase as Jill's tolerance increases. Given the autonomic signs of distress Jill displayed during the assessment, the therapist takes baseline measurements of pulse, respiration rate, or blood pressure to determine Jill's response to the intervention. Other vestibular activities would include anteroposterior rocking with Jill positioned in her wheelchair and positioned sidelying in a wagon. It is important that Jill experience movement in a variety of positions. It is equally important that Jill feel secure while she is being moved.

As Jill's tolerance for anteroposterior movement increases, movements in other directions would be added. Movements to be introduced would include mediolateral, cephalocaudal, nonrepetitive rotation about the body axis (as in rolling prone to supine to prone), diagonal, and finally rotatory movements. Tolerance of each new movement would be carefully assessed.

As Jill's control of her head and trunk position improve (Chapter 7), problems with control of the oral musculature can be addressed. Maintained jaw closure will be difficult to achieve as long as Jill continues to posture with her head and neck extended. The skin overlying the oral musculature can be desensitized by the

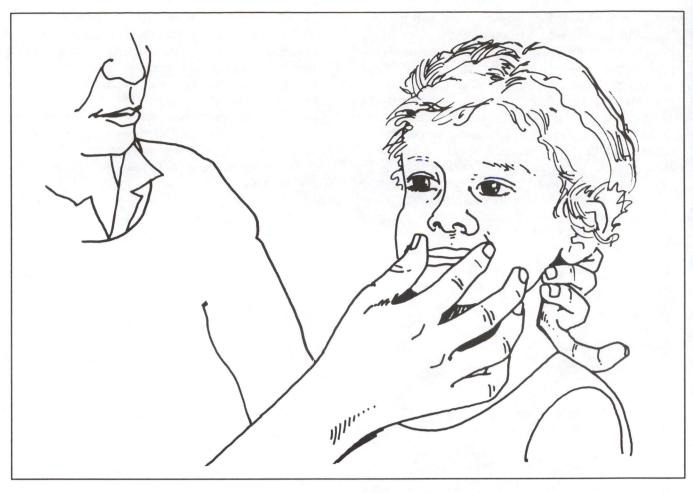

FIGURE 13. *Quick stretch to orbicularis oris to facilitate lip closure.*

therapist's use of maintained manual contact around the mouth. This should assist in decreasing withdrawal responses. The therapist must be sure to approach Jill's face carefully so that a visual startle or withdrawal is not elicited.

Jaw and lip closure can be facilitated by quick stretch (Figure 13) or fingertip vibration of the appropriate musculature. The therapist should desensitize the skin prior to application of these techniques. Functional activities such as drinking from a straw will assist Jill in consolidating her gains (Figure 14). The therapist can use finger pressure to the orbicularis oris to facilitate lip closure or can construct a mouthpiece as suggested by Farber to provide a similar response. [4]

The therapist should attend to the stimulation of intra-oral muscles as well as extra-oral musculature. Oral hygiene swabs can be used to stroke the gums, to stretch the insides of the cheeks, or to resist tongue motions (Figure 15). The therapist must select an instrument that will not harm the child in case a bite reflex is triggered.

Jill's progress in control of her mouth and tongue will be linked with her progress in developing head and trunk control. Activities in these two areas will reinforce her attempts at oral motor control.

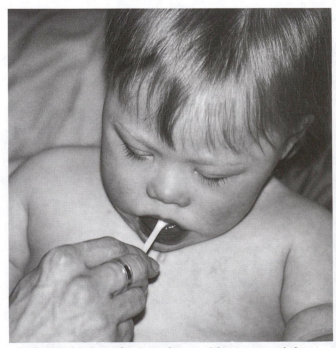

FIGURE 15. *Introduction of an oral hygiene swab for stimulation of intra-oral muscles. Note that the child's head is positioned in flexion to counter the tendency to withdraw from the stimulus.*

Therapeutic Exercise In Developmental Disabilities

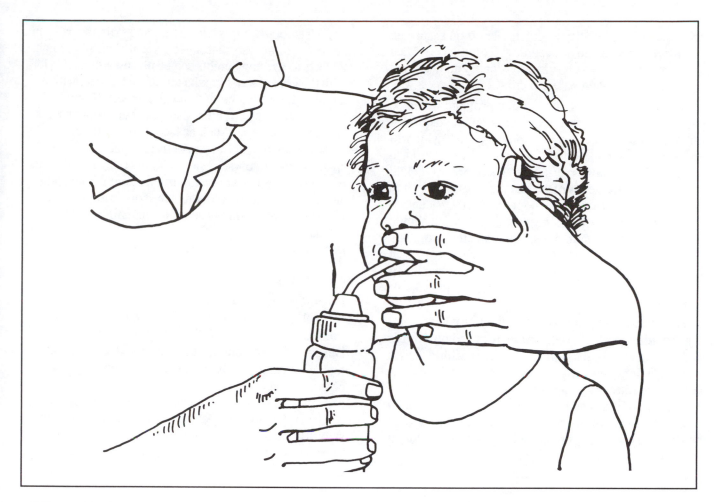

FIGURE 14. *Therapist facilitation of jaw and lip closure to assist Jill in drinking through a straw.*

Case No. 3 — Taylor

Myelomeningocele, Repaired L 1-2, 4 Years

The assessment of Taylor related to his sensory problems reveals a loss of cutaneous and proprioceptive sensation below the level of T-12. The lack of proprioceptive information from hips, knees, ankles, and feet present difficulties in Taylor's attempts to maintain a challenged sitting posture, static all fours position, or standing posture in an orthosis.

Taylor's visual acuity problems necessitate the wearing of glasses at all times. Taylor has figure ground discrimination difficulties and has difficulty locating small objects on a visually distracting background. In standing, when he bends his head to look at the floor through his glasses, his balance is disturbed. This presents difficulty in correct placement of his crutches among objects on the floor.

The therapist must extrapolate information from the overall assessment to suggest the origin of the balance deficit when Taylor looks down in standing. Since somatosensory information from the lower extremities is lacking, Taylor has an increased reliance on vestibular and visual information for balance. The normal head righting and protective extension reactions in sitting suggest that vestibular responses are within normal limits. The therapist concludes that visual perceptual problems are the primary contributors to balance problems in standing with head movement. Taylor must learn to produce the appropriate compensatory movements when his center of gravity is displaced by motion of the head.

General goals for Taylor include educating Taylor and his parents in skin care of the lower extremities due to the lack of sensation, increasing his balance in standing, and increasing visual figure ground discrimination abilities. Following treatment, Taylor will be able to perform the following tasks:

1. Correctly don his shoes and socks eliminating potential pressure areas every time.
2. Maintain correct body alignment in his new orthosis while reciprocally lifting his crutches 10 times in 30 seconds.
3. Maintain standing balance in his new orthosis for 15 seconds with his eyes closed (with crutches).
4. Maintain standing balance in his new orthosis for one minute while moving his head up, down, right, and left (with crutches).

5. In standing, identify numbers placed on shapes on the floor with 80% accuracy. This objective assumes that Taylor can visually identify numbers and shapes on a plain background.

Included in Taylor's intervention program would be education of Taylor and his parents on techniques of providing good skin care. The parents and Taylor will learn to monitor the condition of the skin with each change of his shoes or orthosis. The therapist should evaluate the consistency of the parents' visual inspection of Taylor's legs at each preschool session they attend. If the behavior is ingrained within this setting, it should generalize to other situations. The objective would be stated as follows: Taylor's parents will visually inspect his lower extremities for indications of skin irritation or pressure following every removal of shoes and socks, or orthosis.

Activities addressing balance and figure ground training should be conducted both in the freestanding orthosis and his new orthosis (long leg braces with a pelvic band). Taylor eventually can learn to maintain his balance while hitting a ball with one crutch. A variety of floor backgrounds can be used, progressing from plain to visually distracting patterns. Initially the ball should be stationary with its position being varied for different trials (Figure 16).

As Taylor increases his balance and skill, the ball can be rolled to him so that he can bat it with his crutch. Objects of varying heights can be placed around Taylor with the goal of touching the top of each object with his crutch without knocking over the object (Figure 17). These types of activities also address problems discussed in Chapter 7, such as lack of trunk rotation.

Taylor may benefit from activities such as a wheelchair obstacle course. Manipulation of his chair will increase upper extremity and trunk strength and endurance. Successful completion of the course requires good visual perceptual skills and motor planning. This activity can be a fun reward for successful completion of more difficult tasks during the therapy session.

CASE NO. 4 — ASHLEY
Down Syndrome, 15 Months

Ashley demonstrates a lack of stability in all positions as well as generalized hypotonia (Figure 18). During her evaluation, she was noted to respond to rapid, irregular vestibular input with more appropriate postural tone and stability. Proprioceptive and cutaneous input also improved her ability to maintain postures.

General treatment goals focus on increasing postural stability. An increase in shoulder and hip stability in the quadruped position would be sought. Lengthening of the

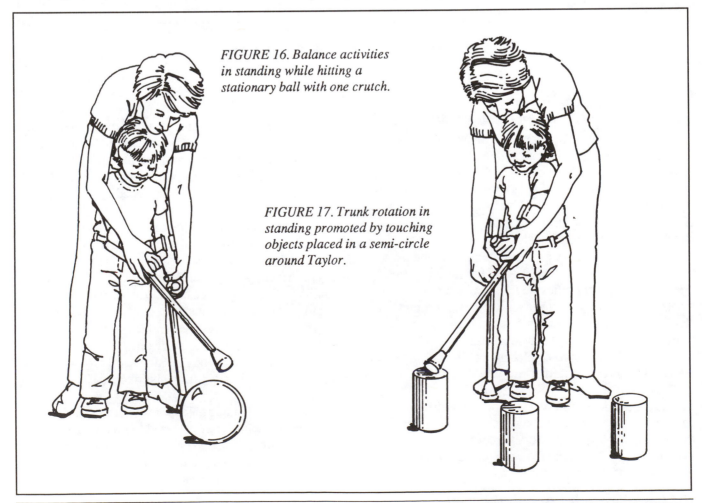

FIGURE 16. Balance activities in standing while hitting a stationary ball with one crutch.

FIGURE 17. Trunk rotation in standing promoted by touching objects placed in a semi-circle around Taylor.

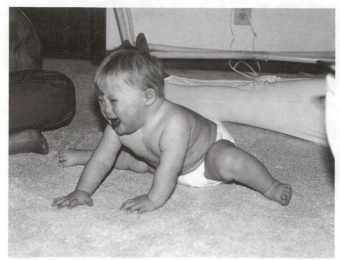

FIGURE 18. Ashley's posture in moving from prone to sitting indicates the exaggerated flexibility present in the hips due to her generalized hypotonia.

capital extensor muscles may permit Ashley to make more appropriate righting and equilibrium reactions. Goals include improving standing alignment and improving sitting posture.

Ashley was noted to be generally apprehensive about movement. Discussion with the parents indicates that Ashley's ongoing series of medical problems have resulted in her being treated by the family as a "fragile" child. Ashley has not had the opportunity to experience motion as a part of typical games parents play with infants. The therapist must not only introduce Ashley to the fun of movement activities, but also reassure her parents that the activities are appropriate for her. Following treatment, Ashley will be able to accomplish the following tasks:

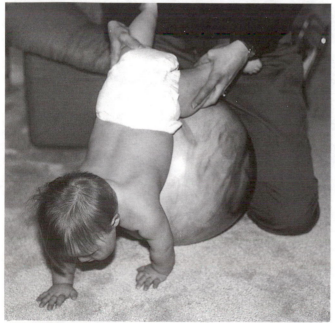

FIGURE 19. Inversion over a ball to promote shoulder girdle stability with weight bearing through upper extremities.

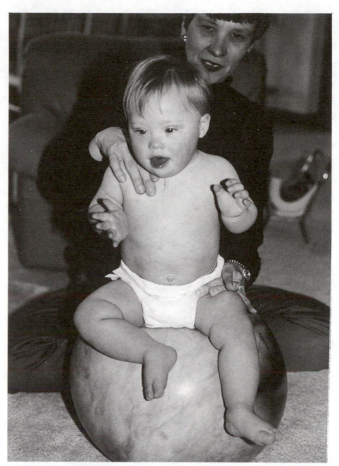

FIGURE 20. Bouncing on ball with therapist assisting in maintaining appropriate postural alignment.

1. Maintain an appropriate alignment in a quadruped position for 30 seconds with no more than one cue from the handler.
2. Maintain appropriate alignment in standing with upper extremities on a support for one minute with the handler providing no more than two cues.
3. Move from standing to sitting to all fours position with no indications of apprehension.
4. Tolerate therapist assisted movements between various developmentally appropriate postures with no indications of apprehension.

Activities in the intervention program are designed to increase postural stability. Ashley can be inverted on a ball leading to weightbearing support through her arms (Figure 19). Sitting on the ball, she can be bounced. This provides vestibular stimulation and approximation through the vertebral column (Figure 20). Ashley should be encouraged to rock in the all fours position while the therapist approximates through the head or pelvis in the long axis of the vertebral column (Figure 21). The therapist may approximate through the long axis of the upper extremities or the femurs to reinforce postural holding contractions through the extremities. Following the inversion activity on the ball, Ashley could be moved into a standing position. Approximation through

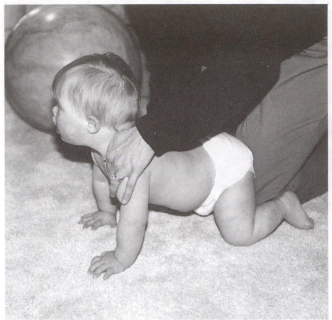

FIGURE 21. Rocking in all fours with therapist approximating through the long axis of the vertebral column to reinforce postural alignment.

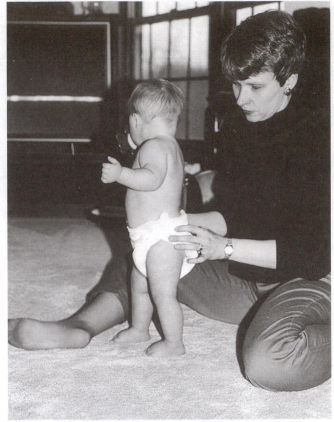

FIGURE 23.

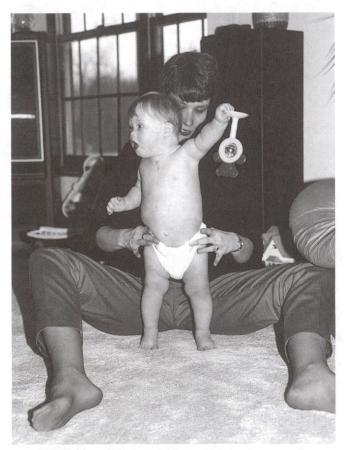

FIGURE 22.

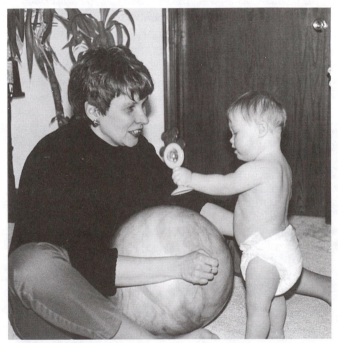

FIGURE 24.

Figures 22, 23 and 24 display practice of standing balance while involved in upper extremity play activities.

the pelvis with the force vector through the correct alignment of the lower extremities should improve Ashley's standing posture. Ashley should be involved in upper extremity play activities as the therapist reinforces correct standing alignment (Figures 22-24). This should assist Ashley in integrating the control she is learning to situations outside of therapy.

Following inversion or other vestibular facilitory techniques, the therapist should assist Ashley in moving between developmental positions. The therapist is assisting Ashley in using the increased postural control developed during the intervention session. ❑

REFERENCES

1. Polit A, Bizzi E: Characteristics of motor programs underlying arm movements in monkey. J Neurophys 42: 183-194, 1979
2. Schmidt RA: Motor Control and Learning, ed 2. Champaign, IL, Human Kinetics Publishers, Inc., 1988
3. Gentile AM: Skill acquisition: action, movement, and neuromotor processes. In Carr JH et al.: Movement Science Foundations for Physical Therapy in Rehabilitation. Rockville, MD, Aspen Publishers, Inc., 1987, pp 155-177
4. Farber SD: Neurorehabilitation - A Multisensory Approach. Philadelphia, PA, WB Saunders Co., 1982
5. Nasher LM: Sensory, neuromuscular, and biomechanical contributions to human balance. In Duncan PW (ed): Balance: Proceedings of the APTA Forum. Alexandria, VA, APTA, 1990, pp 5-12
6. Umphred DA, McCormack GL: Classification of common facilitatory and inhibitory treatment techniques. In Umphred D, (ed): Neurological Rehabilitation, ed 2. St. Louis, MO, CV Mosby Co., 1990, pp 111-162
7. Noback CR, Strominger NL, Demarest RJ: The Human Nervous System. Malvern PA, Lea & Febiger, 1991, p 160
8. McGraw MB: Neuromuscular mechanism of the infant. Am J Dis Child 60: 1031-1042, 1940
9. Ayres JA: Southern California Post-rotatory Nystagmus Test. Los Angeles, CA, Western Psychological Services, 1975
10. Hagbarth KE, Eklund G: The muscle vibrator - a useful tool in neurological therapeutic work. In Payton O, Hirt S, Newton R (eds): Therapeutic Exercise, Philadelphia, PA, FA Davis Co., 1977, p. 138
11. Woollacott MH: Postural control and development. In Whiting, HTA, Wade, MG (eds): Themes in Motor Development. Boston MA, Martinus Nijhoff Publishers, 1986

SUGGESTED READINGS

1. Campbell SK (ed): Pediatric Neurological Physical Therapy. New York, NY, Churchill Livingstone, 1984
2. Carr JH, et al: Movement Science Foundations for Physical Therapy in Rehabilitation. Rockville, MD, Aspen Publishers, Inc., 1987
3. Montgomery PC, Connolly BH (eds): Motor Control and Physical Therapy: Theoretical Framework and Practical Applications. Hixson TN, Chattanooga Group, Inc., 1991
4. Schmidt RA: Motor Control and Learning, ed 2. Champaign, IL, Human Kinetics Publishers, Inc., 1988
5. Scully RM, Barnes MR (eds): Physical Therapy, Philadelphia, PA, J.B. Lippincott, 1989
6. Umphred D, (ed): Neurological Rehabilitation, ed 2. St. Louis, MO, CV Mosby Co., 1990

CHAPTER 7

DEVELOPING HEAD & TRUNK CONTROL

Janet Sternat, PT

◆

To look closely at the head and trunk is somewhat like putting a drop of water under a microscope. What appears at first to be a simple whole is in fact a dynamic system made up of many parts. Through movement, the skin, bones, muscles, and fascia all contribute to what appears to be the static function of maintaining postural alignment. This apparent mechanical alignment, along with neurophysiological control systems and basic synergistic patterns, are the substrates of body-mind expression which incorporate emotional expression with intention.[1-3] The fluidity of this expression depends on many systems of learning and repeated practice becoming neatly stored in the central nervous system (CNS) and defining clearly the body image of our vertical axis.[1,3]

From a hierarchial reflex motor control model, spinal movements and their underlying reflexes are simple enough to delineate.[1] Functional motion analysis is another way to view the movements of the head, neck, thorax, and related parts. The head and trunk should be able to extend, flex, laterally flex, and rotate in a variety of pro- and anti-gravity positions.[4] To accomplish these seemingly fundamental movements, the musculoskeletal and nervous systems are interdependent in a motor-sensory-motor relationship.[5,6] This relationship includes, to a significant extent, internal emotional and excitement levels (arousal) which affect motivation, intent, attention, and muscle tone.[7,8] Specifically, the cerebellum, limbic system, reticular system, and proprioceptors participate in preparing for and monitoring motor activity.[5,8,9,10]

As if the head and trunk are not complex enough, the development of "control" requires the additional perspective of intrauterine progression of fetal movement. The potential for competent movement is a composite of many factors including the practiced movement of the fetus in utero.[11] This is significant especially when viewed with the intrauterine development (as differentiated from post-natal development) of passive muscle tonus which has been found to occur in a caudal to cephalic and distal to proximal direction.[9]

Descriptions of fetal movement support a motor-sensory-motor basis.[11] Trunk and head movements occur initially, followed by isolated and differentiated movements of head, limbs, diaphragm, and then jaw. Limb and head movements were reported to precede tactile exploration of the face which was followed by sucking and swallowing. Spontaneous movement was documented to occur before reflexive movement (see Chapter 1).

The relationship of the neck to head and trunk movement, of the spine and ribs to respiration and posture, of the pelvis to posture and movement, and the interrelationships of muscles to postural tone, dynamic stability, and movement patterns also must be understood. A child must be able to maintain desired postures while freely using distal components of the body (i.e. hands, feet, mouth, and eyes.) Chest movements must be supported and free for respiration to occur and change as demands vary from resting to active states.[8,12] Changes in body position must occur with graded control between supported and upright positions. Adaptive responses must be possible as environmental changes mandate balance reactions or a simple shift of weight.[1,2]

Primary movement responses of the head and trunk are incorporated during development into all variations of movement from automatic postural adjustments to skilled volitional acts. The muscles responsible for controlled movement must work in synergy. The ability to move with grace, power, and lightness, depends on balanced muscle strength, tonus, and patterns of movement that have become incorporated as automatic movement.[1,3,12-14] Opposing muscles must be able to elongate fully, "letting go" through the full excursion of joint range, while other muscle groups are contracting to provide a stable point from which movement can occur.[15,16] The active muscle groups must have sufficient contractile force to carry the body part in the desired direction.

Antagonists must grade the elongation or decelerate the moving part to prevent loss of control.[15,17] Specific muscle groups related to trunk control include the capital flexors and extensors, spinal flexors and extensors, intercostals, and hip flexors and extensors. The latter two groups are mentioned as they pertain to the function of the pelvis. As these muscles work to balance one another, they enable the head and trunk to respond with movements of lateral flexion and rotation.[8,12,13]

In treatment, two goals are primary. One is establishing firm somatic proprioceptive responses that become the basis for sensory perception and interplay with movement.[2] The second is developing the potential for muscle groups to be used in a functionally appropriate manner to respond as movement demands occur from internal states or environmental situations.[1,18,19] Functional movement should be possible with a sense of lightness and ease, as well as incorporating the element of reversibility.[6,14] This amount of control allows for the expression of postural reactions and the integration of innate motor programs within the execution of skilled movements.[8,12,16,20]

CONTROL OF MOVEMENT

Seven basic principles that should be defined as they pertain to motor control include: muscle elongation,

mobilization, body biomechanics, tonus gradation, balanced muscle function, activation, and repetition.

In motor development, shortened muscles must elongate from physiologic flexion to achieve the full variety of postures associated with normal movement.[4] This need for elongation as a preparation for movement continues throughout life.[12]

Elongation is the ability of a muscle to release its hold or tension and lengthen through the full excursion of joint movement. Skin, ligaments, and subcutaneous tissue all have visco-elastic properties which may take over the function of postural holding. When low muscle tone, inadequate strength, or trauma have led to an imbalance of muscle function, these structures may begin to restrict movement and cause pain.[12] Movement restricted by the unnatural holding of muscles, skin, fascia, or ligaments may require specialized preparation that includes soft tissue mobilization, myofascial release, and massage.[12,21]

Biomechanical influences of the body also may produce changes in muscle function and create the malalignment often associated with disorganized motor function.[2] Realignment of the thoracic spine will have a direct effect on trunk flexors through elongation produced by lifting the thorax. Biomechanical influences may be produced passively during handling and positioning or actively during facilitation of specific muscle groups (e.g. promotion of active upper back extension in prone).

The ability to produce normal variations in postural tone is one of the desired outcomes of treatment. To achieve this requires an understanding of the events that produce and change tonus. Internal emotional states and thought patterns have an effect on body tone.[22] These conditions may vary from moment to moment with different levels of excitement, worry, fear, anger, depression, or within a sleep/wake cycle. Each produces a definite effect on the body which can be felt through the muscles and fascia.[12,14,22,23]

External events or stimulation also may have an effect on body tone. Children may respond differently to direct input such as percussion, tapping, bouncing, or jumping. While some children will calm to increased proprioceptive input, others will become more active. Techniques such as slow rhythmic rocking, deep massage, myofascial release, muscle elongation, and soft rhythmic sound, generally result in inhibition. However, a child who does not feel like taking a nap or quieting may instead become quite irritable and tense. The physical environment and the feelings of others in the immediate environment have a direct effect on body tone and child behavior.[24] Events such as changes in barometric pressure, extreme temperatures, or even the attitude and/or expectations of the therapist may help to explain mood swings, comfort level, and body tension.[14,23-25] Muscles have a natural level of tension at rest

Therapeutic Exercise In Developmental Disabilities

which increases with active motion and reduces again when activity ceases. This often is not seen in children with lesions of the CNS, emotional arousal problems, or genetically predisposed extremes of muscle tone (e.g. Down Syndrome or Melnick/Needles Syndrome).

Normally, muscles function optimally and a feeling of lightness and ease of movement results. [12-14] The muscles used to control the head and trunk must work synergistically to achieve this ease in maintaining spinal alignment. [13] Once this balance of muscle function is achieved, the expression of righting reactions and other postural responses becomes possible in all planes of movement. [1,2,16]

A familiar phrase from an unknown source goes, "if you don't use it, you'll lose it". This pertains to most living cells and tissue including the nervous and musculoskeletal systems. [9] It pertains to initial fetal development and continuing growth. Muscles that are inactive and do not produce movement become atrophied and, through disuse, sensory awareness of that body part also is diminished. [23] Movement can be initiated from at least two levels of the brain. [8] On a conscious directed level, new skills can be learned in isolation and executed in component parts. The young child actively may practice parts of higher level skills. For example, reciprocal kicking observed in play uses many of the same muscles required for walking, although it is not the same task as walking. Although this kicking may not always be directed through conscious effort, the child is conscious of, and delights in the movement sensation. Early isolated attempts at movement may become incorporated into patterns of movement as postural control develops (see Chapter 3). After actively practicing weight shifting, the body may be more responsive to changes in position (i.e. weight shift producing the need to realign posture). Automatic and semiautomatic responses are desired for adaptation to the environment and to provide the ability to act on the environment with efficient, fluid execution. Both types of actively produced responses, volitional and automatic, can be used in treatment. The first goal is to establish the ability to move. The second goal is to perfect the quality of movement through practice in a functional context.

In the process of normal development the infant can be observed to produce specific movements thousands of times. This practice enhances communication between the sensory and motor systems of the body. [12] The developmental process may be used during treatment to achieve the goal of changing or enhancing motor output. One hypothesis is that repetitions must be precisely matched to the individual's innate neural programs. When this match is truly made, fewer repetitions are required to result in the desired outcome. For example, a change in tonus may require as few as 30 repetitions if the quality of movement is guided. [12] Holding a position, as in elongation techniques, if done precisely, may require only 30-90 seconds to release unwanted muscle tension. [12,26] The more often a motion is produced, the easier it becomes to produce and eventually to incorporate with more complex patterns of movement. [10]

ASSESSMENT

In order to determine treatment strategies and techniques for the head and trunk, a baseline of accepted function must be determined and assessment procedures delineated. The anatomical and biomechanical components of the trunk and head serve most reliably as a baseline for desired function when combined with factors such as muscle tone, strength, and flexibility. [2,13] The quality and intent of movement is a mere reflection of the individual's nervous system, which is more changeable than previously believed. [2,9,10,19]

Lack of trunk and head control usually is described as trunk or head instability. This instability often is associated with underlying hypotonia. [4,6] To determine tonus state of muscles, the examiner must handle the child. At rest, ease of passive movement should be felt. When the child is excited or stimulated, emotional tone can be expressed as increased muscle tension. During active movement of isolated body parts or of the total body through space, compensatory tone or stability patterns may be noted. [2,4]

When muscle tonus or motor control are insufficient to support posture, predictable compensations result. [4,9] The compensatory stability patterns may be observed or felt during active movement. For example, an increase in muscle tone or exaggerated extension postures might be apparent at the shoulders (elevation and retraction), and spine (cervical and lumbar hyperextension). [2,6,8] The use of a Valsalva maneuver or breath holding might be observed when the upper back extensors or trunk flexors are insufficient to maintain an erect spine. [8] Hip flexor "fixing" or holding might be a substitute for inadequate pelvic control. [13] Fixing also may occur in the pectoral muscles to provide increased shoulder stability. [4] Such compensatory use of muscles generally interferes with efficient movement. [27]

As the use of compensatory patterns continues, additional problems may result, such as shortening of the muscles used for "holding", and weakness of other muscles (due in part to hypotonia or to disuse). A distorted body image and maladaptive patterns of somatic dominance patterns may occur instead of balanced responses for postural holding. [2,23,25]

Problems associated with poor head and trunk control are different in the infant as compared to problems in the older child. Initial problems with sucking and respiration may be early indicators of trunk instability in the infant. [4,6,8,18] Secondary, more obvious problems develop as the infant attempts to use what control is available to gain mobility or an upright position. Sequences of both normal and abnormal chest development have been described.[19]

If problems with head and trunk control remain untreated, they become easier to recognize because of the compounding effects of effort and repeated abnormal use of compensatory movement patterns.[4] Even subtle problems of postural control should be identified early because of the resultant pathological outcome of untreated problems.[2]

Assessment procedures can be simplified by focusing on the mechanics of head and trunk control. More important than procedure, however, is the examiner's reference point. What is normal? That is, what is the human potential for flexibility, balanced muscle function, and motor control without compensation? This reference point will influence the goals set for treatment and the quality of dynamic posture achieved. Normal posture and movement potential have been described in children.[22] These descriptions are useful for illustrating abdominal muscle activation and in demonstrating the potential of the spine and hips for flexibility, especially into hyperextension. Another aspect of trunk control which requires full understanding is the pelvic tilt.[13] Important factors in trunk control are balanced tonus, use of abdominal muscles in respiration and posture, and adequate range of motion of the iliopsoas to allow appropriate function of the abdominal muscles. Ginther has described significant aspects of pelvic development during the first six months of life.[28] Key muscles and their anatomical relationships in the changing movement patterns of the normally developing child are discussed. Other references describe muscular relationships of the shoulder girdle and trunk and relationships of muscles, fascia, organs, and function of the thorax.[29-30]

When normal head and trunk control are understood clearly, the following guidelines will be useful in determination of problems related to deficits in head and trunk control.

GUIDELINE I

Posture should be observed in supine, prone on extended arms, side sitting, long sitting, and bench sitting. Asymmetries should be noted and investigated further. In sitting, collapse of the spine, especially upper thoracic and cervical areas, and the pelvic position should be carefully observed. Deviations, such as an indented sternum, retracted jaw, and structural changes of the ribs should be noted. The child's ability to change positions and to isolate requested movement should be observed. Can the head be lifted from a supporting surface in supine, prone, and sidelying? Are there unnecessary movements in the mouth, extremities, and shoulders when activation is attempted? Can fluctuations of muscle tone be felt as changes of posture occur from supported (resting) to unsupported (active) positions? Breathing

patterns can be observed readily as a part of posture evaluation. A boney looking rib cage often can be a sign of tightness in the intercostal muscles. Pectus excavatum is associated with a forward flexed thoracic spine, shallow rapid breathing patterns even at rest, and flared out lower ribs.[19]

GUIDELINE II

Mobility should be examined from two perspectives. First, actual flexibility of the joints and subcutaneous tissue must be palpated. Are joints hypermobile? Is full range of motion (ROM) possible passively? In particular, the atlanto-occipital, lumbar-sacral, hip, and intervertebral joints must be able to move freely. To obtain full shoulder flexor ROM, the rib cage must be able to elevate for the last 20 degrees of shoulder motion.[19,27] When evaluating spinal rotation, the pelvis should remain stationary while the upper trunk turns, and the shoulders should remain stationary while the head turns on the neck.[2,27] When all segments of the spine are able to move freely, the motions of flexion/extension and rotation combined with the straight planes of motion will have a segmental look. Differentiated movement then becomes possible and the thoracic skeleton has a chain effect on itself and its related parts.[9,14]

A second perspective is the amount of active flexibility. The examiner must inhibit unwanted movement. For example, shoulder elevation must be prevented when the subject attempts to lift the head from supine and the pelvis must be stabilized while an attempt is made to reach from a sidelying position. The examiner must determine whether joint excursion is blocked by shortened muscles, limited by weak agonists, or prevented by muscle holding or fixing".[30]

GUIDELINE III

Movement patterns may be considered to consist of individual components of movement. Functional movement analyses can be used to determine head and trunk responses required in postural reactions and functional motor tasks. Another general rule of thumb is to passively do the work of the muscle(s) by supporting the skeleton in the same configuration of movement after active movement ceases. If the neck is being arched in hyperextension, support the back, neck, and head at the end point, observe the child's breathing and when the muscle activity quiets, and breathing becomes easy, move the part as much as possible into a more natural anatomical position. It is important to observe continually the child's breathing pattern as an indicator of comfort and acceptance.[19]

Assessment should include requests for movement (e.g. look here, roll over) as well as elicitation of movement during handling and function (i.e. removal of clothing). Does the head turn and lift with ease and efficiency? Does the pelvis shift or tilt in anticipation of postural changes or in response to movement facilitation? Is breath holding occurring to attain stability during hand function or during movement of the body through the environment?

GUIDELINE IV

Automatic reactions and skilled movements, such as catching or kicking a ball, are dependent on motor programs for efficient execution.[10] These motor programs consist of innate centrally programmed movements and practiced or learned responses.[1,10,16,17] Skilled observation is necessary to determine the quality of head and trunk control. Does the head right sufficiently during rolling? Are the eyes able to locate objects and monitor the hands without excessive head movement? Does movement occur from the pelvis to position the head and trunk in anticipation of reaching for a desired object or taking a drink from a cup? Are there observable disorganized motor function and vestibular dominance during attempts to balance?[2] Is there lack of automatic proprioceptive control during facilitated weight shifting?[2] Is there a variety of postures observed during play?[2]

TREATMENT

In the same way that head and trunk control have been dissected and defined by the underlying biomechanics, kinesiology, and components of movement, treatment can be analyzed by looking at basic principles. If the basic principles are understood, treatment techniques can be selected from a variety of approaches including neurodevelopmental treatment (NDT), sensory integration (SI), Proprioceptive Neuromuscular Facilitation (PNF), Feldenkrais, Rood, myofascial release, joint mobilization, and massage. Techniques then can be combined to achieve optimal results.

Designing effective intervention is accomplished by discovering and following the child's developmental process and movement sequences. This means a child can be viewed as the leader or guide for intervention. The intervention activities are selected after observing the function already revealed by the child's play, interactions, breathing patterns, or need states. The physical therapist needs simply ask: What activities or handling techniques will enhance what a child is already doing? How can the total body be incorporated more fully into a task or movement pattern?[31,32]

Something as simple as hand placement by the therapist on a child's body part can increase the awareness of that part by the CNS at the conscious and subconscious levels. Touch seldom goes unnoticed by the brain. This contact can lead to a direct change in function of the part by reducing or enhancing muscular effort. It also may yield an avoidance or defensive response if the touch is interpreted by the child's nervous system as threatening.[24,31] It becomes the therapist's responsibility to monitor a child's response to touch and at the same time monitor how the touching is presented from the therapist's own state of arousal, physical comfort, intention of outcome, and skill at establishing physical and emotional rapport. Time is too often a factor which plays a significant part in setting up the emotional tone of the therapist. Rushed work often reduces sensitivity and complicates effective intervention.[33] It is necessary, therefore, for the therapist to develop an intervention plan that matches comfortably with the time allotted for treatment.

In the remediation of problems associated with head and trunk control, the selected techniques will be organized into four categories: techniques used to prepare muscles for activation, techniques used to activate specific muscles, techniques used to elicit normal movement responses, and techniques used to enhance breathing. The ultimate measure of effectiveness is the child's interplay, his acceptance of handling, and then his interest in "taking over" the movement. This includes play with the sensation of movement, practice of isolated movement (e.g. kicking or waving), or use of movement patterns in a functional activity or skill (e.g. climbing, creeping, looking).

MUSCLE PREPARATION

The purpose of muscle preparation is threefold: 1) establishment of improved somatic proprioception, vestibular proprioception, and connectedness;[24,25,32] 2) elongation of shortened muscles;[4,17,34] and 3) development of tonus or stability adequate for active movement.[1,5,12,19]

Techniques used to prepare muscles can be drawn from a variety of treatment approaches. Superficial techniques such as massage,[21] and deeper indirect techniques, such as those used in myofascial release,[22] are often pleasant methods of introducing hands-on contact with children. Maintained pressure on motor points, soft tissue mobilization, stretching, and maintained joint traction are included in methods of releasing "bound down" muscle fibers and fascia.[17,22,34] Where "fixing" or muscle holding is preventing joint excursion, techniques including weight bearing, active elongation, and overall CNS inhibition may be the treatment choices. These techniques are used widely in such approaches as NDT,[35] PNF,[36] and SI.[20]

Treatment principals suggested by Magrun[37] in his neuro-postural approach to changing movement organization include the importance of direct handling to guide learning and create new movement/spatial experiencing prior to direct sensory stimulation.

Other resources for learning more about techniques that enrich proprioception availability include the works written about the Feldenkrais Method, in particular the functional integration aspects.[32,33] Other authors[29,38] explain more fully how therapist contact with a child can more fully develop body scheme through the proprioceptors. By increasing the available body image, a new potential for movement of that part is established, which in turn actively stimulates proprioceptors. This interplay between the muscles, joints, fascia, and the brain is what stimulates cellular growth in early development as well as recovery from trauma and ongoing learning.

The basis of the above techniques is simply the functional relationships of bones and muscles. Further study of these relationships in the work by Boehm,[29] Barral,[30] Ginther,[28] and Kendall and McCreary[27] may produce an understanding of the body biomechanics which then can be directly applied in treatment. Proprioceptive stimulation can be expanded from a simple idea of joint compression to one of linkage in which the thorax is a middle point through which movement occurs with a body sitting, standing, on all fours, or even lying down.

The therapist must keep in mind that the child must interact with his environment for any muscle preparation to become useful.[31] Sometimes simply motivating a child or assisting the child to move is sufficient to improve function. Another concept includes accepting any of the child's movement patterns (quantity as well as quality). It means supplying approval and support for what is already occurring and introducing change only after the therapist understands what is meaningful to the child.[31,33] It means, to avoid correcting a child by saying "don't move that way!" and instead assisting a child to access his world in easier and more meaningful ways using technology (e.g. computers, biofeedback, switches, electric wheelchairs, and visual aides) as soon as the child's interest is present.[39]

Muscle elongation is necessary when muscles have not been elongated from the position of physiologic flexion at birth, or when muscles are chronically shortened. Habitual postures (such as kyphotic upper back or hyperlordotic low back) or muscle tone imbalances are common causes of muscle shortening. Gravitational forces and muscle contractions combine to shape and form the thorax.[18,19] Weakened or habitually contracting muscles can greatly influence the ultimate shape and function of the thorax. The functions of posture, balance, breathing, vision, and communication all are affected directly by the capabilities of and the development of the thorax.[2,18,19,40]

Head, neck, and trunk muscle groups which often require elongation include the following: capital and cervical extensors and lateral flexors; jaw retractors; shoulder internal rotators and elevators; scapular abductors; shoulder extensors; lumbar spine extensors; trunk rotators, flexors, and lateral flexors; and hip flexors and extensors.

When muscle elongation is completed, movement potential is created in the lengthened and opposing muscle groups. For example, elongation of the capital and cervical extensors creates the option of active capital flexion allowing a chin tuck position or head lift in supine. When the pectoral muscles are elongated, the upper back extensors may be facilitated to produce an extended spine in prone or sitting. When the lumbar extensors are elongated, the abdominal muscles may be facilitated to produce controlled movements of the pelvis needed in rolling or weight shifting. When lateral trunk and neck muscles are elongated, muscle groups producing righting and balance reactions can be facilitated. When hip flexor muscles are elongated, gluteal muscles can be facilitated to promote normal pelvic and spinal alignment needed for sitting and standing. Muscles which have been elongated may need strengthening to balance active use of opposing muscles.

The following positions which allow several treatment techniques to be applied simultaneously are suggested for treatment when muscle preparation is necessary. These positions should not be the only positions used. A variety of positions and the child's acceptance of any one position should be considered in any treatment program.

To elongate the capital, cervical, and lumbar extensors the child can be positioned supine on the floor and therapist's knees (Figure 1). Therapist's control is at the

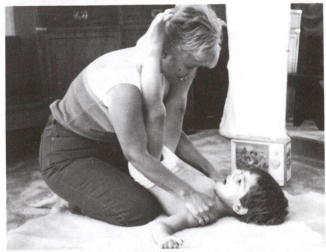

FIGURE 1. *Elongation of capital, cervical and lumbar extensors.*

child's shoulders. Gentle rocking movement is possible at the shoulders as they are depressed. The head should be in a chin tucked position when elongation is completed and the pelvis in a neutral or posterior tilt position. From this position, active head lifting can be encouraged, as well as abdominal activation as the feet are brought towards the midline of the body. While the therapist is sitting on a bench, a small child can be supported entirely on the therapist's lap (Figure 2). The therapist can use an up and down movement of the knees

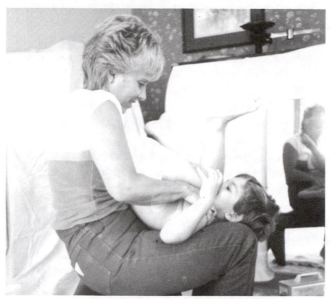

FIGURE 2. *Additional position for elongation of capital, cervical and lumbar extensors.*

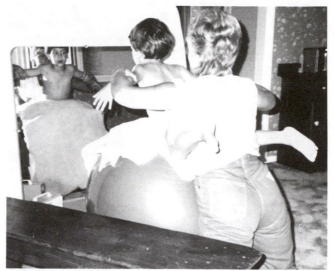

FIGURE 4. *Pivot prone position on therapeutic ball.*

to create a slow back and forth movement of the child's head while depressing the shoulders.

To elongate the pectoral muscles and hip flexors, the child can be positioned supine over a large therapy ball or suspended down the therapist's legs while the therapist is sitting on a bench (Figure 3). Massage or maintained pressure to the motor point will assist these muscles in "letting go." Active elongation of these muscle groups also is possible from a prone position (Figures 4, 5). In both positions, the therapist is controlling at the child's upper arm to promote an active "airplane" or pivot prone position as upper back extensor muscles are activated. The shoulders must be free to externally rotate and the scapula free to adduct.

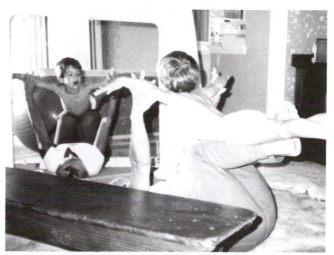

FIGURE 5. *Pivot prone position on therapist's legs.*

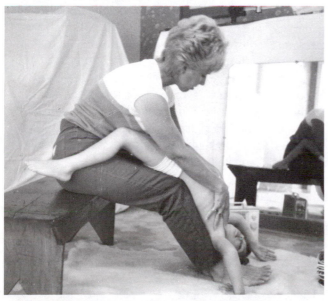

FIGURE 3. *Elongation of pectoral muscles and hip flexors.*

Elongation of the scapulo-humeral muscles is possible with the child sidelying on the floor or across the therapist's lap (Figure 6). The child's weight bearing arm should be flexed at the shoulder and externally rotated. When this shoulder is in full flexion, upper back extension is possible both biomechanically and actively as the child reaches. In sidelying, the inhibition of scapulo-humeral muscles is possible through weight bearing. At the "up" shoulder, the therapist can facilitate shoulder depression and lateral neck flexion. This position can lead naturally into rolling or prone or supine positions.

Elongation of trunk muscles is possible with the child supported in prone or supine. Maintained opposing traction at the iliac crest and rib cage can be used to promote movement into lateral flexion on the opposite side or rotation at the lumbar spine, causing the thorax and pelvis to move in opposite directions (Figure 7). This position is useful to release intercostal muscles. The

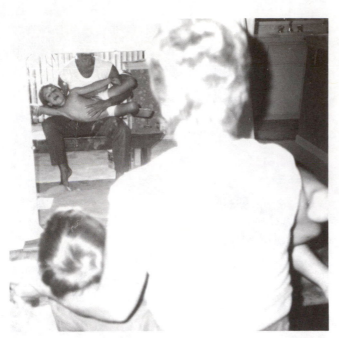

FIGURE 6. Elongation of the scapulo-humeral muscles.

finger tips of the therapist can be used to apply pressure evenly between the ribs. Starting from a lateral position and working toward the sternum, slow movement should free the ribs for expansion with the child's inspiration. Percussion on the chest or in the back thoracic area may increase tonus of the thoracic muscles.

Elongation of the gluteal muscles and hip flexors is possible with the child in prone. The therapist assists the child to move one leg into full hip flexion while the other leg is positioned in full hip extension. Traction may be applied to the extended leg, while the child's weight is used to inhibit extension at the flexed leg. A bolster may be used to support the child's chest and maintain the upper back in extension. Slow weight shifting or gentle rocking may assist muscles in "letting go".

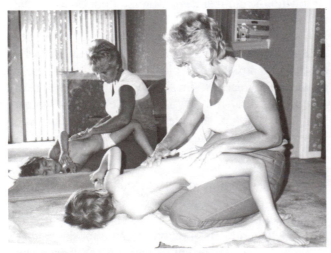

FIGURE 7. Elongation of trunk musculature using rotation.

When muscle elongation is the purpose of treatment, caution should be used to move joints slowly and in a way that is natural to the child. Positions may require holding up to 90 seconds for muscle tension to release.[17,34] Full joint excursion may require several treatment sessions and should never be forced where restrictions are felt or pain expressed. In cases where the muscle length is not interfering with function, but muscle tonus or stiffness has an overriding effect on initiating movement or grading precise movements, the following suggestions are made in relationship to the trunk and spinal muscles.

Differentiation is a key to achieving a resting tone state that is neither too high or too low. This ready-to-move state at rest lends itself to fluid and symmetrical weight shifting followed by ease of limb placing for weight bearing movements of the shoulder and pelvic girdles.[28,29,37] Differentiation can be achieved through rotational movements of the spine,[37] through using opposing movements of any parts[31,33] (head/shoulders, clavicle/pelvis, pelvis/head), or through manual techniques.[30]

Another way to affect tonus is to support the skeletal part or do the work of a particular muscle group. This tends to decrease the muscular activity and free up movement potential. In this way, the skeleton can be realigned to a more anatomically advantageous position (e.g. more midline or symmetrical). When muscle activity is quieted, joint compression or decompression can be implemented. Joint compression can be applied through one or more body parts when bony alignment is achieved and muscle activity is evenly distributed through all joints.[12,31-33]

MUSCLE ACTIVATION

Techniques used to activate specific muscles are generally more "work" for the child. This phase of treatment requires a more dynamic effort from both the therapist and the child, as compared to elongation techniques which require more quiet cooperation (i.e. looking at books or in a mirror, talking, or listening to music). Activation should be fun for the child to result in the necessary repetitions that will strengthen responses. Reaching for objects, singing songs, or pretend scenarios are ways to engage more active interest.[41]

Facilitation of isolated movements of the head and trunk may be necessary before total movement patterns can be elicited. In the head and neck, the following isolated combinations should be addressed: capital flexion with cervical extension, capital extension with cervical extension, and capital and cervical lateral flexion. As the capital flexors are activated, the cervical extensors need to produce a retraction of the neck to align the cervical spine. In supine, this is accomplished with a request for the child to lift his head. The therapist pulls the shoulders into depression, thus inhibiting the trapezius muscles. In sitting, the "chin tuck" position can be accomplished by requesting a downward gaze of the child or by "leaning" the child back against a supporting surface to keep the head and neck aligned (Figure 8).

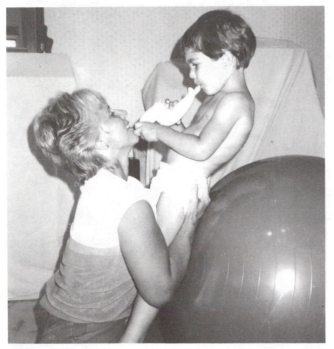

FIGURE 8. Facilitation of "chin tuck" position.

Capital extension with cervical extension produces the desired neck hyperextension required to control head movement in prone. A gymnastic ball provides a surface which supports the trunk while a mirror provides visual feedback (Figure 9). The head is not collapsed on the neck, but extended from the neck which is extended from the thoracic spine. The therapist may have to retract the child's shoulders during this activity to prevent pectoral

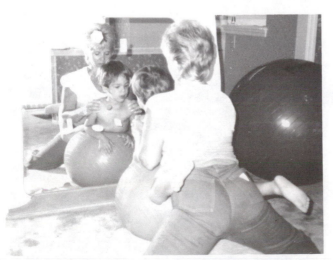

FIGURE 9. Facilitation of cervical extension on gymnastic ball.

shortening. Prone on extended arms is another way to promote head and neck extension (Figure 10). A bolster may be used under the child's chest to offer additional support. Requests to "look at" or visually follow a specific object will engage muscles actively.

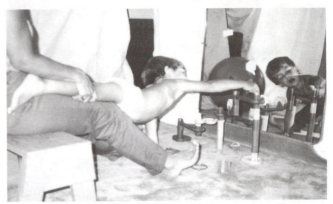

FIGURE 10. Facilitation of cervical extension while prone on extended arms.

The motion of capital/cervical lateral flexion follows control of the head and neck in straight planes (supine, prone, sitting). Lateral flexion precedes rotational ability in erect positions, but neck rotation may be possible sooner when the head and neck are supported, such as in supine.

The child may be positioned sidelying on a firm surface as the therapist controls the pelvis, thorax, and shoulders in straight alignment (Figure 11). The child is requested to lift the head or motion is elicited by a downward pull of the shoulder. Lateral flexion is difficult to achieve in isolation, but important to develop for balance responses.

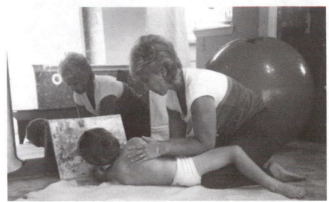

FIGURE 11. Sidelying positioning to facilitate lateral flexion.

Isolated movements of the shoulders may be used to activate the trunk muscles. Serratus activation results in a forward push which brings the shoulder forward for dynamic weight bearing. Pushing by the child can be requested in any extended arm position from supine to sitting (Figure 12). Back support is necessary for freeing the shoulders to move forward. This release requires the

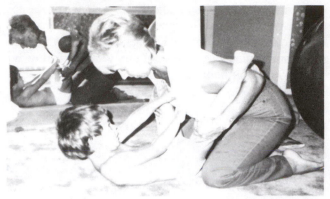

FIGURE 12. Serratus activation during forward pushing. Child's hand should be flat on therapist's chest.

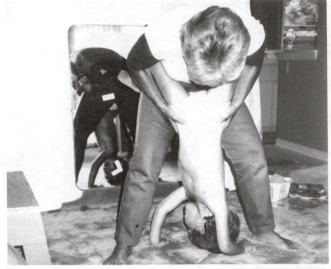

FIGURE 14. Recruitment of upper back extensors in the suspended position.

abdominals to work as trunk stabilizers, versus trunk movers.

The shoulder flexors, when used to raise the arms, recruit the upper back extensors to provide dynamic support of the upper trunk. Raising the arms can be requested in a sitting or suspended position (Figures 13, 14). A more difficult request is for the child to reach across his chest, which recruits trunk rotators (Figure 15). The therapist must assist shoulder flexion in this activity to free the opposite arm (serratus) to reach. The pelvis may require stabilization.

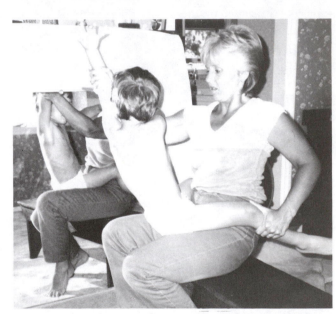

FIGURE 15. Recruitment of trunk rotators during sitting.

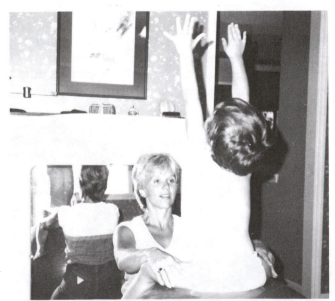

FIGURE 13. Recruitment of upper back extensors during sitting.

Isolated activity of the trunk muscles is important. Abdominals can be activated from supine, working against gravity, by encouraging the child to play with his feet. Placing the child's legs in an extended position (hips flexed, knees extended) and asking him to push upward also will facilitate trunk activation. The therapist must control the hips in flexion and knees in extension while providing a stable surface to push against. The

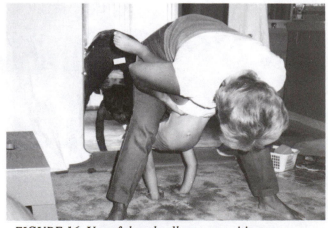

FIGURE 16. Use of the wheelbarrow position to facilitate upper back extension.

Therapeutic Exercise In Developmental Disabilities

child may lift his head as the abdominals become active. The extensor muscles of the back can be activated against gravity in a pivot prone position. This might be accomplished over a gymnastic ball or the therapist's legs. It is also possible to facilitate upper back extension in a suspended position, which may lead to a more dynamic wheelbarrow activity (Figure 16).

In children 5 to 6 years of age, the pelvic tilt can be taught in isolation. This includes anterior and posterior movement, as well as a rotational movement where the points of the pelvis rotate similar to a flat disc going around on its rim.[12] The pelvic tilt is accomplished most easily in supine, but should be mastered in all positions, including standing.

MOVEMENT RESPONSES

Many treatment techniques used to activate muscles require the ability to weight shift. After trunk muscles have been sufficiently prepared, the pelvis can be used to facilitate automatic reactions. Readiness assumes adequate postural tone and sufficient mobility and strength in key muscle groups to allow movement to occur. Proprioception must be intact in the trunk and visual fixation should not substitute for proprioceptively based head and body righting (see Chapter 6). The child must be free to move and willing to respond to movement.

Weight shift can be produced on dynamic surfaces. While sitting on a therapist's lap, the child can be moved by the slow elevation of one of the therapist's knees (Figure 17). This produces a graded shift of the pelvis. The child's arm position can vary, but the objective is to keep the spine erect and fluid. The therapist's hands can be used to facilitate abdominal muscles or provide support at the shoulders while guiding the desired movement.

Movement while sitting the child on a gymnastic ball requires advanced skills of the therapist and much preparation of the child. The weight shift is elicited by

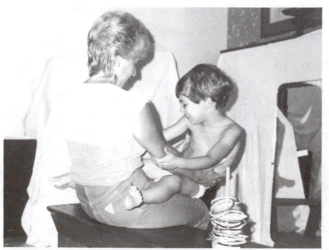

FIGURE 17. Weight shifting during sitting.

movement of the ball while the child's legs are held in contact with it (Figure 18). The legs are abducted at the hips and externally rotated. The child may be requested to bounce initially to increase body tonus. Shifting is done slowly and held at a point where it is possible to obtain a body response. Weight shift is accompanied by the therapist moving the weight bearing leg into external rotation.

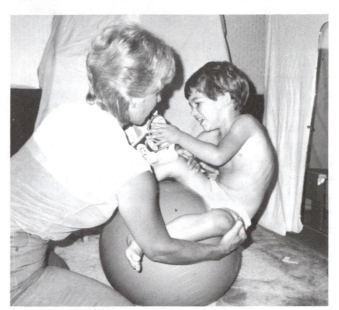

FIGURE 18. Weight shifting on gymnastic ball.

Weight shift also can be produced on stable surfaces. The therapist's lap can be used as a stable surface. In prone over the therapist's lap (child's head toward therapist's feet), the pelvic shift can be accomplished with the knees held level and steady, but moving off to one side. The child may be requested to look back at the therapist. The therapist holds onto the pelvis so that elongation of one side (side to which knees shift) occurs. This requires the child's shoulders to be free to move and the therapist's trunk to rotate as the knee movement is produced. One hand of the therapist assists to produce shoulder depression and lateral flexion while elongation occurs on the opposite weight-bearing side.

BREATHING

Massery[18,19] and Davis[40] studied breathing, pulmonary function, respiration, and phonation as related to aspects of trunk development and intervention. Abdominal muscle strength and freely moving intercostal muscles are two factors required for airway pressure to build up for secretion clearing and sustained phonation.[39,40] Ways of assessing breathing patterns are through hand placement on the child's chest or shoulders. This hand placement enhances particular phases of breathing or promotes graded exhalation.

This brief section on breathing at the end of treatment is to alert you to its usefulness as a place to start treatment as well as to its importance as a functional outcome of major importance. Breathing is essential in sustaining life, enriching development through the oxygenation of CNS cells, and communication itself. This aspect of the treatment of head and trunk is not to be overlooked or diminished in importance by the space allotted in this Chapter. Changes in breathing can signal comfort and distress during intervention and care should be used at all times to monitor intervention, handling, and rapport (see Chapter 9).

Palpation and observation are easier when the child's clothing is removed. The use of a sheep skin may add comfort when bare skin comes in contact with cool or rough surfaces. A mirror may be useful not only to engage the child's interest, but also as visual feedback for the therapist. Selected toys and materials should be incorporated at the child's interest level, but avoid over stimulation by keeping toys simple and at a minimum.

During any treatment session, the therapist's hands can be used to apply sensory input to direct or support the musculoskeletal system and to perceive what changes are occurring in temperature, underlying muscle tension, or movement. The therapist's hands can communicate to the child a sense of caring and confidence more directly than words can communicate.

CASE STUDIES

Suggested treatment applied to the specific cases which follow includes ideas presented in the text as well as more general techniques which might be useful. Hand placement and amount of support will vary as individual needs change from session to session and child to child.

CASE NO. 1 — JASON
Cerebral Palsy, Hemiparesis, 18 Months

Assessment reveals the following problem with trunk and head control. An asymmetrical posture is evident with a slight anterior tilt of the pelvis. The pelvis is retracted on the right. The hip flexors are shortened on the right more than on the left. The lateral trunk flexors are shortened on the right which contribute to the asymmetry. Weakness is evident in shortened muscle groups. When Jason is active, tone or muscle stiffness increases in the trunk which limits dissociation of pelvis and shoulders. Equilibrium reactions are expressed poorly due to poor quality of trunk control which results in poor ability to weight shift, especially on the right side. Head righting is adequate for protection, but asymmetry is apparent, associated with shoulder retraction on the right. Capital flexion is poor in isolation and does not balance use of capital extensors during functional movement. Extensor muscle groups dominate movement

patterns used to gain upright postures. Trunk rotation is limited to the left more than the right.

Treatment Goals are to:
1. increase mobility of the hips and thoracic spine.
2. increase ability to shift weight to the right.
3. increase ability to activate cervical and abdominal muscles.

Short-term objectives: Jason will
1. sit independently on a bench showing symmetrical position of pelvis with weight on the right ischium equal to weight on the left ischium, 100% of the time.
2. rise from supine to sitting using rotation to the right or left, 50% of the time.
3. climb using reciprocal movement in the lower¡ extremities, 100% of the time.
4. move actively through full range of motion in all joints of trunk, neck, and the hips, 100% of the time when required by the task.

Treatment Recommendations:

To prepare Jason for movement activities, the following muscles require elongation: hip flexors, lateral trunk flexors, capital extensors, and the scapular abductors. Passive movement of the thoracic spine must be possible for rotation to occur.

When muscle elongation is possible, active responses should be facilitated in the capital flexors and trunk flexors and extensors. Treatment positions should include supine (playing with feet), prone (as on the therapy ball or bolster), and in sitting (such as on the therapist's lap or therapy ball).

Functional activities which might be incorporated into Jason's play include swinging, climbing, and jumping. In a hammock, Jason could be positioned prone with a pillow to support the trunk. The therapist might push from underneath the hammock while Jason reaches out with extended arms. Jason also might sit on a suspended hoppity hop ball and swing. Climbing and jumping can be encouraged by piling blankets and pillows in front of a couch.

CASE NO. 2 — JILL
Cerebral Palsy, Spastic Quadriparesis, Mental Retardation, 7 Years

Assessment reveals the following problems with trunk and head control. Jill's upper spine is collapsed forward into a kyphotic posture with head and neck hyperextension. She has poor ability to lift her head in prone, to maintain it in upright, or to turn it in unsupported positions. Jill cannot sit without support. Tightness and limitation of movement are exhibited in capital extensor, pectoral, shoulder girdle, hip flexor, and lumbar spine muscles. A deformity is noted in the chest by an indented sternum.

Treatment goals are to:

1. improve postural control of upper back extension, abdominal function, and freedom of the thorax for breathing.
2. increase flexibility in shoulders, shoulder girdle, and hips.
3. improve head control and symmetrical posture.

Short-term objectives: Jill will

1. support and turn her head with equal ability to the right or left while sitting with assistance, 100% of the time.
2. lift her head in prone on elbows position and maintain the position for 5 seconds.
3. prolong an ah-ah sound with manual chest vibration for 3 to 5 seconds.

Treatment Recommendations:

To prepare muscles for activation and to achieve upright postures, elongation of the following muscles should be accomplished: cervical extensors, pectorals, lumbar extensors, hip flexors, and trunk flexors.

Jill may require supported positions initially during facilitation of inactive muscle groups. Vibration and percussion to the chest and upper back may be one way to normalize trunk tone or decrease general stiffness. Jill should be encouraged to vocalize during these techniques. Visual stimulation (looking in a mirror or at preferred toys) may assist in producing head movement while Jill is prone or suspended supine on a therapy ball. With Jill's arms extended over her head to extend the upper back and the therapist supporting her in sitting, a bouncing movement can be produced to increase muscle activation. In sidelying, Jill can be requested to track or reach for preferred toys while shoulder elevation is being inhibited by the therapist.

Functional activities might include positioning in sidelying while Jill is being shown a book or picture cards. In prone over a wedge or bolster, Jill might be encouraged to track preferred toys (small cars, a ball, or bubbles). Jill may be supported in sitting and assisted to use her arms while engaging in songs or in attempts to activate toys.

CASE NO. 3 — TAYLOR
Myelomeningocele, Repaired, L 1-2, 4 Years

Assessment reveals the following problems with head and trunk control. Taylor's abdominal muscles are weak. There is poor ability to activate abdominals in supine against gravity. Any attempt to rise to sitting results in the legs adducting. Breath holding is used to stabilize the trunk during movement of the upper extremities, which blocks the ability to rotate the spine (upper back moving on the pelvis). Active extension of the trunk is accomplished with retraction of the shoulders and hyperlordosis of the lumbar spine. In sitting,

upright posture is maintained by Taylor's "hanging on ligaments" rather than through active use of gluteal and abdominal muscles. Rolling is completed with poor leg dissociation. Equilibrium reactions are not expressed through the hips. In a hands and knees position, lordotic posture is evident, and shoulder support is inadequate as evidenced by winging scapulae and elevated shoulders.

Treatment goals are to:

1. improve voluntary control of intercostal muscles, abdominal muscles, and back extensors.
2. increase strength in abdominal and gluteal muscles.
3. mobilize pelvis (lumbosacral, sacroiliac joints).
4. develop trunk control in quadruped and sitting to improve balance reactions.

Short-term objectives: Taylor will

1. maintain a kneeling position with minimal support while maintaining normal spinal alignment.
2. do a pelvic tilt during bridging exercises.
3. rotate from quadruped to sitting and back while keeping hands on a stable surface.
4. use upper extremities without breath holding and reach forward in unsupported sitting.

Treatment Recommendations:

Muscle preparation requires elongation of the lumbar spine extensors and intercostal muscles. Muscle activation is needed in the capital and cervical extensors, and capital and cervical lateral flexors. The shoulder muscles must be elongated to produce a push (serratus), as well as abdominal muscles for control of movement from supine and during weight shifting on a stable surface.

Functional activities can vary from specific exercises to play skills. Bridging could be used to play "draw bridge" while toys are going under the raised hips. A hammock could be used to swing in prone or in sitting positions. A therapy ball might be used for prone support while Taylor is batting at a suspended balloon. Taylor could be encouraged to kick at a suspended hoppity hop ball or blow at bubbles floating by while lying on his back.

CASE NO. 4 — ASHLEY
Down Syndrome, 15 Months

Assessment reveals the following problem areas. Ashley's shoulders are elevated. She uses accessory neck muscles to assist the head when trying to produce capital flexion. Capital extensor muscles are shortened. Touching areas around the neck and shoulders is tolerated poorly. Postural support is poor due to weakness in trunk extensors and flexors. Movement variation is limited by lack of rotational components. Ashley generally is apprehensive about movement from a supporting surface or when movement is unexpected, such as in "rough housing".

Treatment goals are to:

1. increase tolerance to touch around shoulders and neck.
2. increase strength in trunk muscles, especially to promote control of upper back extension and flexion against gravity.
3. increase tolerance for handling and interest in movement.
4. increase independent ability to interact with movement equipment (e.g. swing, rocking horse, tyke bike).

Short-term objectives: Ashley will

1. get on/off a tyke bike with assistance.
2. express comfort and pleasure with rough housing in a suspended position.
3. tuck chin and extend legs while being pulled to sit, 50% of the time.

Treatment Recommendations:

Muscle preparation should include elongation of the capital extensors and shoulder elevators. Because Ashley also shows an aversion for tactile input, caution must be used when directly contacting sensitive areas. Ashley should be encouraged to use her own hands to touch various parts of her body.

Muscle activation should include isolated movements of the head and neck, facilitation of back extensors and trunk flexors, and the promotion of weight shifting on a dynamic surface.

Functional activities should include the introduction of tactile materials. Encourage Ashley to play in a bin of lentils or chestnuts, plastic balls, or in a cardboard box with pillows and blankets. Provide as needed, hugging, blowing, and touching to all parts of her body. Overall body massage with cream or rubbing with terry/flannel towels may be used. Provide a small gymnastic ball to play catch or roll over in playful rough housing. ❏

REFERENCES

1. Cohen B: The Alphabet of Movement: Primitive Reflexes, Righting Reactions, and Equilibrium Responses, Part 2. Northhampton, MA, Contact Quarterly, 14: 1989
2. Magrun W.M.: Clinical Observation of Posture. Videotape, Tucson, AZ, Therapy Skill Builders
3. Nadis S: The Energy Efficient Brain. Omni Magazine, 2:1992
4. Bly L: The Components of Normal Movement During the First Year of Life and Abnormal Motor Development. NDTA, Chicago, IL, Monograph, 1983
5. DiJoseph L.: Motor Behavioral vs. Motor Control: Holistic Approach to Movement. Rockville, MD, AOTA Sensory Integration Special Interest Section Newsletter 7:1984
6. Dubowitz V: The Floppy Infant, ed 2. Lavenham, Suffolk, England, The Lavenham Press Ltd., Spastic International Medical Publications, 1980
7. Brazelton TB: Neonatal Behavioral Assessment. Lavenham, Suffolk, England, Spastics International Medical Publications, 1973
8. Casaer P: Postural Behavior in Newborn Infants. Lavenham, Suffolk, England, The Lavenham Press Ltd., Spastics International Medical Publications, 1979
9. Gilles FH, Leviton A, Dooling EC: The Developing Human Brain, Growth, Epidemiology, Neuropathology. Boston, MA, John Wright PSG, 1983
10. Restak R: The Brain. New York, NY, Bantam Books, 1984
11. Prechtl H: Continuity of Neural Functions from Prenatal to Postnatal Life. Netherhall Gardens, London, Spastics International Medical Publications, 1984
12. Feldenkrais M: Awareness Through Movement. New York, NY, Harper & Row, 1977
13. Batson G: Reeducating or strengthening: Relooking at the pelvic tilt. King of Prussa, PA, Physical Therapy Forum, October 2, 1985
14. Seifert M: Gerda Alexander's Eutony: Its theory, its practice and its teaching. Novato, CA, Somatics Journal, Spring-Summer, 1985
15. Wells KF: Kinesiology: The Scientific Basis of Human Motion, ed 4. Philadelphia, PA, WB Saunders Co., 1978
16. Campbell S: Pediatric Neurologic Physical Therapy. New York, NY, Churchill Livingstone, Inc., 1984
17. Alter J: Surviving Exercise. Boston, MA, Houghton Mifflin Co., 1983
18. Massery M: Respiratory Rehabilation Secondary to Neurological Deficits: Understanding the Deficits. Chest Physical Therapy and Pulmonary Rehabilitation, ed 2. Chicago, IL, Year Book Medical Publishers, Inc., 1987
19. Massery, M: Chest Development as a component of normal motor development: Implications for pediatric physical therapists. Washington, D.C., Pediatric Physical Therapy, 3:3-8, 1991
20. Ayres AJ: Sensory Integration and Learning Disorders. Los Angeles, CA, Western Psychological Services, 1983
21. Anderson B: Stretching. Bolinas, CA, Shelter Publication, 1980
22. Prudden B: How to keep your Child Fit from Birth to Six. New York, NY, The Dial Press, 1983
23. Upledger JE, Vredevoogd JD: Craniosacral Therapy. Seattle, WA, Eastland Press, 1973
24. Boehme R: When Children Cry in Therapy. Milwaukee, WI, Teamtalk, July, 1991
25. Feldenkrais M: Bodily Expressions. Petaluma, CA, Somatics, Spring-Summer, 1988
26. Hanna T: The Body of Life. New York, NY Alfred A. Knopf, Inc., 1983
27. Kendall F, McCreary E: Muscles, Testing and Function, ed 3. Baltimore, MD, The Williams And Wilkins Co., 1983
28. Ginther C: Significant Aspects of Pelvic Development in the First Six Months of Life. Milwaukee, WI, Teamtalk, Winter, 1991-1992
29. Boehme R: How Do I Get Scapular Stability in My Patients? Milwaukee, WI, Teamtalk, March 1991
30. Barral J: The Thorax. Seattle, WA, Eastland Press, Inc., 1991
31. Reese M: Jill, Notes Towards a Case Study. Feldenkrais Journal, No. 3, 1987
32. Goldfarb L: Emily's New Crutches. Feldenkrais Journal, 6:43-48, 1990
33. Casey J: Introduction to Feldenkrais Method. Excellcare Quarterly, Winter 1991
34. Tappan FM: Healing Massage Techniques. Reston, VA, Reston Publishing Co., 1980
35. Scherzer AL, Tscharnuter I: Early Diagnosis and Therapy in Cerebral Palsy. New York, NY, Marcel Dekker, Inc., 1982
36. Knott M, Voss, D: Proprioceptive Neuromuscular Facilitation: Patterns and Techniques, ed 2. New York, NY, Harper and Row, 1968
37. Mangrun W: A Neuro-Postural Approach to Movement and Posture Disorgaization in Learning Disabilities: Direct Physical Handling, Advanced Therapeutics. Syracuse, NY 1990
38. Alexander G: Eutony. Great Neck, NY, Felix Morrow, 1985
39. Martin S: Floor sitting with sandbags: An adjunct to physical therapy. Pediatric Physical Therapy 2:192-195, 1990
40. Davis LF: Respiratory/Phonatory Function. New York, NY, Thieme Medical Publishers, 1987
41. Rosenholtz S: Songs! Movements! Fun!, Rosewood Publishing, San Mateo, CA, Audiotape, 1991

CHAPTER 8

DEVELOPING
POSTURAL CONTROL

Susan K. Effgen, Ph.D., PT

◆

For a child to explore his environment, whether by rolling, crawling, or walking, a series of continual movements and postural adjustments must be made. Postural adjustments are necessary if a child is to move freely and appropriately, and adjust rapidly to the demands of the environment. As a child matures he displays a number of distinct movements and reactions which orient his head and body in space, protect him when he falls, and assist him in maintaining balance.

The traditional view of the development of postural reactions is the reflex-hierarchical model. This model is no longer the only model proposed to account for development of movement and postural control.[1] Contemporary models, such as the systems model of motor control, distributed control model, or dynamical systems model also are used to explain movement.[2] The development of movement results from the complex interaction and evolution of numerous subsystems, not all of which are fully understood.

Although a specific model for the development of postural control is in the theoretical stage, the fact that postural reactions occur in normal infants and tend to follow a relatively set sequence, cannot be disregarded. Lack of development of these reactions may indicate neuromotor delay or disability and typically are assessed

to aid in the diagnosis of central nervous system CNS) disorders. Therefore, it is important to understand the evolution of these reactions, to test for their presence or absence, and to develop treatment strategies to encourage independent and efficient movement. What must be understood is that the development of postural control is no longer considered to depend solely on the maturation of the CNS.[1,2] The evolution of postural movements is not invariant. Many subsystems interact and the environmental context plays a critical role in motor development. Postural control is an evolving area of research in neuroscience and we must be prepared to evaluate new theories and determine their appropriateness and impact on our intervention procedures.

DESCRIPTION AND ASSESSMENT
OF POSTURAL REACTIONS

The description and study of postural reactions and control are difficult because of varying terminology and a diversity of concepts. As more has been learned about the development of postural reactions, a shift from the static, stimulus-response paradigm to a more dynamic, function oriented concept has occurred. The child must interact with numerous demands of the environment.

Experience with different aspects of the environment facilitates the emergence of a range of postural responses. Conversely, lack of experience delays the maturation of these responses, as will CNS impairments.

As described in Chapter 1, the motor pattern has replaced the reflex as the basic functional unit of neuromotor organization. Motor patterns can be elicited by sensory stimuli or by internal processes within the CNS. Descriptions of postural responses in this chapter refer not only to patterns of movement that result because of imposed changes in position of the body, but also to movement patterns that may be initiated by the child in the context of functional motor behaviors.

Initially, a child develops righting reactions which allow him to orient his head in space so the eyes and mouth remain in a horizontal plane regardless of the body's position. The righting reactions assist in restoring the body alignment to a neutral anatomical position when segments of the body are rotated. As righting reactions fully develop in a particular posture, the protective reactions emerge in that posture. [3,4] Protective reactions generally are extension movements of the extremities in the same direction as the displacing force. Depending on the child's position, there can be extension of one or both arms or legs. Generally the extended limb should bear weight and "protect" the body from falling.

As protective reactions develop in a position, equilibrium reactions emerge in that position. [3,4] Equilibrium reactions counteract an opposing force and attempt to maintain a stable posture over the base of support. When an equilibrium reaction fails, a protective reaction should occur.

Postural reactions are divided traditionally into three groups: righting, protective, and equilibrium or balancing reactions. They each will be reviewed. They should not, however, be considered separate, distinct entities, because they are interdependent and represent interactive subsystems.

RIGHTING REACTIONS

Righting reactions orient the head in space so that the eyes and mouth are in a horizontal plane or the body parts are restored to a normal alignment following rotation. They allow us to right from any position in space. Righting reactions have been classified according to the receptor stimulated, the proposed regulating area of the brain, or the response given. Righting reactions depend on a number of different stimuli and receptors to function, including visual, vestibular, and somatosensory. The righting reactions can be divided into two separate groups: vertical righting and rotational righting reactions. Both types of righting reactions develop simultaneously.

VERTICAL RIGHTING REACTIONS

The ability to orient the head to vertical should be present in a number of different positions. If a child is held upright and tilted 30 to 45 degrees in a lateral, anterior, or posterior direction (Figure 1), alignment of the head to vertical with the mouth horizontal is the expected response. Maintaining the head in alignment with the body is a partial response. The stimuli are mainly visual and vestibular with some somatosensory and perhaps cognitive input. The child should be able to right his head by 2.5 to 6 months of age. [3,5-7] Visual input can be occluded by blindfolding, therefore providing only vestibular and somatosensory input. The head should still right to vertical. This response also has been called labyrinthine righting. [6]

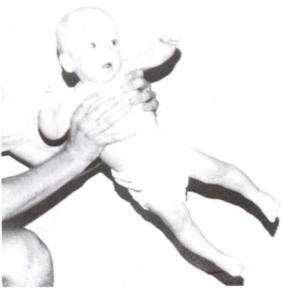

FIGURE 1. *Vertical neck righting reaction in infant when suspended upright and tilted laterally.*

Vertical righting reactions in prone occur when the child extends his head. These are present by 1.5 to 4 months of age (Figure 2). [3,5,8,9] Lifting the head to 45 degrees is considered a partial response. Capital hyperextension is seen frequently in the child with neurologic dysfunction. A normal child develops head extension in prone and then develops additional trunk and extremity extension. By 3 to 10 months of age, the child should be able to extend his entire trunk and pelvis when suspended in prone so an upward concavity is observed. [5,8] This posture frequently is called the Landau reaction, however, Milani-Comparetti and Gidoni termed the response "body in sagittal plane". [5] The development and presence of vertical righting in prone is an excellent example of the complex interactions of multiple subsystems required for an infant to display a response. By six months of age, an infant has the cognitive ability to

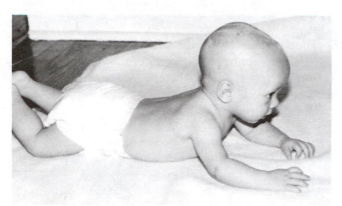

FIGURE 2. Head righting reaction in prone position.

cooperate in this movement . If the infant is unhappy or tired, he can overcome the physiological input and choose not to extend. An overweight infant may not have the muscle force production needed to volitionally lift his body against gravity. In a comprehensive study of 51 low risk infants, Touwen found the Landau response was highly inconsistent and a definite developmental sequence could not be established.[8]

In supine, a righting reaction also can be observed. The child should lift his head from the supporting surface by 5 months of age (Figure 3).[5] This is not a frequent, spontaneous activity and gently pulling the child up to sitting and observing for chin tuck may be necessary for testing.[3] Haley reported that, when testing in this manner, a complete chin tuck throughout the entire movement to sitting did not occur in a sample of normal infants until 8 to 10 months of age.[3]

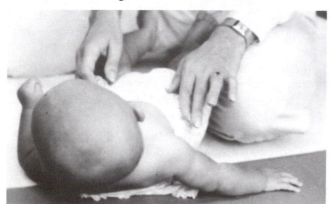

FIGURE 3. Head righting reaction seen in the supine position.

Head righting also should be present in sidelying and other positions. If the infant can sit or stand with proper head position, it can be assumed the righting reactions have developed to allow for these more mature positions. In fact, once the infant can freely sit or stand, he consciously may choose to suppress the righting reactions in any position.

When testing righting reactions, a consistent degree and speed of tilt, and length of time allowed for a response should be used. Unfortunately, little information is in the literature to indicate optimal speed for providing the stimulus or time needed for a response. The impact of behavior and attentiveness also must be considered.

ROTATIONAL RIGHTING REACTIONS

The rotational righting reactions[10] or body righting reactions[11] have many different, confusing, and contradictory names. It is, therefore, best to describe the stimulus and response to avoid misleading terminology. The rotational righting reactions restore the body parts to normal alignment following rotation of some body segment. In the neonate, when the head* is turned or the leg+ is flexed and adducted, the infant rotates like a log, nonsegmentally. This nonsegmental roll can be seen as late as 6[6] to 12[12] months of age, after which it is considered an immature response. A mature response occurs when the head‡ is turned or leg§ is flexed and adducted, and the child rolls showing distinct rotation between the pelvis and shoulder girdle with head and trunk rotation around the central body axis. The stimulus for the rotational righting reactions is somatosensory, due to asymmetrical body contact, joint proprioception, and muscle stretch. As the head is turned, there are also vestibular and visual inputs.

---

* A log roll in response to head turning has been called the neck righting reflex of the body,[6,12] and neonatal neck righting.[11]

+ A log roll in response to leg turning has been called the body righting reflex of the head[12] and neonatal body righting.

‡ A segmental roll in response to head turning has been called neck righting acting on the body[15] and body righting acting on the body.[6]

§ A segmental roll in response to leg turning has been called body righting acting on the head,[11] body derotating,[5] and rotation in trunk.[27]

PROTECTIVE REACTIONS

Protective reactions, also called parachute[5] or propping reactions,[13] consist of extension movements of the extremities generally in the same direction of a displacing force which shifts the body's center of mass past the limits of stability. They can be facilitated by vestibular input caused by movement in space, somatosensory input to the weight bearing skin surfaces or changes in joint angles, and visual or auditory input from the impending displacing force.

Protective reactions can be elicited in many different positions. If the child's body is thrust downward, feet first from the upright vertical position, leg extension and abduction are expected by 4 months of age.[5] If adduction and internal rotation occur, a pathological condition is suspected. When a child is moved forward toward the ground in a head first position, arm extension and abduction should result by 6 to 7 months of age (Figure 4).[5,6] Horizontal linear acceleration, as experienced on a scooter board, also can produce protective extension in the extremities.

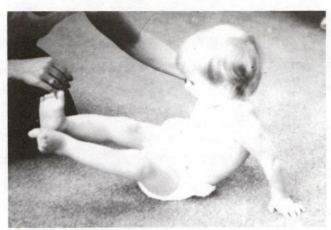

FIGURE 5. Backward protective reaction noted in sitting.

reaction might occur instead of a protective reaction. If the speed of the force is too rapid and there is not enough time for a protective response, a fall will occur. Too slow a force may result in an equilibrium reaction or a conscious decision that a protective response is not necessary. Facilitating a protective reaction in a child who has already developed equilibrium reactions is difficult. He will use equilibrium movements initially and only may display a protective reaction when pushed past the limits of stability. Protective reactions are highly context dependent.

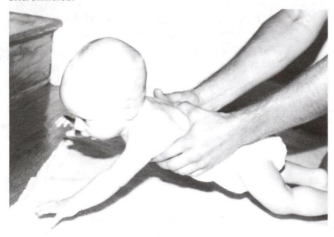

FIGURE 4. Protective reaction when infant is moved forward towards the ground.

In sitting, a child can be pushed gently in all directions to facilitate protective reactions of the arms. The sequence of observation of the protective reactions in sitting is experience and context dependent. Recent information suggests they develop laterally or sideways by age 6 to 11 months[3,5,8] then forwards,[3] and finally backwards by 9[5] to 12 months of age (Figure 5).[14] A study by Touwen indicated that lateral protective reactions improved along with a parallel increase in sitting duration.[8]

Critical to the facilitation of a protective reaction is the amount, speed, and point of application of the force and the child's anticipation. If the force is applied at the shoulders, less force is needed to shift the center of mass than if applied at the pelvis. If the child anticipates the stimulus, he may prepare his body and an equilibrium

EQUILIBRIUM REACTIONS AND BALANCE

As with righting and protective reactions, numerous terms have been used to describe the ability of an individual to maintain his upright posture when his center of mass is shifted, either due to a push, pull, tilt, or perturbation. Further complicating the definition of equilibrium reactions is a distinction between shifts of posture on a stable or unstable base of support. The terms postural fixation[15] or balance[15] have been used to describe reactions on a stable based support, where the body moves over the support surface. Equilibrium reactions[3], tilting reactions[5], and balance[15] are used to describe movements on an unstable base of support such as a tilt board, ball, foam rubber surface[16], or moving platform[17], where the supporting surface moves under the body.

When the body's center of mass is shifted or displaced on either a stable or unstable base of support, the muscular response can be invisible, detected only by palpation or electromyography (EMG). There may be an observable countermovement of the head, neck, trunk, or extremities. The movement is generally in a direction opposite the opposing force, unlike protective reactions which are in the same direction as the force. When pushed or tilted laterally, the observable responses can include a spinal concavity on the side pushed or elevated. Rotation of the upper trunk and head toward midline and counter-rotation of the lower trunk may occur.[10] Extension and abduction of the extremities on the elevated side or side being pushed may occur to help bring the body alignment back to center. Abduction and extension of the extremities on the depressed side or in the direction of a push also might occur in preparation for a protective reaction if the limits of stability are surpassed. When pushed or tilted forward so the anterior support surface is lowered, extension of the legs and trunk occur. When pushed or tilted in a posterior direction, hip and trunk flexion occurs. The amount of flexion or extension will depend on numerous factors such as the position of the child, the amount of sensory input, and the ability of the child to respond.

To test equilibrium reactions on a stable base of support, the child is pushed gently. The amount of force is critical since a rapid push which puts the center of mass beyond the body's limits of stability will produce a protective reaction or fall. Observation of counter movements and muscle palpation determine if subtle responses are occurring.

Equilibrium reactions can be tested on an unstable base of support, such as a lap, chair, ball, vestibular board, or moving platform. A vestibular board, with blocks limiting the degree of tilt, provides more standardization as does moving platform posturography[16]. Speed of tilt and length of time allowed for a response are important variables. Equilibrium reactions should not be tested only in the cardinal planes of motion, but also in the functionally important diagonal planes which should result in rotational responses.

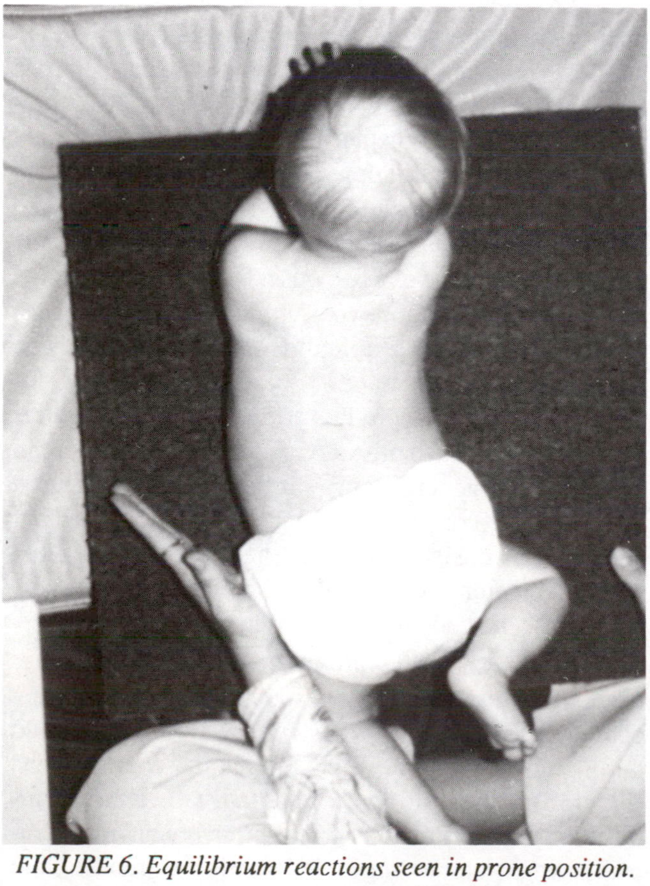

Equilibrium reactions develop in a position after the child learns to assume that position independently.[4,18] Generally equilibrium reactions develop on a stable base of support before an unstable base of support in that position. Equilibrium reactions usually occur first in prone (5 to 9 months) (Figure 6), then supine (7 to 11 months), sitting (7 to 8 months) (Figure 7), quadruped (8 to 12 months), and standing (12 to 21 months).[3,5] Haley suggested equilibrium reactions in sitting might occur before those in prone and supine.[3] The age of achievement of these reactions is related to the achievement of motoric skills in that position and interaction with the environment, therefore, variability can be expected.[4,19]

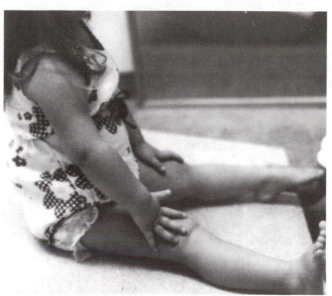

FIGURE 7. Equilibrium reactions seen in sitting position.

A number of recent studies have investigated the effect of different and varying sensory inputs on equilibrium reactions. Nashner and colleagues found that in adults and children over 7 years of age, while standing, the primary source of postural stability was somatosensory input. The vestibular and visual systems were secondary monitors of postural stability with a major role in resolving sensory conflict. Under conditions of sensory conflict, the vestibular system generally predominated.[20] In children under 7 years of age, the visual system was dominant in maintaining postural control.[21-23] It has been proposed that, in young children, the proprioceptors provide only "rudimentary and imprecise information"[22] and that practice is necessary to fine tune the somatosensory system. Forssberg and Nashner suggested that vestibular responses in young children are immature due to either the receptor apparatus or higher central nervous system centers.[21] Thus, the visual system predominates until other systems mature and sensory integration occurs.[21,24]

FIGURE 6. Equilibrium reactions seen in prone position.

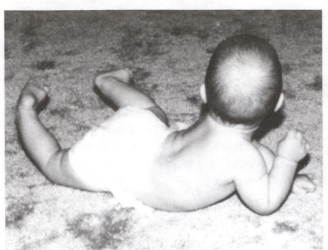

FIGURE 8. Equilibrium reaction during functional activity of rolling.

During 4 to 6 years of age, somatosensory inputs gain greater importance. It is during this time span that variability of postural responses is seen, as transition to the adult pattern of postural control occurs.[23]

In children and adults, there is a pattern or synergy of muscle activation in response to movement of the base of support in standing. The distal leg muscles activate before the proximal muscles[21,23] with the pattern described as a reverse pendulum.[20] The muscular responses are larger in amplitude and longer in duration in children than adults.[21,23] In standing, when there are small movements in the support surface, the ankle muscles activate to maintain the body upright. This is termed an ankle strategy. When there are large, fast movements of the support surface or when the support surface is very narrow, as when standing on a balance beam or small step, the hip muscles respond. If this hip strategy is insufficient to maintain upright posture, a stepping reaction occurs.

Children having Down syndrome appear to respond in a manner similar to normal children. They have, however, slower onset latencies[24] and develop postural reactions later than normal children.[18,25] The association between postural reactions and motor milestone achievement is similar for normal infants and those having Down syndrome.[18] Children with different types of cerebral palsy generally do not have postural responses comparable to normal children. Their problems in postural control may be due to delay or disruption of normal development of central sensory or motor organizing mechanisms or due to disruption of peripheral sensory inputs.[26] Investigations are revealing the wide range and variability of characteristics of responses in children with cerebral palsy.[26]

ASSESSMENT OF POSTURAL REACTIONS AND BALANCE

In order to elicit a postural reaction, we generally stimulate the visual, vestibular, and/or somatosensory systems. To occlude the visual system, a child can be blindfolded. Unfortunately, especially with a young child, blindfolding can lead to a change in behavioral state and cooperation.[4] Instead of blindfolding, visual input can be reduced by testing in a darkened room, drawing the child's attention to a toy,[8] or using testing equipment that provides a stable visual surrounding.[21,23-26] Without sophisticated equipment, vestibular or somatosensory stimuli can not be eliminated. Vestibular input, however, can be limited by decreasing the amount of head movement and avoiding rapid accelerations, decelerations, or stops. Somatosensory input can be decreased slightly by placing the child on foam rubber pads.[19] As discussed previously, it is important to be consistent in the force, amount of tilt, or speed used to elicit a response.

The somatosensory system should be evaluated to determine if all its many components are functioning properly. Are vibration and joint perception in the feet and legs intact? Does the child have proper eye/head stabilization? Does the child have the motor planning skills necessary to reach out and protect himself when pushed by a playmate, or use the correct strategy when stepping onto a moving walkway?

To provide more objective assessment, a number of measurement tools have been developed.[5-7,9,16,27,28] Discussion of several assessment tools which include evaluation of postural reactions and movement are presented in Chapter 2. Whether using a published assessment tool or an individually developed tool, consistency and standardization of testing and grading procedures are imperative. The easiest grading system indicates the presence or absence of a response. Due to the limitations of a simple dichotomous (present/absent) system, grading systems describing variations of responses have been developed. The Movement Assessment of Infants, for example, has specific grading criteria for four categories of responses for each postural reaction.[27] At a minimum, the following general four point scale should be used when grading a response: present or normal, present but abnormal, inconsistent or partial, and absent. In addition, subjective comments should be included regarding the responses, antecedents, and consequences.

Finally, because we are interested in how postural reactions are used in active movement, an important component of assessment is observation of the child during independent movement in natural environments (Figure 8). Is the child able to maintain balance in various positions and during transitions of movement in quadruped, sitting, and standing? If balance is lost, can the child regain his equilibrium? Are protective reactions used appropriately and efficiently?

When assessing postural reactions, it is difficult for one therapist to simultaneously stimulate the child, objectively grade, and then record the response. Stimulating the same response several times for observation has the negative outcome of habituation, fatigue, and decreased cooperation. Ideally, assessments should be videotaped. Videotapes provide a permanent record of the child's responses which can be replayed and objectively graded by independent observers. Videotaping also allows for determination of the strategy a child is using for equilibrium reactions. If it is not possible to videotape, it is preferable to have two therapists present during the evaluation. One can elicit the reactions while the other grades and records the responses.

The child's emotional state should be considered during any assessment. An active alert state is best for testing. The cognitive capabilities and degree of cooperation of the child should be considered. A child may refuse to display a postural reaction. The inability to perform a movement must be distinguished from a refusal. A child also might be habituated to the activity so it becomes a game and the desired response, although neurologically within the child's capability, is suppressed. This is seen frequently when the backwards protective reaction is facilitated in sitting. The child may consider it a game to be pushed and to fall backwards, confident of being caught by the therapist.

Musculoskeletal components should be evaluated to determine if the child has adequate range of motion to perform the movement. Lateral trunk mobility is necessary for lateral equilibrium reactions in all positions. Sufficient hip, knee, and ankle mobility are necessary for appropriate balance strategies in standing to overcome anterior, posterior, or lateral displacements. Shoulder flexion, extension, and abduction as well as elbow and wrist extension are necessary for functional protective reactions. Trunk and extremity muscle force production must be sufficient to overcome gravity and environmental perturbations.

TREATMENT RECOMMENDATIONS

After a careful assessment and evaluation of the child's postural reactions and movement, a program specific to the child's needs should be developed. Treatment of postural reactions cannot be done in isolation and must be compatible with all areas of motor development.

The ultimate goal in activating postural reactions is to have an automatic response. Maintaining stability and responding to environmental stimuli require a speed of execution above voluntary reaction times.[24] Although initially a conscious approach might be used to learn a postural reaction or to activate a muscle group, coordinated, mature postural reactions will not occur until they are automatic and do not require conscious control.

Generally it is best to start intervention at a point where the child will have some success and where you believe reinforcement of specific reactions or movements might be necessary. Methods of eliciting postural reactions and control are limited only by the therapist's imagination. The consistency required for objective assessment make for dull, functionless intervention. Creativity is necessary in treatment to encourage child participation. Remember to praise or reward the child for hard work and correct responses, but be judicious with praise since most children know when they really have worked hard or correctly. Constant praise also may be deleterious to motor learning (see Chapter 3).

There are many ways to organize treatment . Levels of response competence used by educators are well suited for physical therapy.[29] Initially there is acquisition of the skill or behavior. This is followed by fluency or proficiency in that skill or behavior. Fluency makes a behavior more functional. The skill or behavior then must be maintained in a phase labeled maintenance. This is followed by the very important level of generalization of the skill or behavior. Generalization includes not only generalization to different environments such as the home and classroom, but also generalization to different trainers, therapists or teachers, and different cues, materials, formats, or stimuli. (Table 1)

When working on acquisition of postural reactions or control, a number of issues must be considered. Will you practice the target behavior? If you do, how frequently will you practice it? Will you use massed or distributed practice? How often will you provide the child with knowledge of the results of their response, if not clearly evident? Will you tell the child what you are doing and direct him in performing the desired response? If you do, you are using a cognitive processing approach. A cognitive approach will not lead directly to a fully functional response since the speed of execution is slower than is necessary for an automatic, involuntary postural response. However, attention to task may be essential initially for motor learning.

When practicing the target behavior, you must decide whether you will vary the environments or materials used if variety will help later with generalization of the response. It is not yet known whether it is best to first acquire the response under the same conditions and to later program for generalization.

Your evaluation should indicate what other problems to address in your treatment program. For example, is the child deconditioned? Deconditioning is present frequently in children with chronic health problems or after recovery from long illnesses or surgery. A reconditioning program similar to that used for any deconditioned child should be implemented.

TABLE 1

LEVELS OF RESPONSE COMPETENCY

Level	Example
Acquisition	Child learns to sit independently.
Fluency/Proficiency	Child can reach for a toy while sitting and not fall over. If he does fall, he will have protective extension.
Maintenance	Child can still sit one week after initially learning to sit.
Generalization	
Generalization of environment	Child can sit on the floor in the therapy department and on the floor at home.
Generalization of trainer	Child will sit when placed by father or therapist.
Generalization of materials or stimuli	Child will sit on a hard wood floor or a carpet and not fall over when gently pushed.

Therapeutic Exercise In Developmental Disabilities

Are there musculoskeletal problems? If there are, these need to be addressed. Range of motion must be adequate to allow the desired response to occur. Shoulder flexion, extension, and abduction, as well as elbow, wrist and finger extension are necessary for upper extremity protective extension. Hip flexion and extension, knee extension, and ankle dorsi and plantar flexion are needed for appropriate hip or ankle strategies in standing. The child must have sufficient muscle strength to resist the forces of gravity and environmental perturbations. Weak muscles should be strengthened within the context of functional skills.

The treatment program must consider sensory impairments and inappropriate or insufficient use of the sensory systems. Some children rely solely on the visual system. While this might be functional under some situations, it can not be relied on for optimal postural control, especially under conditions of sensory conflict or darkness. To decrease visual input, you might blindfold a cooperative child, use a head dome[16], or decrease the light in the room. Proprioception can be decreased by placing the child on a foam surface. Eye-head coordination might be improved by exercises to encourage visual tracking with the head stable, and visual fixation on a stable object while moving the head first slowly and then rapidly.[16,19]

Motor planning and coordination are also important components of postural reactions and control. The child should learn to slowly and then rapidly shift his base of support in all directions in sitting, quadruped, and standing. After he can independently do this, the movement should be imposed on him by an outside source such as a push or a tilt. Reaching for toys just out of reach or hitting a ball suspended from the ceiling are fun ways to encourage protective extension or balance. The child may have to be taught how to coordinate a hip or ankle strategy while standing on various surfaces. Sophisticated equipment is available to assist in motor planning activities related to balance and equilibrium. Some of this equipment is calibrated for the light weights of young children, others are not.

In conclusion, treatment of children with deficits in postural control and balance is very complex. Multiple systems are involved and each system may need to be treated directly and then as part of an interaction of several systems to achieve an automatic, coordinated, functional response.

Case Studies

Case No. 1 — Jason
Cerebral Palsy, Right Hemiparesis, 18 Months
Assessment Of Postural Reactions

Righting Reactions: Jason rights his head in all planes and displays rotational righting reactions in all directions when moved passively and during active movement.

Protective Reactions: In sitting, Jason has left anterior, lateral, and posterior protective reactions in response to tilt. The right arm initiates movement forward and sideward, but without full extension and weight bearing. There is no right protective response backward.

Equilibrium Reactions: When laterally pushed on stable base of support in prone and supine, a trunk response is present to either side. In sitting, when pushed in an anterior or posterior direction or toward the right, a trunk response is present. When pushed toward the left, or when rotation is required, the trunk musculature does not respond adequately. In standing, when displaced in any direction, the left musculature responds, but even mild displacement cannot be counteracted and Jason will use a protective stepping reaction when possible or fall. When tilted on an unstable base of support in prone and supine, the trunk response is adequate on the left and partially present on the right. In sitting, when tilted in an anterior or posterior direction or toward the right (right side is down) the response is present, although delayed. It is absent when tilted toward the left and if rotation is required. Jason cannot stand on the tilt board independently.

General Goal: Jason will display protective reactions when pushed over in sitting by his twin brother and during active movement when balance is lost.

Short Term Objectives:
1. When Jason creeps he will extend the right elbow to -5 degrees, 80% of the time.
2. Jason will extend the right arm and weight bear on it 80% of the time when pushed forward or to the right side in sitting.
3. Jason will extend the right arm and weight bear on it 80% of the time when pushed backwards in sitting.
4. Jason will display a protective reaction of the right arm when he loses his balance and falls to the right when walking.

Treatment Procedures: Initial preparation before working on the specific objectives might include trunk relaxation activities by placing Jason in sidelying and gently rotating the pelvis and shoulders in opposite directions. He also could be placed in supine with hips and knees flexed and his legs rotated from side to side. In quadruped Jason should be encouraged to weight bear equally on both extended arms. He should weight shift onto the right arm and reach for a toy with the left arm. Proper creeping posture should be encouraged.

While sitting on the floor, Jason should bear weight equally on both ischial tuberosities. Work on reaching activities emphasizing the right arm and trunk rotation. The deltoid, triceps, and wrist extensors can be facilitated using tapping. Ask Jason to place the right hand on hand prints placed in a forward, lateral, and eventually posterior direction on the floor and encourage weight bearing with elbow extension. Then, gently push Jason in various directions helping with arm extension as necessary, progressing to less assistance and more rapid and forceful pushes. Initially provide verbal instruction. After he has acquired the ability to protect himself when instructed, surprise him with a push or have him reach outside his base of support so that he falls to the right.

General Goal: Jason will display equilibrium reactions on his right side when pushed toward the left or in a diagonal direction, when sitting or standing on a stable surface.

Short Term Objectives:

1. Jason will display an equilibrium reaction in sitting 80% of the time when reaching for a toy towards the left at his limits of stability.
2. Jason will display an equilibrium reaction in sitting 80% of the time when reaching for a toy diagonally toward the left in an anterior or posterior direction at his limits of stability.
3. Jason will display equilibrium reaction in standing at all times when pushed toward the right side by his twin brother.
4. Jason will display an equilibrium reaction in standing at all times when pushed toward the left side by his twin brother.
5. Jason will display an ankle strategy when standing and reaching forward for a toy at all times.

General Goal: Jason will display an equilibrium reaction on his right side when tilted with the left side down 20 degrees while sitting on an unstable surface.

Short Term Objectives:

1. Jason will display an equilibrium reaction 100% of the time when slowly tilted with the left side down 20 degrees when sitting on a rocking dome.
2. Jason will display an equilibrium reaction 80% of the time when rapidly tilted with the left side down 20 degrees when sitting on a rocking dome.
3. Jason will display an equilibrium reaction, or if necessary a protective reaction, all of the time when crawling on and off furniture.

Treatment Procedures: The initial preparation for the second and third Goals could be the same as in the first Goal. After initial preparation, activities encouraging eccentric and concentric contraction of the right trunk musculature should be attempted. These include placing Jason in prone and supine on a vestibular board and tilting it at greater speeds than usual, playing "Row, Row, Row Your Boat," or reaching up to the left or right for a favorite toy which is suspended with theraband to provide resistance. In sitting, slowly elevate Jason's legs or move a car under his raised leg, so minimal equilibrium responses are required. Getting on and off furniture should first be done with low set pieces progressing to standard height furniture. Activities specific to improving equilibrium on an unstable base might include prone on a scooter, prone or sitting on a swing, and use of a vestibular board, therapy ball, or see-saw.

Since Jason has tight right hip and lateral trunk flexors, active right hip extension and lateral trunk flexion to the left should be encouraged. "Swimming" prone over a bolster or reaching for a suspended toy with the left arm while sidelying on the right can be tried. His toes could be painted or puppets placed on his right foot to encourage active dorsiflexion as preparation for learning an ankle strategy in standing. In standing, Jason can practice reaching forward for a toy, first flexing at the hips and progressing to flexing only at the ankles.

CASE NO. 2 — JILL
Cerebral Palsy, Spastic Quadriparesis
Mental Retardation, 7 Years
Assessment Of Postural Reactions

Righting Reactions: Jill can maintain her head in neutral when held vertical. However, she cannot right her head when tilted in an anterior, posterior, or lateral direction. Jill can raise her head momentarily in prone, but not in supine. Head extension with rotation in prone results in a log roll.

Protective Reactions: These reactions are not present in response to imposed or volitional movement.

Equilibrium Reactions: These reactions are not present in response to imposed or volitional movement.

General Goal: Jill will be able to right and maintain her head in vertical in response to changes in her center of mass.

Short Term Objectives:

1. Jill will be able to maintain her head in a vertical position for one minute with capital flexion when placed while in supported sitting.
2. Jill will be able to right her head to a vertical position 80% of the time when tilted slowly 45 degrees to the left or right.
3. Jill will be able to right her head to a vertical position 80% of the time when tilted slowly 45 degrees forward.
4. Jill will be able to right her head to a vertical position 80% of the time when tilted slowly 45 degrees backwards.
5. Jill will be able to right and maintain her head in vertical when being lifted or carried.

No objectives with regard to protective or equilibrium reactions are presented for Jill at this time due to her severe motor deficits.

Treatment Procedures: The initial treatment of Jill would involve relaxation to achieve complete cervical range of motion. Gentle rocking, swinging on a swing, and soft music might be used. She could be placed astride the therapist's lap, and while proper support given to the trunk, a vertical head position and active contraction of the cervical muscles can be encouraged. She could be placed in prone and encouraged to lift and turn her head from side to side, avoiding capital hyperextension. In supine, she can be pulled gently to sitting. If she cannot initiate or maintain head flexion, work at the end of the range near sitting, where gravity offers less resistance. Slowly moving in a small arc of motion in supported sitting will encourage both concentric and eccentric muscle contractions. In supported sitting, either in a chair, rocking chair, or on the therapist's lap, Jill can be tilted from side to side and forward and back. It is best to start with 5 to 10 degrees of slow tilt, giving adequate time for a response. If no response occurs, Jill's head could be positioned and a holding contraction required. Once she can right her head following 5 to 10 degrees tilt, then progress slowly to larger degrees of tilt and more rapid movement. Make the activities fun and meaningful by having her look out a window or in a mirror when she is vertical.

CASE NO. 3 — TAYLOR
Myelomeningocele, Repaired, L 1-2, 4 Years
Assessment Of Postural Reactions

Righting Reactions: Taylor rights his head in all directions when tilted in vertical and during active movement . Rotational righting reactions are present when the head is used to facilitate a response, but not the legs.

Protective Reactions: All upper extremity protective reactions in sitting are present to passive tilt and during active movement. Standing reactions are not testable.

Equilibrium Reactions: In prone and supine, on a stable and unstable base of support, the upper trunk response is present. In sitting on stable and unstable bases of support, the upper trunk response is present, however, the quality of the response is poor. Taylor responds slowly and frequently has insufficient muscle strength or endurance to maintain an upright posture without reverting to a protective response. No equilibrium reactions were tested in standing.

General Goal: Taylor will have increased endurance and speed of response in his equilibrium reactions.

Short Term Objectives:

1. In 2 out of 3 trials, when Taylor reaches laterally to the limits of his base of stability for a toy, he will remain upright without using a protective reaction in sitting.
2. In 2 out of 3 trials, when Taylor reaches diagonally to the limits of his base of stability for a toy, he will remain upright without using a protective reaction in sitting.
3. Taylor will maintain an upright position when tilted in an anterior or posterior direction while playing on a see-saw.
4. In 2 out of 3 trials, Taylor will maintain an upright position in sitting when tilted 20 degrees laterally without using a protective reaction.

Treatment Procedures: Initial preparation might include active trunk extension in prone, upper trunk flexion in supine, and lateral flexion in sidelying. These antigravity movements will help increase muscular endurance of those muscles necessary for equilibrium reactions. Once Taylor can perform these antigravity movements, resistance can be added and diagonal patterns encouraged.

When placed in sitting, he should be encouraged to reach for toys placed on the floor and hung at ear level in an area around his body. When he reaches for a toy, provide resistance either by theraband attached to the hanging toys or using heavy toys on the floor. You also can push him gently in all directions making certain his center of gravity doesn't shift so much that he must use a protective reaction. Try pushing while he is holding onto a toy with both hands. Tilting reactions on an unstable base of support, such as a ball, should be done first in prone then supine to strengthen muscles involved. The amount of tilt and speed should be varied as would occur naturally in the environment. Taylor can be placed in sitting on your lap, a see-saw, an inverted dome, or a therapy ball and slowly tilted. In addition to anterior, posterior, and lateral tilting, diagonal tilting should be provided.

CASE NO. 4 — ASHLEY
Down Syndrome, 15 Months
Assessment Of Postural Reactions

Righting Reactions: All vertical and rotational reactions are present during passive tilt and active movement.

Protective Reactions: In sitting, Ashley has anterior and lateral responses, but an inconsistent response in a posterior direction to tilt and falling backwards.

Equilibrium Reactions: Equilibrium responses are present in prone and supine on a stable base of support. In sitting on a stable base of support, anterior and posterior responses are present, but lateral equilibrium responses are delayed and inconsistent. Quadruped on an unstable base of support could not be tested. No equilibrium reactions are present in standing.

Equilibrium responses are present on an unstable base of support in prone and supine and to anterior and posterior tilt in sitting. Lateral response to tilt in sitting is delayed and inconsistent. In quadruped on a stable base of support, Ashley can counteract minor displacements in anterior or posterior directions, but not laterally or diagonally.

General Goal: Ashley will develop all protective and equilibrium reactions in sitting and quadruped so she can sit without falling and can creep over and around objects safely.

Short Term Objectives:

1. In all trials, Ashley will display a posterior protective reaction in sitting when reaching backwards to get a toy just beyond her base of stability.

2. In all trials, Ashley will display a posterior protective reaction in sitting when pushed backwards in a diagonal direction by another child.

3. In 1 out of 2 trials, Ashley will display a lateral equilibrium reaction in sitting when reaching laterally for a toy.

4. In all trials, Ashley will display a lateral equilibrium reaction in sitting when pushed laterally on a stable base of support.

5. In all trials, Ashley will display lateral equilibrium reactions in sitting when tilted 20 degrees on an inverted play dome.

6. Ashley will be able to reach laterally for a toy while quadruped on the floor for one trial in each direction.

7. Ashley will be able to counteract a forward diagonal push in quadruped for one trial each to the right and left.

8. Ashley will be able to counteract a backward diagonal push in quadruped for one trial each to the right and left.

9. Ashley will be able to creep over a 4 inch high pillow on the floor.

Treatment Procedures: Ashley responds to vestibular input with more normal tone and stability, therefore, vestibular activities such as playing prone on a scooter board, swinging on a swing, or rocking in a rocking chair should be used. After initial sensory preparation, Ashley should be placed in sitting with a neutral to slightly posterior pelvic tilt. Her abdominal muscles could be tapped to facilitate their activity. In sitting, have her reach for toys laterally and posteriorly. In addition, she can be pushed gently laterally or her legs elevated to facilitate an equilibrium response. Equilibrium reactions on an unstable base of support can be done on a therapy ball, vestibular board, your lap, or a see-saw. Diagonal patterns with resultant trunk rotation should be emphasized. Fixation or rigid stabilizing postures of her legs should be discouraged, as should an extremely lordotic posture. Creeping over and around various objects should be encouraged as should reaching for toys placed at various heights while she is in quadruped. ❏

REFERENCES

1. VanSant AF: Motor control, motor learning, and motor development. In Montgomery PC, Connolly BH (eds): Motor Control and Physical Therapy. Hixson, TN, Chattanooga Corp., 1991, pp 13-30

2. Contemporary Management of Motor Control Problems, Proceedings of the II Step Conference. Lister M (ed): Alexandria, VA: Foundation for Physical Therapy, 1991

3. Haley SM: Sequential analysis of postural reactions in non-handicapped infants. Phys Ther 66:531-536, 1986

4. Bobath K: The Neurophysiological Basis for the Treatment of Cerebral Palsy, Clinics in Developmental Medicine, No. 75, Philadelphia, PA, JB Lippincott, 1980

5. Milani-Comparetti A, Gidoni EA: Routine developmental examination in normal and retarded children. Dev Med Child Neurol 9:631-638, 1967

6. Fiorentino MR: Reflex Testing Methods for Evaluating C.N.S. Development, ed 2. Springfield, IL, Charles C. Thomas, 1973

7. Bayley N: Bayley Scales of Infant Development. New York, NY, Psychological Corp, 1969

8. Touwen B: Neurological Development in Infancy, Clinics in Developmental Medicine, No. 58, Philadelphia, PA, JB Lippincott, 1976

9. Knobloch H: Manual of Developmental Diagnosis. New York, NY, Harper & Row, Publishers, 1980

10. Gilfoyle EM, Grady AP, Moore JC: Children Adapt. Thorofare, NJ, Charles B. Slack Inc., 1981, pp 57-77

11. Tower G: Selected developmental reflexes and reactions - A literature search. In Hopkins HL, Smith HD (eds): Willard and Spackman's Occupational Therapy, ed 6. Philadelphia, PA, Lippincott, 1983, pp 175-187

12. Peiper A: Cerebral Function in Infancy. New York, NY, Consultants Bureau, 1963, pp 156-210

13. Saint-Anne D'Argassies S: Neurodevelopmental symptoms during the first year of life. Dev Med Child Neurol 14:235-246, 1972

14. Coryell JF: Temporal Relationship Between Postural Reactions and Motor Milestones in 12 Month old Infants. Read at 1986 Annual Conference of the American Physical Therapy Association, Chicago, IL, June 8-12, 1986

15. Barnes MR, Crutchfield CA, Heriza CB, Herdman SJ: Reflex and Vestibular Aspects of Motor Control, Motor Development and Motor Learning. Atlanta, GA, Stokesville Publishing Co., 1990, pps. 379 & 451

16. Shumway-Cook A, Horak FB: Rehabilitation strategies for patients with vestibular deficits. Neurologic Clinics 8:441-457, 1990

17. Nashner L, Black FO, Wall C: Adaptation to altered support and visual conditions during stance: patients with vestibular deficits. J of Neuroscience, 2:536-44, 1982

18. Haley SM: Postural reactions in infants with Down syndrome. Phys Ther 66:17-22, 1986

19. Shumway-Cook A, McCollum G: Assessment and treatment of balance deficits. In PC Montgomery, BH Connolly (eds): Motor Control and Physical Therapy. Hixson, TN, Chattanooga Corp., 1991, pp 123-140

20. Nashner L: Analysis of stance posture in humans. In Towe AL, Luschei ES (eds): Handbook of Behavioral Neurobiology: Volume 5, Motor coordination. New York, NY, Plenum Press, 1981, pp 527-565

21. Forssberg H, Nashner L: Ontogenetic development of postural control in man: Adaptation to altered support and visual conditions during stance. J Neurosci 2:545-552, 1982

22. Lee DH, Aronson E: Visual proprioceptive control of standing in human infants. Perception and Psychophysics 15:529-532, 1974

23. Shumway-Cook A, Woollacott MH: The growth of stability: Postural control from a developmental perspective. J Motor Beh 17:131-147, 1985

24. Shumway-Cook A, Woollacott MH: Dynamics of postural control in the child with Down syndrome. Phys Ther 9:1315-1322, 1985

25. Effgen SK: An Analysis of the Effects of Visual and Somatosensory-Vestibular Input on the Postural Reactions of Infants Having Down Syndrome. Doctoral Dissertation, Atlanta, GA, Georgia State University, 1984

26. Nashner LM, Shumway-Cook, Marin O: Stance posture control in selected groups of children with cerebral palsy: Deficits in sensory organization and muscular coordination. Exp Brain Res 49:393-409, 1983

27. Chandler LS, Andrews MS, Swanson MW: Movement Assessment of Infants: A Manual. Rolling Bay, WA, Movement Assessment of Infants, 1980

28. Folio R, Fewell RR: Peabody Developmental Motor Scales and Activity Cards. Allen, TX, Teaching Resources, 1983

29. Alberto PA, Troutman AC: Applied Behavior Analysis for Teachers, ed 3. Columbus, OH, Merrill Publishing Co., 1990

CHAPTER 9

RESPIRATORY AND ORAL-MOTOR FUNCTIONING

Rona Alexander, Ph.D., CCC-SP

◆

Speech is a complex and highly sophisticated means by which information can be exchanged or communicated among individuals.[1] It requires the effective and efficient integration of a variety of features, including pitch, loudness, resonance, duration, vocal quality, articulation, rate, and rhythm. The integration of these features for proficient speech functioning has its foundation in the development of a basic motor control system. This motor control system is influenced by an extensive number of anatomical, physiological, kinesiological, neurological, neuromotor, sensory-motor, perceptual, acoustical, cognitive, and environmental factors.[2,3]

Speech cannot be viewed as a total reflection of a child's level of language functioning. As described by Bloom and Lahey, language consists of an element of content or meaning (i.e., semantics of a message).[4] Content or meaning is represented by a linguistic form (i.e., an expressive mode of communication used according to specific phonological, morphological, and syntactic rules). Language use or function is specific (i.e., the purpose of a message and the context of the utterance). As children interact in their environment, they develop a base of language competence which is the interaction of language content, form, and use. Although speech is significant because of its general acceptance as our primary form of expressive language, it must not be

equated with overall language competence. Speech should not be regarded as the only form in which knowledge can be communicated to others.

This chapter will present information specifically relevant to the assessment and treatment of oral-motor and respiratory-phonatory functioning because of their intricate relationship to and effect on general movement development. However, this emphasis should not negate the importance of assessment and treatment of receptive and expressive language functioning by a qualified speech-language pathologist when developing programming for children with developmental disabilities.

EARLY ORAL-MOTOR AND RESPIRATORY-PHONATORY FUNCTIONING

To understand the significance of oral-motor and respiratory-phonatory functioning in pediatric assessment and treatment, it is necessary to understand their role in normal development. From birth, the normal, full-term infant uses the oral, pharyngeal, laryngeal, esophageal, and respiratory mechanisms for feeding, breathing, crying, sound production, and sensory exploration. Liquids presented by bottle or breast are ingested using a negative-pressure sucking pattern. This sucking pattern is created by a combination of jaw, tongue, and cheek/lip movements. These movement patterns directly are related to the newborn's physiological flexion and small intra-oral space.[5] The newborn can breathe through the nose and suck simultaneously, since liquids are moved back over a cupped tongue and pass around the sides of the epiglottis directly into the esophagus. This process avoids the high-positioned laryngeal area which is protected by the hyoid bone, pharyngeal musculature, and the close approximation of the uvula and epiglottis (Figure 1).

Once the infant begins to turn and lift the head with neck extension against gravity, the influence of physiological flexion on the mouth is reduced, resulting in wider ranges of jaw and tongue activity. Suckling now becomes the active oral pattern of the infant and is composed of large up/down and forward/backward movements of the jaw and large, rhythmical, forward and backward movements of a thin, cupped tongue. Minimal muscle activity occurs in the cheeks and lips. Oral movements for sucking still will occur when the infant's head is held in a more stable flexed position by the feeder.

The newborn's respiratory functioning at rest is largely positional because the pharyngeal airway is kept open by the pharyngeal musculature. There is close approximation of the back of the tongue to the soft palate.[6] The rib cage is at almost a 90 degree angle to the spine and is limited in its active mobility (Figure 2). On inhalation, abdominal or belly breathing occurs as the diaphragm contracts and lowers causing expansion of the abdominal wall and lower ribs. With effortful crying, movement, or stress, strong contraction of the diaphragm may pull the anterior ribs and sternum downward and posterior while expanding the abdominal wall and pushing the lower ribs outward.

A direct relationship exists between sound production and body movement starting at birth. Sounds are produced spontaneously on expiration and crying is nasal in quality. Short duration and low intensity vegetative sounds are produced by the infant, especially during feeding.

The infant's development of more controlled movement against gravity throughout the first year of life establishes a basis on which more functional oral-motor, respiratory-phonatory, and sound production activity can be produced. Changes in oral-motor and respiratory-phonatory functioning also have a significant influence on general movement development. This is apparent in the development of well-controlled head and neck flexion, which depends on the active use of the suprahyoid and infrahyoid muscles that have primary control of jaw, tongue, and hyoid movements.[7]

Developmental changes in the respiratory system have a profound effect on general movement, as well as on oral-motor and respiratory-phonatory functioning. As the child of 4 to 6 months of age begins to use the abdominal musculature in supine and is held passively upright against gravity in sitting, the ribs are drawn downward, creating an angle between the ribs and spine of less than 90 degrees. This stabilization of the rib cage by the abdominals in a more downward direction will modify the anatomy of the rib cage. The intercostals and levator costarum then are prepared for future active use in more adult abdominal/thoracic respiratory functioning. Abdominal activities will provide the musculature of the head, neck, shoulder girdle, mouth, and pharynx with a base of stability from which more integrated, controlled movements can be developed.

Oral-motor development is affected by a variety of factors, including anatomical changes and growth; the introduction of new varieties of oral sensory stimulation (e.g., semi-solids, solids, toys); the child's active coordinated movement against gravity; and changes in the respiratory mechanism. The 6-month-old child reflects the interaction of these factors in use of the cheeks, lips, and tongue in bottle or breastfeeding for more active negative-pressure sucking. However, the wider range of movements which compose suckling continue to predominate in spoonfeeding and cupdrinking, facial expression, and sound production. Although solid foods generally will be handled using sucking or suckling movements, some new movements of the tongue and jaw may appear as a munching pattern develops. Sound production will modify to include a greater variety of vowels and consonants with changes in duration, loudness, intonation, and vocal quality.

By 12 months of age, the child has developed more highly coordinated general movement abilities. These skills provide an integrated neuromotor and sensory-motor foundation from which more precise oral-motor and respiratory-sound production coordination can be produced and developed. Movements of the jaw, tongue, cheeks, and lips for sucking, and fine coordination of these movements with breathing are now predominant in bottledrinking, breastfeeding, and spoonfeeding. Greater sucking activity is evident in cupdrinking, although excessive jaw activity is compensated for by use of tongue protrusion under the cup for stability. The tongue exhibits lateral movements as it transfers and maintains food on the sides of the mouth in coordination with cheek musculature activity inward for chewing. The jaw uses a variety of up and down, diagonal, and circular-diagonal movements as it breaks up the solid food in preparation for swallowing. More controlled abdominal/thoracic respiratory functioning and oral-pharyngeal functioning provide a foundation for long chains of sounds, with varying consonant-vowel combinations and occasional single word productions.

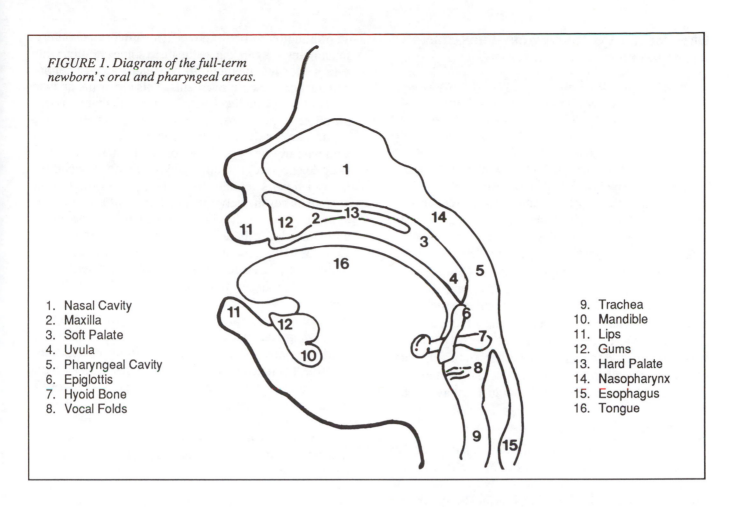

FIGURE 1. Diagram of the full-term newborn's oral and pharyngeal areas.

1. Nasal Cavity
2. Maxilla
3. Soft Palate
4. Uvula
5. Pharyngeal Cavity
6. Epiglottis
7. Hyoid Bone
8. Vocal Folds

9. Trachea
10. Mandible
11. Lips
12. Gums
13. Hard Palate
14. Nasopharynx
15. Esophagus
16. Tongue

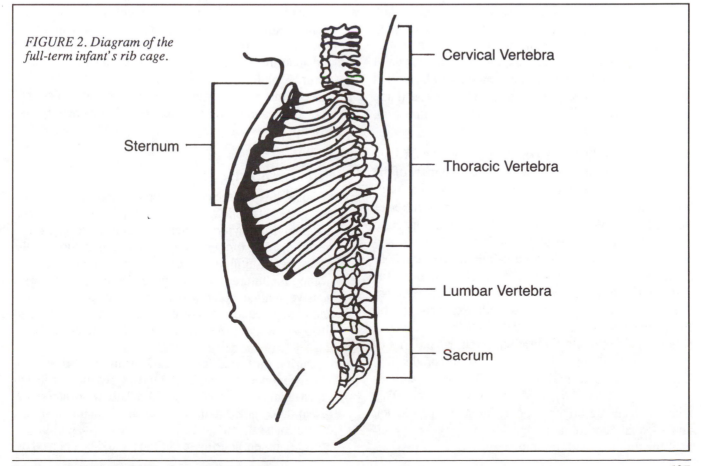

FIGURE 2. Diagram of the full-term infant's rib cage.

Cervical Vertebra

Sternum

Thoracic Vertebra

Lumbar Vertebra

Sacrum

ORAL-MOTOR AND RESPIRATORY-PHONATORY DYSFUNCTION

As is true in normal infants, infants with neuromotor involvement begin to function using the oral-motor and respiratory mechanisms at birth. The type and severity of their motor involvement, however, may result in abnormal extensor activity. Stability at the head, neck, mouth, and shoulder girdle may be provided through the use of abnormal head and neck hyperextension, tongue retraction (i.e., the pulling back and holding of the tongue body in a more posterior position in the oral mechanism), and humeral extension with adduction and internal rotation. With the head and neck in a hyperextended position, the cheeks and lips will be drawn back into retraction and the jaw will depress or thrust open and retract. Compensatory shoulder elevation and oral movements such as lip pursing (i.e., purse-string positioning of the lips and cheeks), tongue thrusting (i.e., strong forward pushing of a thickly bunched tongue), tongue retraction with anterior tongue elevation against the hard palate, jaw thrusting with protrusion, or exaggerated jaw closure may develop as the infant attempts to function in feeding, sound production, and general movement activities.

The infant may not be able to suck or suckle liquids efficiently from the bottle or breast due to cheek-lip and tongue retraction. He may be able only to swallow with strong head and neck hyperextension and tongue thrusting, which result in choking, coughing, or gagging. Jaw thrusting and exaggerated jaw closure may occur due to jaw instability whenever the nipple or spoon is presented. The variety of oral movements which the child can use for vowel and consonant sounds will be limited to those which can be produced when there is head and neck hyperextension, tongue retraction, jaw thrusting, and cheek-lip retraction.

Respiratory-phonatory coordination will be affected directly by abnormal or inadequate development of the head, neck, shoulder girdle, and extrinsic tongue musculature. Problems that may develop include prevention or restriction of active stability and mobility of the upper rib cage, active use of the abdominals in expiration, and active thoracic expansion for inhalation. Compensatory shoulder elevation and use of a shortened rectus abdominus for stability may result in severe retraction of the sternum and anterior ribs with excessive lateral flaring of the lower ribs on inhalation. This will influence abnormally the quality, duration, pitch, rhythm, loudness, and rate of phonation and early sound production. Immobility or deformities of the rib cage as well as immobility of the laryngeal area will develop. This restricts adequate breath support for sound production and adequate coordination between respiration, laryngeal functioning, and oral-motor activity.

Although early oral-motor and respiratory-phonatory functioning may appear adequate in some children with neuromotor involvement, there is generally an abnormal quality to their movements. This abnormal quality may interfere with the development of fine motor coordination required in activities such as chewing, cupdrinking, and speech. When abnormal lumbar extension with hip flexion, abduction, and external rotation (frog-leg posture) is maintained for abnormal stability, the hip flexors remain in a shortened position. This posture places the pelvis in an anterior tilt and does not allow for active abdominal muscle activity. Therefore, a shallow belly breathing pattern may be retained. Changes in the contour and alignment of the structures of the rib cage as well as activity of its musculature will be limited, giving the thoracic area a more barrel-shaped appearance. Longer, controlled exhalations for sound production and speech cannot be developed. If compensatory humeral extension with adduction is used to reinforce spinal extension in prone, sitting, or standing, additional compensations at the head, neck, and mouth may result which interfere with development of coordinated oral-motor control.

When adequate thoracic and lumbar extension and abdominal muscle activity do not develop, some children attempt to stabilize the trunk using the hip adductors and hamstrings. This may result in abnormal hip extension and adduction. To shift the center of gravity forward in sitting and standing, compensatory humeral extension with adduction, abnormal upper trunk flexion, and compensatory head and neck hyperextension are used. Limitations in the expansion of the upper thoracic area and abnormal contraction of the rectus abdominus may occur. Mobility of the ribs, sternum, and abdominal musculature for respiratory coordination with feeding, phonation, and sound production activities may be restricted.

INTERVENTION FRAMEWORK

Subsequent to the completion of a thorough clinical assessment of a child's oral-motor, respiratory-phonatory, and sound production function, recommendations are made regarding further testing and instrumentation. Oral-pharyngeal motility or videoswallow studies may be needed for future treatment programming. A comprehensive treatment plan will include delineation of goals and objectives for both direct patient treatment by the therapist and carryover activities such as mealtime feeding.

During mealtime feeding, the primary goal always will focus on nutritional intake and its presentation in the safest manner possible for the child. If there are any signs of aspiration noted in the clinical assessment, the introduction of new strategies (e.g., changes in positioning or body alignment) during mealtime should be delayed or

Therapeutic Exercise In Developmental Disabilities

limited. Further testing is essential to determine the relationship of head/neck/trunk alignment, food texture, and food presentation to the child's risk for aspiration before implementing a program change.

Direct patient treatment should improve function through active preparation and handling. These strategies are based on our knowledge of the normal and abnormal developmental process. Treatment must reflect our understanding of the relationship between general movement, oral-motor, and respiratory-phonatory development. We must recognize as well the importance of repetition for learning and our abilities to analyze the specific movements required for task accomplishment. Once specific objectives begin to be accomplished in direct treatment, they can be incorporated into carryover activities.

ASSESSMENT PROCEDURES

When assessing a child's oral-motor and respiratory-phonatory-sound production functioning, information should be obtained on the movements of the child's oral mechanism during feeding, sound production, and general movement. The quality and coordination of these oral movements and the effect of postural control, movement, and sensory stimulation on oral-motor and respiratory-phonatory-sound production functioning also should be assessed. In addition, the coordination of respiration with feeding, sound production, and general movement must be observed. The child's use of different modes of communication during movement, play, and feeding activities are important components of the assessment. This information is gathered through careful questioning of the parent or caregiver, observation of the child with the caregiver during various activities, and, when appropriate, direct testing by the evaluator. [8]

Analysis of the child's oral-motor and respiratory functioning during feeding activities is a significant part of the assessment. Questions should be posed to the caregiver to obtain information on feeding and respiratory history as well as on mealtime length, nutritional intake, preferred food textures, feeding utensils, positioning used, and the child's feeding activity. Such a judgment probably would be based on the child's nutritional intake and not actually on the quality of oral musculature activity.

Careful observation of the interactions of the caregiver and child, the procedures used, and the child's oral-motor and respiratory function during feeding is an essential component of the assessment process. Special emphasis should be placed on describing the initial position of the child for feeding and any changes that occur in this position over time. How food and liquid are presented, the child's response to these presentations, the oral movements used during feeding, and the coordination of respiration with oral movements also are noted.

After observing the child and caregiver, direct testing may be appropriate to analyze movements already observed or to try to modify functioning through changes in handling, positioning, food textures, or food presentation. Handling to stimulate more active anti-gravity postural control and movement may be provided to evaluate the child's potential for changes in oral-motor, respiratory-phonatory, sound production, and general communication functioning. Direct testing by the evaluator should be placed on obtaining maximum information through discussions with the parent or caregiver and observation of the caregiver and the child during general movement, feeding, and communication activities.

Recommendations made by the evaluator based on the findings of the clinical assessment generally pertain to additional evaluation consultations and instrumentation procedures needed as well as goals for treatment programming. If aspiration is suspected based on the child's history (e.g., chronic respiratory illnesses, frequent coughing, choking, or gagging during feeding, consistent wet, gurgly vocalizations, and increased respiratory distress during feeding), an oral-pharyngeal motility or videoswallow study should be conducted. These studies more directly evaluate if, when, and under what conditions aspiration occurs prior to implementing any changes in the child's feeding process. [9] Gastroesophageal reflex (GER) is the return flow of the stomach contents into the esophagus. GER may be suspected if the child has a history of excessive spitting-up or vomiting during or after meals, increased irritability after specific amounts of nutritional intake, poor weight gain, fussiness in regard to changes in food types or textures, or aspiration pneumonia. The child's primary physician should be contacted if GER is suspected for discussion of the possibility of further testing or referral for evaluation by a pediatric gastroenterologist. If GER exists, the child will be resistant to changes in food textures. This may limit the possibility of improving oral-motor function for feeding as well as the potential for increasing the child's nutritional intake for weight gain.

TREATMENT PROGRAMMING

Treatment to improve oral-motor function and respiratory-phonatory coordination must address goals and strategies which help the child develop the motor components required to more successfully use the oral, pharyngeal, laryngeal, esophageal, and respiratory mechanisms for feeding, crying, sound/speech production, and communication. Emphasis must be placed on developing functional activity of the cheeks, lips, tongue, and jaw as well as their coordination with respiration. Strategies for direct treatment services leading to progressive improvement in function may not be immediately incorporated into activities such as mealtime feeding if their use initially interferes with overall nutritional intake. Therefore, a well-coordinated program for improved function in both direct treatment and carryover activities should be designed.

Underlying all treatment for improved oral-motor function and respiratory-phonatory-sound production coordination is the developmental relationship between active movement in these areas and coordinated anti-gravity movement in general. Dynamic handling during direct treatment is necessary to facilitate more normal active movements of the head, neck, mouth, shoulder girdle, spine, rib cage, pelvis, and hips. Appropriate handling will lead to the development of active functional movements which can be repeated and generalized to a wide variety of activities. Proper body alignment through positioning may provide a base of central stability for better oral-motor, oral-pharyngeal, and respiratory functioning during carryover activities such as mealtime feeding. This alignment will not provide a foundation for the generalization of integration of these new movements to other activities (e.g., general movements, sound/speech production). Dynamic handling which facilitates the integration of active anti-gravity movements and proper body alignment through positioning plays an important role in the child's overall treatment program.

When problems with aspiration and GER do not exist, there are strategies that may be implemented during mealtime feeding to support the primary goal of nutritional intake. These strategies often include the establishment of proper positions for feeding, the modification of food textures and feeding utensils being used, and the incorporation of other methods or procedures for food presentation. There is not one piece of equipment or way to adapt equipment which is successful in establishing good feeding positions for all children. However, proper positioning for better function at mealtime requires good body alignment. This includes neutral head flexion with neck elongation; symmetrical, stable shoulder girdle depression with scapulo-humeral dissociation; and symmetrical trunk elongation. Also included are neutral positioning of a stable, symmetrical pelvis; hip stability with neutral abduction and rotation; and stable, symmetrical positioning of the feet flat on a surface (Figure 3). Any deviation from this central base of good body alignment due to physical deformity or inappropriate equipment will restrict the positive effects of positioning on function during mealtime.

Although proper positioning will have a significant effect on mealtime feeding, the wide variety of sensory experiences which occur during mealtime may continue to make feeding difficult. Thickened textures of food and liquid, rather than thin or pureed food and liquid, may provide sensory-motor information which stimulates more active oral-motor functioning.[10,11] The selection of appropriate feeding utensils can be essential

FIGURE 3. Examples of proper body positioning for improved oral-motor and respiratory functioning during mealtime.

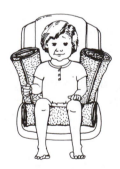

A. A young child positioned in a car seat with adaptations using towel rolls for feeding.

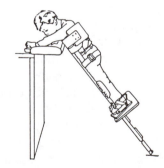

B. A young child positioned on a prone board in standing for mealtime.

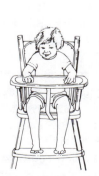

C. A child positioned in a high chair with adaptations for greater hip stability and symmetry during feeding.

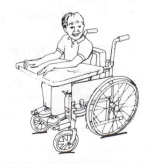

D. A child positioned in his wheel chair with an adapted seat insert, cut-out tray, and hip stabilizing straps for mealtime.

Therapeutic Exercise In Developmental Disabilities

to the encouragement of greater functional activity of the cheeks, lips, tongue, and jaw during mealtime. Examples are a narrow spoon that fits within the child's oral cavity without touching the side teeth or a small cup without a spouted-lid. The presentation of food and liquid by the feeder must be modified so that visual, auditory, and tactile input do not result in abnormal postures. Abnormal postures may reduce nutritional intake and restrict or limit oral activity and its coordination with respiration. Strategies directed toward mealtime feeding are important but narrow in focus. Strategies for direct treatment at times other than mealtime are of primary significance to the modification of overall oral-motor and respiratory-phonatory-sound production functioning. As function is modified through direct treatment, changes may be made in positioning and procedures used during mealtime for generalization of these new activities.

Preparation through handling is necessary for developing the motor components required for coordinated oral-motor and respiratory-phonatory functioning. Handling is combined with specific activities to facilitate the development of neutral head flexion with neck elongation (chin tuck position); stable shoulder girdle depression with scapulo-humeral mobility. Active rib cage mobility and stability with abdominal musculature activity are important. Additionally, handling should facilitate active lip closure, rounding, and spreading as well as active up and down, forward and backward, diagonal, and circular-rotary jaw movements in ways similar to those used in the normal developmental process. Special emphasis in treatment must be placed on handling which enhances respiratory coordination with oral function. Facilitation of active thoracic and lumbar spinal extension in supine, prone, and through transitional movements will help elongate shoulder girdle and abdominal musculature. This may lead to development of greater rib cage mobility and stability. As the child begins to sit and move in and out of sitting and standing, the abdominals actively hold the rib cage from below. This abdominal holding results in elongation of the musculature between each rib and between the ribs and spine. Thus, the rib cage can expand on inhalation and provide a foundation for longer controlled exhalation. This allows more adult abdominal/thoracic respiratory functioning. In addition, active shoulder girdle and rib cage mobility and stability, along with active abdominal musculature, provide a basis for coordinated oral-motor and oral-pharyngeal movement.

Modifying oral tactile sensitivity is another important aspect of treatment. Deep pressure tactile stimulation presented on the face and within the oral area can prepare the mouth for more normal sensory-motor activity. The effects of abnormal feedback the child has used to learn abnormal and compensatory oral movements may be diminished through the use of appropriate stimulation.

Deep pressure stroking on the face toward and through the lips helps to elongate cheek and lip musculature. The child then may be able to initiate more active cheek, lower lip, and upper lip movements. Subsequent presentation of cupdrinking, bottledrinking, spoonfeeding, or stimulation for bilabial sound production then is introduced. A consistent program of deep pressure rubbing on the biting surfaces of the gums or teeth can help reduce the occurrence of tonic bite. Tonic bite may occur in response to the presentation of the spoon, cup, bottle, the child's own fingers, toys, and solid foods.

The strength of the gag response and the range and quality of tongue movements in sucking and suckling activities can be modified. One technique is the use of rhythmical, well-graded downward and slightly forward, deep pressure stroking of the tongue body prior to feeding and sound production stimulation. This tactile input to the tongue also has a significant influence on respiratory function as well as the development of more coordinated head flexion and neck elongation.

Remember that there is a progression of motor components developed by the normal child. This progression leads to the efficient use of cheek, lip, jaw, and tongue movements and their coordination with respiration for feeding, crying, sound production, and speech. Treatment of oral-motor and respiratory-phonatory function must allow the child to develop functional skills based on knowledge of motor components or sequences required in the normal process. Strategies for direct treatment and carryover activities must be well-balanced and well-coordinated if the child is to function effectively and efficiently in the oral-motor, respiratory-phonatory, and speech areas.

CASE STUDIES

CASE NO. 1 — JASON
Cerebral Palsy, Right Hemiparesis, 18 Months

At rest, Jason exhibits subtle cheek/lip retraction on the right, an asymmetrical contour to his tongue, and a slight pull of his jaw laterally to the right. With general movement activities, cheek/lip retraction and lateral jaw deviation to the right increase with some asymmetry of the tongue evident. Drooling which increases with movement, especially walking, is noted from the right side of the mouth. Drooling often is noted in children with hemiparesis due to asymmetry in oral activity and poor sensory regard on the more involved side within the oral cavity.

Jason relies heavily on gestures and movement for communication. As with most children his age, he has a small number of real single words. His overall use of vocalizations and jargon with gestures for communication is limited, especially when he is ambulating. His vocalizations are nasal in quality and reveal minimal variety in intonation and inflectional patterns unlike what would be expected at his age.

Jason produces a variety of vowel sounds while his consonants are limited in quantity and have some distortions. He is unable to produce good quality lip activity for bilabial productions (m, b, p, w) due to his cheek/lip retraction.

Jason eats a variety of foods. He chews solids only on the left side of his mouth and uses his hand to move solids initially placed on the right to the left. His tongue lateralizes more to the left than the right. Jason uses his lips to surround the spoon for food removal, although with imprecise closure. Another sign of his lack of good sensory information is that food remains on the lips, especially on the right. When cupdrinking, Jason places the cup far back between his teeth and uses slight head/neck hyperextension to compensate for his cheek/lip retraction. He occasionally loses some liquid when the cup is removed. His lack of good tongue activity is revealed in the gulp-like quality of his swallowing.

Jason reveals some problems with coordination of breathing and oral activity. He gasps for breath after drinking a cup of liquid. His vocalizations are somewhat limited in length. He has some observable asymmetry of his rib cage with greater flattening of the upper thoracic area on the right. Rib flaring is evident revealing his lack of good, consistent use of abdominal musculature.

Jason's general treatment goals should include:
1. improved oral sensory awareness, especially to the cheeks, lips, and tongue on the right.
2. increased symmetrical activity of the cheeks and lips for lip closure and lip rounding.
3. increased symmetry and variety of tongue movements being used.
4. improved coordination of respiration with oral-motor activity.

Following treatment, Jason will be able to:
1. produce the consonant sound for "b" and "m" with good quality of lip closure in 4 of 8 attempts.
2. maintain good lip closure on the cup rim while drinking 4 ounces of liquid.
3. take 3-4 sips of liquid from a cup before pausing to breathe with no subsequent gasping noted, 2 of 4 times.
4. lateralize the tongue when solid food is placed on the right, 2 of 5 times.

Sample Activities

Initially, it is essential to facilitate active symmetrical flexion and extension, elongation and lateral flexion, and rotation through the rib cage and spine (see Chapter 7). While on a moveable surface, Jason is encouraged to play using transitional movements (e.g., supine to sidelying to sitting or prone to sidelying to sitting), while tactile input is presented to the rib cage and abdominals. Longer, more varied sound productions are stimulated

simultaneously through singing and other sound play activities.

Well-graded oral tactile stimulation emphasizing the cheeks and lips, biting surfaces of the teeth/gums, and tongue is presented. Following this stimulation, thickened liquid is presented by cup to be drawn into the mouth using the cheeks and lips. Pieces of crunchy cereal are placed on the biting surfaces of the teeth/gums, more often on the right, for chewing while encouraging active lateral tongue movements.

Case No. 2 — Jill
Cerebral Palsy, Spastic Quadriparesis, Mental Retardation, 7 Years

Jill uses head/neck hyperextension and tongue retraction with shoulder girdle evaluation in all her attempts to move, communicate, and eat. She has severe cheek/lip retraction and jaw thrusting with retraction, which probably began early as a consequence of the position of her head, neck, and tongue, but which now have become significant problems in themselves.

Her rib cage generally is immobile. The sternum is fixed in retraction by her shortened, tight rectus abdominus. Although the lower ribs appear flat in contour, the upper ribs appear rounded in the front and flat laterally. This appearance is due to restrictions placed on the ribs by her abnormal humeral extension/adduction/internal rotation. Jill has a shallow belly breathing pattern with retraction of the sternum and anterior ribs on inhalation. Greater retraction of the anterior rib cage is evident as she attempts to move, communicate, and eat. On inhalation, her rib cage expands laterally with severe flaring.

Jill sits in a wheelchair with adaptations for feeding. She continues to exhibit asymmetry, head/neck hyperextension, humeral extension/adduction/internal rotation, hip extension/adduction/internal rotation, and significant problems with coordinating her respiratory function in this position. Therefore, her body alignment in her adapted wheelchair does not provide an optimal foundation for oral-motor, oral-pharyngeal, and respiratory functioning.

While feeding, Jill remains in some degree of head/neck hyperextension with humeral extension/adduction/internal rotation and shoulder girdle elevation. Her tongue is thick in contour and retracted, with only a small range of forward and backward movement noted in spoonfeeding and cupdrinking. Cheek/lip retraction is noted during all feeding activities, although she attempts to compensate with lip pursing at the initiation of cupdrinking. Initially when food is presented, jaw thrusting with retraction occurs. She uses some exaggerated jaw closure on the spoon and cup rim for stability. Tongue thrusting is evident in the final part of the swallow of semisolids and liquids. Small horizontal shifts of the tongue are noted to the left with solid food presentation. Generally, Jill uses her head/neck hyperextension and small-range, suckling movements of the tongue to move food and liquid back for swallowing. Respiratory coordination during cupdrinking is poor with much coughing and choking. Jill has never had an oral-pharyngeal motility or videoswallow study to determine if she aspirates.

Jill attempts to say a few words such as "bye," "hi," and "mom." However, her attempts to say these words are greatly restricted by the excessive abnormal extension she uses to initiate sound.

Emphasis should not be placed on modifying Jill's oral-motor activity and body position during feeding and drinking tasks until an oral-pharyngeal motility study is conducted and analyzed. Information from the study must be used to determine the appropriateness of the goals, objectives, and strategies directed toward feeding activities in treatment and mealtime. If aspiration is noted due to problems in pharyngeal motility, changes in oral-motor function will not eliminate aspiration. If the head/neck and body position used by Jill now are found to prevent aspiration from occurring, changes in her alignment during feeding could place her at a greater risk for aspiration.

Jill's general treatment goals should include:
1. improve coordination of respiration with oral-motor activity in feeding and sound production.
2. increase forward and backward and up and down tongue movements with reduced tongue retraction during feeding and sound production activities.
3. increase cheek/lip activity with reduced cheek/lip retraction and lip pursing during cupdrinking, spoonfeeding, and sound production activities.

Short-Term Objectives:
Following treatment, Jill will be able to:
1. initiate vowel productions without abnormal extension throughout her body in 3 of 5 attempts.
2. close her lips on the cup rim when it is presented 50% of the time without lip pursing.
3. sustain a mid-vowel sound production for up to 3 seconds in 3 of 5 attempts.
4. use forward and backward (suckling) movements of her tongue with a thin, cupped tongue contour to move semisolids back in the oral cavity during spoonfeeding in 6 of 10 attempts.

Sample Activities
In sitting, administer slow, passive trunk rotation while providing deep pressure inward and downward to the lateral rib cage and abdominals to increase spinal and rib cage mobility. Jill may be sitting on a bench or straddling a roll between the legs of a therapist. Activities to stimulate mid-vowel sound production then can be presented.

In sidelying, facilitate slow movement in and out of sidelying with deep pressure inward and downward to the rib cage and abdominals for greater rib cage and scapulo-humeral mobility. This may be done while on a mat or large ball. Follow with activities to stimulate long mid-vowel sound productions.

Provide well-graded deep pressure input to the cheeks, lips, and tongue to establish a better sensory-motor base for cheek/lip and tongue activity. Follow with spoonfeeding of a thickened semisolid for greater lip closure upon presentation and for greater rhythmical forward and backward tongue movements to move the food back for swallowing.

CASE NO. 3 — TAYLOR
Myelomeningocele Repaired L 1-2, 4 Years

Taylor's oral-motor activity during spoonfeeding, cupdrinking, and solid food intake appears to be within normal age limits. He uses a variety of communication modes including speech. His mean sentence length of 3 to 4 words and the sounds he produces during spontaneous speech appear to be within normal age limits.

Taylor should have a thorough evaluation of his language functioning by a qualified speech-language pathologist. Children with myelomeningocele and hydrocephalus often appear to have normal language functioning according to tests of intelligence and vocabulary comprehension which require specific verbal responses. Many speak excessively using cliches and phrases learned by rote. These children may be unable to identify words during testing that they produce in spontaneous speech. This suggests the existence of very specific expressive and receptive language deficits. Taylor does not have adequate abdominal activity to support sustained exhalation and good respiratory coordination. He appears to run out of air after about 3 words and can sequence only about 3 sips from a cup before stopping to breathe.

Taylor's general treatment goals should include improved coordination of respiration with oral-motor activity for greater sustained exhalation during functional activities. Other goals will depend on results from the evaluation of Taylor's language functioning.

Short-Term Objectives:
Following treatment, Taylor will be able to:
1. produce sentences of 3 to 4 words on one exhalation without running out of air, 60% of the time.
2. drink 4 to 5 sips of liquid from a cup before stopping to breathe, 75% of the time.

Sample Activities
Incorporate suggested activities from occupational and physical therapists to strengthen/stimulate greater activity of upper extremities, spine, and abdominal muscles. For example, while in supported sitting on a bench or roll, have Taylor push with straightened arms

against the wall. Activities to stimulate speech production on more sustained exhalation, longer cupdrinking sequences, or other specific language tasks can be introduced as greater active movement is noted. For example, sentences of 3 to 4 words in length can be presented for repetition with Taylor using only 1 exhalation.

CASE NO. 4 — ASHLEY
Down Syndrome, 15 Months

Ashley has generally low muscle tone providing a poor base for oral-motor and respiratory-phonatory functioning. A suckle pattern is used in all feeding activities. The tongue is thick in contour and always protrudes from the mouth. The hole in the nipple has been slightly enlarged to allow for greater liquid intake during bottledrinking. She has to pause quite often to breathe during bottledrinking.

Cupdrinking has been introduced, but only during snack time. Ashley only likes pureed foods by spoon. She has been given some solids (crackers, cookies), but her lack of positive response to them has not encouraged their consistent presentation. No signs of aspiration or GER are evident in her medical history or during observations of her feeding and bottledrinking.

Ashley's rib cage is flat, yet high in position. Retraction of the anterior rib cage, especially at the sternum, during belly breathing increases in severity with effortful crying, movement, and attempts at vocalization. Her vocalizations are breathy, nasal, soft, and short. She is a mouth-breather and struggles for breath if her mouth is held in a closed position. This is not unusual for children with Down syndrome. Their small oral mechanism size does not appear to provide enough space for the tongue to sit in the oral cavity without closing off the oropharyngeal and naso-pharyngeal areas when the mouth is closed.

A thorough pre-linguistic/cognitive/language evaluation needs to be conducted because of Ashley's present lack of goal-directed play activities and her history of chronic otitis media with a mild conductive hearing loss. She should have periodic reevaluations of her hearing status by a qualified audiologist.

Ashley's treatment goals should include:
1. improve coordination of respiration with oral-motor activities in feeding and sound production.
2. increase active use of cheeks and lips during feeding and sound production.
3. develop active up and down and lateral movements of tongue during feeding and sound production.

Short-Term Objectives:
Following treatment, Ashley will be able to:
1. bring her lower lip up and out under the cup rim when the cup is presented in 3 of 6 attempts.
2. use up and down tongue movements with the tongue positioned more within the oral cavity during spoonfeeding of thickened textures, 50% of the time.

3. move her tongue laterally to touch solids placed on her side gums/teeth in 3 of 5 presentations.
4. produce vocalizations of 3 to 5 seconds in length with less nasality and greater loudness, 50% of the time.

Sample Activities

Facilitate active transitional movements, such as sidelying to sitting, sitting to quadruped, and kneeling to standing, while providing deep pressure tactile input to the lower rib cage and abdominals. Activities to stimulate vocalizations of greater loudness and length can be presented in conjunction with movement.

Provide well-graded deep pressure tactile input to cheeks/lips, tongue, biting surfaces of teeth/gums, and hard palate while facilitating transitional movements to increase coordination of oral-motor and respiratory functioning with general movement. Follow with the introduction of cupdrinking of thickened liquids and the presentation of solids.

Introduce different food textures (thick semisolids, cereal, crackers) as part of play. While performing active transitional movements, hands, feet, trunk, face, and mouth can be brought in contact with different food textures to encourage increased tolerance for these new tactile experiences. ❑

References

1. Sander E: When are speech sounds learned? J Speech Hear Disord 37:55-63, 1972

2. Netsell R: Speech motor control development. In Reilly A (ed): The Communication Game. Somerville, NJ, Johnson & Johnson Baby Products Co., 1980

3. Lass N, McReynolds L, Northern J, et al (eds): Speech, Language and Hearing. Philadelphia, PA, WB Saunders, 1982, vol 1

4. Bloom L, Lahey M: Language Development and Language Disorders. New York, NY, John Wiley & Sons, 1978

5. Bosma J: Introduction to the symposium. In Bosma J, Showacre J (eds): Symposium on Development of Upper Respiratory Anatomy and Function: Implications for the Sudden Infant Death Syndrome. Washington, DC, US Government Printing Office, 1975

6. Bosma J: Structure and function of the infant oral and pharyngeal mechanisms. In Wilson J (ed): Oral-Motor Function and Dysfunction in Children, Chapel Hill, NC, University of North Carolina, 1978

7. Kapandji I: The Physiology of the Joints: The Trunk and the Vertebral Column. New York, NY, Churchill Livingstone, 1974, vol III

8. Alexander, R: Oral-Motor and respiratory-phonatory assessment. In Gibbs B, Teti D (eds): Interdisciplinary Assessment of Infants: A Guide for Early Intervention Professionals. Baltimore, MD, Macmillan, 1990

9. Fee M, Charney E, Robertson W: Nutritional assessment of the young child with cerebral palsy. Infants and Young Children 1:33-40, 1988

10. Alexander R: Developing pre-speech and feeding abilities in children. In Shanks S (ed): Nursing and the Management of Pediatric Communication Disorders. San Diego, CA, College Hill Press, 1983

11. Morris S: Treatment of children with oral-motor dysfunction. In Wilson J (ed): Oral-Motor Function and Dysfunction in Children. Chapel-Hill, NC. University of North Carolina, 1978

CHAPTER 10

DEVELOPING AMBULATION SKILLS

Janet M. Wilson, M.A.C.T., PT

◆

Walking is an extremely complex pattern of movement which is the culmination of neuromuscular, biomechanical, and kinesiological changes during the first twelve months of life. The stepping movements of normal infants which are present at birth tend to disappear or become difficult to elicit between the second and eighth months of life. After the eighth month, locomotion reappears as supported walking. At this age, children walk voluntarily and can support their body weight on a single leg but still need assistance to maintain equilibrium. Ultimately, the child is able to move against gravity and progress on his feet independent of external support.[1-5] Walking requires acquisition and perfection of those components of postural control responsible for stable posture against the force of gravity. Postural control includes weight shifting and adequate equilibrium to remain upright while moving, as well as righting reactions which allow the child to attain the upright posture. Walking also requires appropriate range of motion and joint stability to allow reciprocal movements, while the head, neck, and trunk retain normal alignment in relation to each other. In addition, walking requires activation and selective control of specific patterns of muscle coordination, synergistic movements, and reciprocal innervation. These patterns must be executed at the appropriate time and in the proper sequence to permit changes in pace and direction and to cope with environmental demands. Finally, walking requires strength, endurance, and changes in energy level to be efficient in daily experiences.

Walking, in all of its complexity, has been hypothesized to depend on central control at various levels in the central nervous system (CNS), including the spinal cord, brain stem, midbrain, and cerebral cortex.[6] Walking also is affected by the brain's ability to react instantaneously to peripheral sensory information to modify and adapt the needs of the body to the environment.[7] When walking develops satisfactorily, little attention is given to the seemingly effortless acquisition of this complex skill. When walking is delayed or develops abnormally, however, great anxiety may occur in both parents and professionals.

DEVELOPMENTAL DISABILITIES: POTENTIAL FOR AMBULATION

In most types of disabilities, there is a relationship between the physical findings and the observed gait. Usually the functional consequences of joint pain or specific muscle weakness can be predicted quite accurately. However, in children with CNS dysfunction, analysis of gait problems and their outcome is less predictable. The reasons for this are twofold. First, damage to the CNS during the prenatal period produces different functional outcomes depending on the age of the infant at the time of insult. For example, it is not accidental that the incidence of spastic diplegia is greater among survivors of extreme prematurity than in full term babies who experience asphyxia.[8] The area of the neonatal brain which is most vulnerable to asphyxia, hemorrhage, or ischemia is that which is most active metabolically at the time of the insult.[8,9] In a newborn of less than 32 weeks gestation, asphyxia or intracranial hemorrhage is likely to cause damage to tracts in the periventricular area and the internal capsule, including axons projecting to motoneurons to the lower extremities and trunk. This type of damage results in the typical outcome of spastic diplegia. Second, damage to the brain perinatally results in an abnormal CNS that must direct the growth and development of a musculoskeletal system which is undergoing developmental changes in the early years.[10] Therefore, by the time the child interacts with the forces of gravity for standing and walking, the resultant sensorimotor patterns may look quite different than those observed in the same child at an earlier age.[11]

Certainly not all children with developmental disabilities have potential for independent walking. Children with myelodysplasia with lesions above L4 - L5 will ambulate only with orthoses, crutches, or walkers.[12-14] In a study of 68 children with myelodysplasia, DeSouza and Carroll reported that none of the children with thoracic level lesions who also lacked power in the muscles crossing or distal to the hip joint were community ambulators.[15] Of children with high lumbar lesions, with power in the hip adductors or flexors or in the extensors of the knee, 10 percent were community ambulators. Thirty-three percent of children with low lumbar lesions with power in the knee flexors, dorsiflexors of the ankles, or hip abductors, and fifty percent of children with sacral lesions who had power in the plantarflexors of the ankle or toes or in the extensors of the hips were community ambulators. While the eventual ambulatory status seemed to depend primarily on the neurosegmental level of the lesion, the motor power within a given neurosegmental level and the extent and degree of orthopedic deformities also were significant factors.

Hoffer and colleagues followed 56 children and reported that none of the children with thoracic level lesions walked, while all with sacral level lesions became community ambulators.[14] In children with lesions at the lumbar level, 45 percent were functional ambulators. In addition, those who achieved functional ambulation did so prior to nine years of age.

Uncomplicated mental retardation must be extremely severe to prevent ambulation. The mental age for walking has never been determined,[16,17] however, Shapiro and colleagues reported that 92 percent of profoundly retarded children (I.Q. less than 25) walked if retardation was not accompanied by other neurologic dysfunction.[18] The median age for this group was 20 months. Only 11 percent of a group with cerebral palsy and profound mental retardation walked. The median age for this group was 63.5 months. Donoghue et al reported on 336 institutionalized children with severe mental retardation.[19] They found fewer walkers (about 9 percent) in those cases complicated by cerebral palsy (walked at a mean age of 5.4 years), while 80 percent of the Down syndrome group walked at a mean age of 3.2 years. Seventy percent of the children in the uncomplicated mentally retarded group walked at a mean age of 4.2 years. The majority of children who succeeded in walking did so by five years and nearly all of the remaining children walked by seven years. Melyn and White reported on noninstitutionalized Down syndrome children who had an average age of walking of 26 months for boys (range 7-74 months) and 22.7 months for girls (range 8-72 months).[20] The significant difference in age of onset of walking in children with Down syndrome reported by Melyn and Donoghue probably is related to the samples under study. Donoghue reported on institutionalized children who experienced changing staff, high staff absence rates, and suboptimal conditions for development. The children examined by Melyn remained at home and attended developmental day care programs.

Of all children with developmental disabilities, the most complicated group for prediction of ambulation potential is children with cerebral palsy. Because of the nature of the problem (i.e., brain damage to an immature brain directing a developing sensorimotor system), the final clinical picture may not be clear for several years. Consequently, therapists should be cautious about making predictions regarding ambulation potential because the outcome may either be better or worse than the initial impression. Some children who appear to be only mildly involved, showing good reciprocal movements of their legs, and the ability to stand with support at twelve months, may develop more severe problems once they interact with gravity. Walking may be delayed until the age of five or six years.[21] Some babies who appear to be severely affected following a difficult birth and perinatal course may make a good recovery and progress at a nearly normal rate in motor milestones.[22]

Several authors have described the development of ambulation in children with various types of cerebral palsy.[11,23-26] Molnar and Gordon, reporting on 233 children, found that 78 percent achieved some degree of functional walking.[23] Largo and colleagues found that the type of cerebral palsy and the severity of tonal abnormalities were correlated with the development of locomotion skills.[25] The mean ages for attaining all forms of locomotion (i.e., crawling, creeping, cruising, and walking) were higher in a group of preterm infants with cerebral palsy than in either normal preterm or full term infants. In addition, some of the movement patterns used by the group of children with cerebral palsy were specific to that group. In the group of children with mild or moderate spastic diplegia, the delay in attaining ambulation was not significant (14.7 months). The locomotion skills of children with moderate to severe spastic diplegia or quadriplegia, however, were delayed significantly.

Molnar also found that the type and severity of cerebral palsy were useful guides in predicting ambulation.[23,26,27] She found that most children with spastic hemiplegia walked by two years and all walked by three years. Children with ataxia attained walking later, but all walked by eight years. Children with spastic diplegia were found to have a favorable outcome for ambulation: 65 percent walked unassisted, 20 percent required assistive devices, and an additional 15 percent relied on wheelchairs and did not walk. However, of the ambulators, the majority walked by three years. Children with spastic quadriplegia had the most variable outcome: 25 percent never became ambulatory because of upper extremity impairment, intellectual deficits, or both; 33 percent walked only with assistive devices; and only 30 percent ambulated independently. Children with athetosis had a favorable outcome for ambulation with 75 percent becoming ambulatory, with or without aids, and 50 percent of these walked by three years of age. Molnar compared sitting and ambulation and found that sitting by two years was a good predictive sign for eventual ambulation in children with spastic diplegia, quadriplegia, and athetosis. Badell-Ribera also confirmed that, in children with spastic diplegia related to prematurity, the control of sitting and crawling at one and a half to two and a half years was predictive of the eventual level of ambulatory function.[24]

Other investigators have tried to link the potential for walking to motor patterns specific to cerebral palsy. Bleck used the persistence of five primary tonic reflexes (asymmetrical and symmetrical tonic neck, moro, neck righting and extensor thrust) and absence of two postural reactions (parachute and foot placement) as indicators of eventual walking.[28] He gave a score of one to each of the five primitive reflexes that was present or to each of two postural reactions that was absent. He found that of 49 children with a score of 0, only three failed to walk, while of the 17 children with scores of 2 or more, only 1 walked. Molnar and Gordon, using the persistence of primitive reflexes to predict walking, found that 27 of 99 infants with cerebral palsy, when seen at twelve months of age, had persistent primary reflexes. Of these children, only 22 percent ultimately walked.[23]

Predicting ambulation for children with cerebral palsy is a difficult and often unrewarding task. Various aspects of motor control have been shown to correlate with delayed onset of walking, but the relative contribution of persistent primary reflexes, absent postural reactions, abnormal patterns of movement, and abnormal muscle tone cannot be determined. Additional factors, including motivation, intelligence, interest, self-image, spatial abilities, family interest, support systems, and accessible school and home environments are all important considerations in the final outcome of ambulation.

ASSESSMENT PRINCIPLES AND PROCEDURES

Interdisciplinary, multidisciplinary, and transdisciplinary approaches are current service delivery models for children with developmental disabilities.[29-31] The physical therapist's role may vary with the child's age, developmental level, degree of involvement, system of service delivery, and physical setting, but always should include an assessment of standing and walking. Standardized assessments may be used to determine how well the child is doing in comparison to normal peers. However, because ambulation onset and abnormalities of gait are common problems, the physical therapy assessment requires detailed analysis of posture, movement, and coordination related to standing and walking. Efforts to summarize descriptive findings in an objective manner will assist the therapist in determining changes that result from intervention or maturation. Gait analysis should provide information important for treating or managing ambulation problems. Assessment described in this chapter will focus on collection of information for program planning. While a developmental motor assessment includes additional information about posture and movement, only those elements related to gait will be presented.

READINESS FOR WALKING

The following areas of motor control, postural alignment, and balance are analyzed to determine whether the child is ready to walk.

Skill Level: Children must be able to get into a standing position. Holt described several strategies that normal children use to get to this point of readiness, including crawling and pulling to stand, hitching or scooting on their bottoms, and simply pulling to stand from prone.[21] These represent normal progressions of motor skills. The strategies children with developmental disabilities use may differ from any of these and are described in this section

In addition, the child's ability to stoop and regain standing is noted, as well as his ability to cruise along furniture, walk holding a support, or walk holding the parent's hands.

Automatic Postural Reactions: Evaluation of appropriate balance in those positions preparatory for walking and for changing positions is essential. A child needs to be able to maintain various positions against the force of gravity as he moves into standing as well as use equilibrium reactions to regain the upright position if he loses balance. If the center of gravity is displaced outside the base of support, the child uses protective extension to catch himself as he falls. How safely the child moves in the upright position helps to determine whether the child is ready to ambulate independently or with external support.

Postural Tonus: When moving to standing and during standing, there must be sufficient postural stability for upright alignment. The lower extremities must support the body weight while allowing weight shift and balance reactions. The child must not be too stiff to permit movement or too floppy to prevent upright postural control.

Range of Motion: There must be adequate range of motion (ROM) in the trunk and lower extremities for the child to move from sitting or prone through half-kneeling and into standing. There must be adequate ROM to allow trunk, hip, and knee extension with ankle dorsiflexion for standing. Muscle contractures or joint deformities will interfere with the child's ability to move into standing and to attain optional standing alignment.

Strength: Children must have enough muscle strength to rise to standing using the legs. Children who do not have adequate strength must pull up with their arms. There must be sufficient strength, particularly in the hip abductors and extensors and the knee extensors, to permit these movement patterns. Unfortunately, if weakness is suspected, muscle testing often is not very helpful for children with developmental disabilities. These children often cannot isolate and contract a muscle to determine its strength, but can recruit it only during a movement pattern. They may not be able to execute the complete pattern of muscle activity necessary to rise to standing even if they can demonstrate adequate strength on testing. Strength for walking includes testing for repetition, endurance, speed, and velocity. Some children may be able to walk only at one speed and cannot exert enough force to speed up or slow down as the task demands.

Selective Control: In addition to having adequate strength and ROM, children must be able to isolate and combine movements of single muscles with many others at the appropriate time and in the correct sequence. Some children have a very limited movement repertoire with predictable patterns of movement and weight bearing when trying to attain or maintain standing. Some children initiate movement in the same way in all situations and are unable to accommodate to changes in the environment. Stopping, starting, changing directions, and slowing down or speeding up require precise control of agonists and antagonists. Individual muscles

must change from patterns of cocontraction to reciprocal innervation quickly and smoothly. During the various phases of swing and stance the muscles around individual joints must combine and recombine in intralimb and interlimb coordination.

Postural Alignment: In standing, the child's alignment should be observed in both frontal and sagittal planes. Normal alignment balances the body above the base of support so that little muscular effort is required. In the frontal plane, the weight is distributed equally over both feet and the center of gravity lies between the feet. The base is sufficiently narrow to place more of the body weight on the lateral sides of feet. During the first two years of life, the hips have 40 degrees of anteversion and the femurs are outwardly rotated so that the knees do not face forward and weight is on the medial side of the feet placing them in pronation. After the second year, the femurs derotate and hip anteversion is only 25 degrees. The legs are aligned with the feet and knees facing forward. The pelvis is level and in neutral rotation. [32-34]

In the sagittal plane, the center of gravity lies just ahead of the lateral malleolus, the knees and hips are fully extended and the trunk is erect. The feet are flat on the floor. During the first eighteen months of life, the pelvis is in an anterior tilt and the hips are not extended fully so the child appears to lean forward. While some children maintain excessive pelvic tilt for several years, the hips are fully extended by the second year. Standing with an excessive anterior pelvic tilt, forward leaning trunk, and hip flexion places more of the body weight on the metatarsal heads and the center of gravity is outside the base of support. To compensate, the child will either hyperextend the knees or flex the knees to realign the body over the base of support. If the child is unable to make muscular adaptations to these changes in alignment, he will need crutches or a walker to balance. [35]

GAIT ANALYSIS

An analysis of the walking pattern is done for several reasons: to determine abnormalities; to show progress or deterioration over time; to determine social suitability and acceptability, and to assist in determining therapeutic, surgical, or orthotic intervention. There are many ways to record gait patterns, ranging from descriptions of clinical observations to computerized gait analysis. Investigators have used computerized gait analysis to understand the pathomechanics of abnormal gait, [36-42] as a tool to guide surgery, and to evaluate treatment outcome. [43-52] Computerized motion analysis determines changes in position of various anatomical points that occur with movement. This is combined with data on ground force reactions and on the firing sequences of different muscles by combining high speed cinematography, electromyography, and force plate signals.

Therapeutic Exercise In Developmental Disabilities

For adequate assessment and treatment, observational analysis of the child's gait is extremely important. However, making reliable observational analyses are difficult and considerable clinical experience and judgment are required.

Components of Gait: Perry described the following eight stages of gait which occur during a single stride. [6] Swing phase accounts for approximately 40 percent of the gait cycle and is made up of three phases: initial swing, mid-swing, and terminal swing. "Toe-off" is the common designation for the onset of initial swing. The limb lifts from the floor with initial advancement of the thigh to achieve toe clearance and forward propulsion. The foot is in 15 degrees equinus, the knee flexed to 35 degrees, and the hip flexed to 20 degrees. The pelvis is level but with backward rotation of five degrees. The key action in this phase is sufficient knee flexion to bring the leg forward to allow the foot to clear the floor.

In mid-swing, the limb advances to achieve a vertical tibial position. The ankle dorsiflexes to neutral, the knee flexes an additional 35 degrees, and the hip flexes an additional 10 degrees. The pelvis remains level, but forward rotation begins on the swing side.

In terminal swing, there is continued tibial advancement toward full knee extension. The foot is ahead of the body and the knee begins to extend for stride length. The hip and ankle continue to flex until the hip reaches 30 degrees and the ankle is in a neutral position. Isolated knee extension with hip and ankle flexion is required. Deceleration of the thigh and maintenance of foot position prepare for heel contact. The pelvis rotates forward on the swing side five degrees.

Stance phase makes up 60 percent of the gait cycle and has five separate components: initial contact, loading, midstance, terminal stance, and pre-swing. Initial contact occurs when the foot touches the ground. Adequate heel strike depends on ankle movement to 90 degrees, full knee extension, and hip flexion to 30 degrees. Failure to attain any of these movements causes the toe to approach the floor. Trunk forward motion continues at heel strike. The pelvis is level with forward rotation maintained.

During loading, the hip is flexed 30 degrees while the knee flexes 15 degrees to absorb the hyperextensor thrust at the knee caused by the momentum of the trunk coming forward. The ankle again moves into 15 degrees of plantarflexion and the pelvis begins to rotate backward.

During the single support period of mid-stance, the foot is stationary and flat on the floor. Advancement of the trunk is continued due to forward momentum which results in ankle dorsiflexion. The hip and knee are fully extended while the pelvis is level and in neutral rotation.

Terminal stance is the final period of single support. The heel rises from the floor as the trunk passes over the toe. The hip is flexed 10 degrees, the knee extended, and the ankle plantarflexed. The pelvis is rotated forward on the swing side.

Double support occurs during pre-swing with the stance limb in contact with the floor while the swing limb accepts body weight. Thirty-five to forty degrees of knee flexion should occur during the last moments of toe contact, thus preparing the limb for knee flexion during swing. The pelvis is level and rotated forward on the swing side and the ankle is plantarflexed to 20 degrees.

Various authors have described changes in gait in the developing child. [2-5, 53] Leonard and colleagues studied gait development during the periods immediately before and after the acquisition of independent locomotion. [53] Normally developing children and children with cerebral palsy were studied to evaluate the influences of supraspinal input on the development of locomotion. They found the locomotive patterns of the children with cerebral palsy were similar to those of normal infants during the stage of supported walking but as they matured, some of the characteristics of the infant stepping pattern such as synchronous muscle activity with excessive cocontraction were retained. The normal plantigrade features of adult walking did not develop in these children. They concluded that the development of locomotion reflected maturational changes in the CNS. Changes involving increased specificity of cortical and subcortical connectivity precede and continue throughout the period of gait acquisition. Locomotion generator circuits seem to depend on descending influences within the hierarchial reflex model. The maturation of locomotion is considered to be a process in which spinal circuits become progressively more influenced by higher centers. In addition, it appears that supraspinal centers become increasingly more integrated and involved in the active coordination of locomotor movements.

The changes in gait characteristics most frequently reported in subjects less than two years of age were greater hip and knee flexion, more ankle dorsiflexion, and backward rotation of the pelvis with external rotation of the hip accompanied by foot pronation during stance. On swing, excessive hip flexion and decreases in knee and foot flexion were noted. As the child matured, the gait pattern showed greater reproducibility, greater smoothness in changing from extension to flexion of the hip and knee, decreased external rotation of the hip and base of support, increased walking speeds, and decreased duration of stance phase with an increased duration of swing phase.

EFFECTIVENESS OF CONTROL

In addition to analyzing the gait cycle, once walking is achieved, the effectiveness of control must be assessed. This includes how the child gets into a walking position independently, initiates walking, stops and starts at will, varies his speed and force depending on the demands of the setting, varies stride length, changes directions, walks on various even and uneven surfaces, climbs stairs or ramps, and falls. A measure of speed can be obtained by timing the child walking a set distance. Comparison of performance over time can be made to determine whether a child is able to increase speed or distance without deterioration of the gait pattern. It is important to determine if the speed and quality of walking during the evaluation correspond to his normal pattern. Some children perform optimally when tested and demonstrate their best pattern, yet this does not represent their typical pattern.

Determining the distance which can be walked comfortably provides a clue to the effort involved. If walking is slow and laborious, walking may not be functional. Distance can be expressed as household ambulation, short distances in the community, or complete community ambulation. Walking for the first time in a new setting (i.e., at the mall or outside in the yard) can be used to rate progress in functional terms. Rose, Medeiros, and Parker found that children with cerebral palsy who used either walkers or canes had a slower rate of ambulation and higher energy expenditure than normal children who ambulated without assistive devices. [54] Stallard and colleagues reported that heart rate decreased and speed of ambulation increased when children with spina bifida used orthoses. [55] Several studies suggested that the closer the gait pattern is to normal, the less energy expended. [55-58]

Assistive devices, such as walkers, crutches, or orthoses, used during ambulation should be described along with their purpose and children's changes in function. Some children may not be able to walk without assistive devices, while other children may walk in the house, yet use crutches or walkers when outside or walking long distances.

TREATMENT PRINCIPLES AND PROCEDURES

Treatment is designed to develop, improve, or refine movements, stability, or alignment which are preventing development of walking skills. The following suggestions should assist the therapist in program planning.

First, therapy should be designed to elicit active movement from the child. The therapist either initiates the movement and then allows the child to complete the pattern or guides the child during the performance of self-initiated movement. Control of movement is maintained by the therapist, but the child should lead the treatment and initiate the activity. [59] For example, stability with an extended hip is an important aspect of the stance phase of gait, yet a young child with hemiplegia often pulls to stand by placing his hemiplegic leg forward. He uses this pattern because he is unable to shift his weight onto his hemiplegic side and stabilize on a fully extended hip. The therapist might place toys on a low bench to motivate the child to move into kneeling.

Then as the child initiates rising to stand to get a toy the therapist shifts the child's weight onto the hemiplegic side, allowing him to maintain this stable position and freeing his noninvolved leg to be placed forward in half-kneeling. Moving the non-hemiplegic leg while weight bearing on the hemiplegic side is an important pattern for walking, as well as for rising to stand.

Second, locomotion activities should be designed to provide motivation and to direct movement. For example, once a child can stand at a small bench or table, toys can be placed at one end to encourage the child to cruise. As he moves toward the toys, the therapist can facilitate weight shift onto the weight bearing side and abduction of the non-weight bearing side through handling techniques. Cruising to get a toy provides purpose and motivation for walking.

Third, a single treatment should progress from positions in which the child has the most normal tone and movement patterns to ones that are more challenging. For example, a child with spastic diplegia often has difficulty with alignment of the trunk and pelvis. In floor sitting, the pelvis is tilted posteriorly and the child sits with a rounded spine. In standing, the pelvis and lumbar spine may be lordotic with the hips flexed. Therapy may begin with the child sitting on a small bench, ball, or bolster which reduces the pull of the hamstrings and hip extensors and allows the child to sit with the pelvis vertical and the back extended. Small movements which displace the child's center of gravity over his base of support will assist in controlling the pelvis and spine. From this position, the therapist may assist the child in rising to stand and facilitate normal standing alignment (Figures 1 & 2).

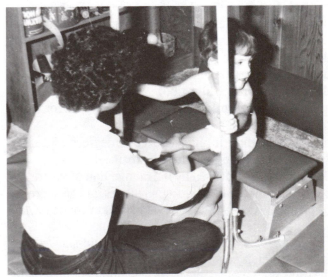

FIGURE 1. The child is placed on a small bench, knees flexed 90 degrees so that spasticity in the hamstrings and adductors is minimized. With the aid of the parallel poles, he is able to bring his center of gravity over his base of support without rounding his thoracic spine.

Therapeutic Exercise In Developmental Disabilities

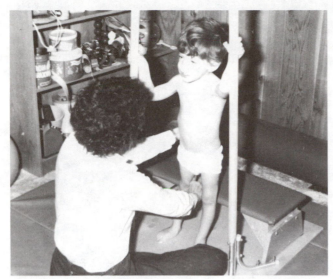

FIGURE 2. *With assistance he now is able to shift his feet and rise to standing with better alignment.*

Fourth, movement in one position should prepare for movement in another position. Activities are used early in a treatment session which allow the child a feeling of control in positions where movement is easier, prior to attempting movement in positions which are difficult or new. For example, gaining control of knee flexion with ankle dorsiflexion is difficult for many children with developmental disabilities. Yet, this control is an extremely important component of normal gait. Active knee flexion with dorsiflexion can be done in many different positions before the child uses this pattern during walking. Early in the treatment session a child may work in supine with the knees flexed and feet placed flat on the floor. The child then "bridges" by extending his hips while maintaining knee flexion. The child can work for this specific movement pattern without worrying about balance. (Figures 3 & 4) This same pattern can be repeated later with the child standing between parallel poles and placing one foot forward on a small bolster or bench. Issues regarding part to whole transfer during motor tasks were discussed in Chapter 3.

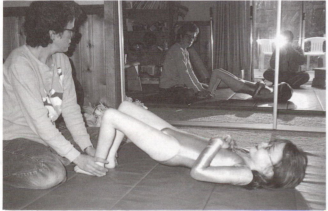

FIGURE 3. *Bridging combines hip extension, knee flexion, and ankle dorsiflexion.*

Fifth, as the child is able to perform movements independently, the therapist should provide time in treatment for free movement. It is important for the child to feel movement produced through his own efforts without the control of the therapist. Only in this way will the child incorporate these movements into his daily living. For example, when beginning to develop balance for standing and walking, a child may be too insecure to attempt this skill at home. The therapist may have to provide motivation and physical support for a child to move from one support to another. The supports can be arranged so that the child has to weight shift and momentarily stand, but take no steps. As the child gains confidence, the distance between supports can be increased so a step or two must be taken before reaching the support.

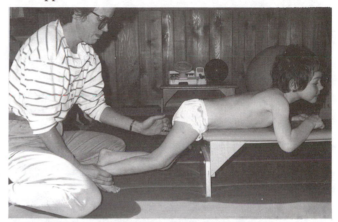

FIGURE 4. *Prone on the bench, this child practices reciprocal hip and knee extension with ankle dorsiflexion and weight on metatarsal heads.*

As a normal child nears two years of age, his need for upright mobility increases with his desire to explore and expand the environment. Even if the child with a disability has good potential for independent walking, adaptive equipment and assistive walking devices should be considered to meet his current needs for mobility. Restricted mobility may have an effect on the child's personality and perpetuate dependency and emotional immaturity. The child who knows the independence of standing and walking can be successful in establishing interactions with the world beyond his immediate family. For example, a young child with myelodysplasia may walk eventually with crutches but initially may lack balance, confidence, and control for walking. By selecting a walker which encourages appropriate postural alignment and provides external balance, the child will have the opportunity to explore while gaining skill and motivation for independent walking. [13]

Sixth, individual treatment sessions should be designed to evaluate the effectiveness of treatment within the session. This can be done informally by motivating the child to demonstrate an activity, movement, or posture at the beginning of treatment and again at the end to determine if changes have occurred. Knowing that change has occurred is motivating to the child and reinforcing for the therapist. For example, initially, the therapist might ask the child to walk a specific distance. Depending on the goals for that treatment session, the therapist could time speed, observe the components of gait, measure the distance walked without support, or observe control of stopping or starting. At the end of the session, the therapist can make the same observations and report to the child or parent the differences observed. While this is an informal evaluation of effectiveness, it can be incorporated easily into one treatment program and charted objectively.

FACILITATION OF GAIT

Facilitation of walking frequently is part of the treatment of children who are developing ambulation skills. Facilitation of gait is used either to assist a child who is delayed in attaining ambulation or to correct the gait of a child who has begun walking abnormally.[29] Even though a child does not have all the readiness skills, treatment must include putting all these components

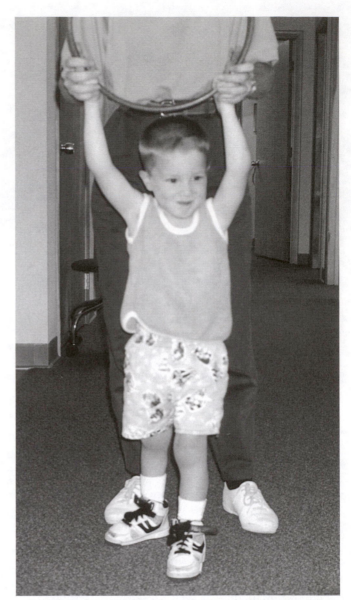

FIGURE 6. Facilitation from the hands with arm extension can aid trunk extension and forward weight shift.

together during gait if the child is expected to transfer these individual components to independent walking.

There are many ways to facilitate walking. These techniques easily are described and visualized but difficult to execute. All facilitation must be done with knowledge of the normal gait pattern for the age of the child, the ability to analyze where in the gait cycle the child performs abnormally, and the skill to translate the child's rhythm and timing through the therapist's hands. Most therapists find facilitation of gait to be the most difficult therapeutic technique to perfect.

Walking requires a constant change in weight bearing. Before the initial step is taken, the weight must be shifted to the stance leg to unload the opposite leg for swing. It is possible to facilitate weight shift onto the support leg prior to taking a step and with each subsequent step, alternating from the right to the left. The therapist needs to note which leg the child uses to initiate

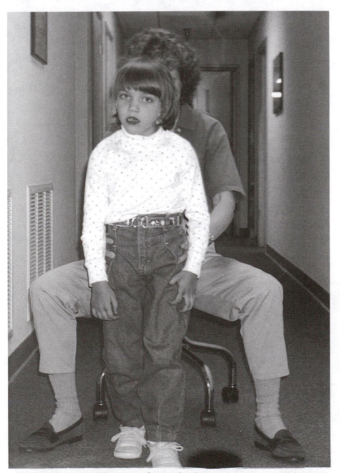

FIGURE 5. Facilitation from the lateral aspects of the pelvis.

Therapeutic Exercise In Developmental Disabilities

the swing phase. The therapist facilitates a lateral shift to the opposite side. This unloads the swing leg and allows the child to step. The amount of lateral weight shift is very small and within the child's base of support. Too much lateral weight shift will provoke an exaggerated equilibrium or righting response of the head and trunk or even a protective stepping reaction of the lower extremity. In either case the child will not be aligned over the base of support and normal stepping will not occur.

Lateral weight shift can be facilitated from the lateral sides of the trunk, the lateral sides of the thighs, the shoulders, or even the arm and hand (Figures 5 & 6). Facilitation from the arm and hand is particularly difficult because it is the arm and hand on the stance side that moves forward initially. It is easier to produce movement from points further away from the child's center of gravity and care must be taken not to displace the child outside his normal support base.

Once swing has been initiated, it is possible to change the step length or amount of rotation of the swing leg by facilitating from either the anterior thigh or the posterior aspect of the thigh on the swing side (Figure 7). Again, it is important to facilitate only the length of step that is within the child's ability and natural walking rhythm.

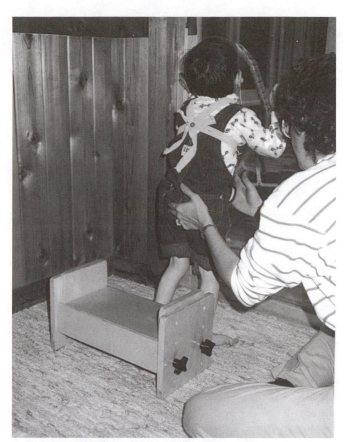

FIGURE 8. *Facilitation from the lower abdomen and sacrum is used to encourage side stepping at the mirror.*

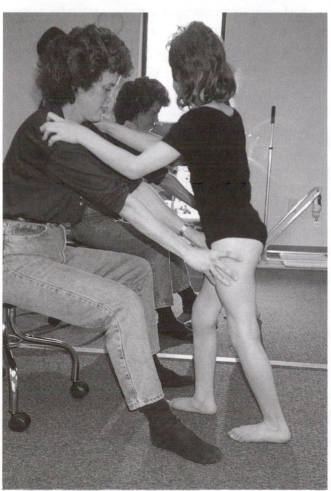

FIGURE 7. *Facilitation from anterior thigh to increase step length.*

It is important to facilitate forward weight shift at the termination of swing phase, if the child has the common problem of difficulty in keeping the trunk and hips aligned over his feet and tends to push backward. This facilitation is usually done with one hand on the lower abdomen and the other on the sacrum (Figure 8). The hand on the abdomen is the facilitating hand.

As swing phase terminates, there is a diagonal weight shift toward the leg that is accepting weight. This is often a time when the entire side rotates forward. The foot hits the ground toe first with the entire limb rotated inward. A more normal foot placement and alignment of the body over the limb are achieved by facilitating rotation around the body axis. Rotation can be elicited with both hands on the lateral aspects of the pelvis so that one hand facilitates forward rotation and the other backward. Remember the total rotation of the pelvis from neutral is only five degrees.

Another appropriate method is with one hand on the lateral aspect of the pelvis and the other on the opposite shoulder or by using both shoulders. The amount of rotation at the shoulders is greater than the rotation at the pelvis so combining the shoulder and pelvis or handling from the shoulders takes considerable skill and practice (Figure 9).

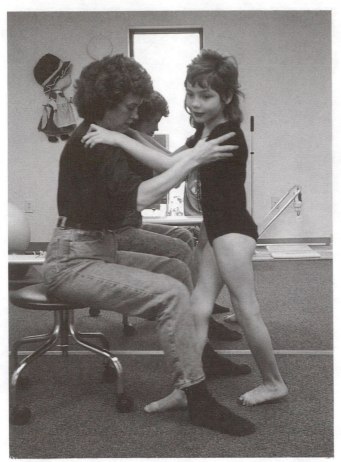

FIGURE 9. *Facilitation from anterior shoulders to add rotation between shoulders and hips.*

Facilitation of individual components of gait, such as heel-strike or knee extension at terminal stance, is possible but is beyond the scope of this chapter. Since facilitation must be done in the rhythm, timing, and speed that are normal for the particular child, many therapists and parents find facilitation of gait to be easier if the child is on a treadmill. The treadmill can be set for the comfortable pace of the child and eliminates disturbances from uneven ground, changes of directions, stopping, or general distractions. If necessary, the child can hold hand rails so that balance is not an issue when working to change gait characteristics (Figure 10).

CHANGING AMBULATION OUTCOME

Most therapists at one time or another have been challenged to change ambulation in children. There is limited information available, however, regarding the possibility to change ambulation outcome in children with developmental disabilities. Functional walking allows increased access to educational programs, community settings, and social acceptability. Therapists often list walking as a long or short term goal without adequate information to make realistic predictions. Specific therapy methods, use of assistive devices, surgical intervention, and use of orthotics and casts are variables some researchers have used to demonstrate changes in ambulation.[60-67] Logan and colleagues[61] and Levangie et al[62] evaluated the changes in ambulation elicited by changing the type of walker used by children with cerebral palsy. These two studies showed that children who used posterior walkers with 4 wheels, had improved posture and gait characteristics including stride length, decreased double support, and increased velocity as compared to walking with anterior walkers.

Wilson and colleagues reported changes in dependence on assistive devices following neurosurgery.[63] Forty-three children with spastic diplegia were followed for 2 1/2 years following selective dorsal rhizotomy. Pre-operatively, this sample was very similar to the children with spastic diplegia reported by Molnar and Gordon.[23] Twenty-one percent were non-ambulatory, 56% walked with assistive devices, and 23% walked unaided. By 2 1/2 years post-op, all were ambulatory. Fifty-four percent walked unaided and 46% used assistive devices (walkers, crutches, or canes). These data show changes in ambulation when compared to Molnar and Gordon who reported that while 65% walked unaided, 20% used assistive devices, and 15% did not walk at all.[23] Storrs and McLane's report on ambulation changes in children with myelodysplasia who underwent selective dorsal rhizotomy revealed that 3 children who had

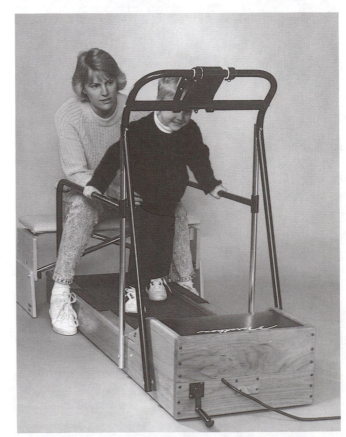

FIGURE 10. *Gait can be facilitated on the treadmill. The treadmill can be used for side stepping and backward walking as well.*

Therapeutic Exercise In Developmental Disabilities

lost the ability to ambulate because of spasticity returned to independent ambulation. Four other children maintained their ambulation level. [64]

Another study using instrumental gait analysis to document and compare changes suggested that selective posterior rhizotomy reduces spasticity and improves gait dynamics, but does not change patterns of muscle activation during walking. [68] Clinical outcomes following selective posterior rhizotomy have been variable. [69]

Other researchers have investigated changes with orthoses. Stallard and colleagues reported that speed of ambulation could be increased when children with myelodysplasia used orthoses. [55] Thomas et al reported that in children with myelodysplasia who wore orthoses, reduced hip, knee and ankle flexion, decreased muscle activity and decreased muscle coactivation were seen. [65]

Some investigators examined changes in ambulation using physical therapy combined with short leg casts. Bertoti reported increases in stride length and symmetry in those children who used short leg casts and Neurodevelopmental Treatment (NDT). [66] Watt and colleagues demonstrated changes in ankle dorsiflexion and foot-floor contact following NDT therapy and short leg casts. [67]

SUMMARY

Children with developmental disabilities often have delays or difficulties in ambulation. Many will never achieve independent ambulation. Understanding the problems confronting children as they attempt to achieve ambulation helps in planning programs, setting goals, and counseling families toward realistic expectations. Assessment includes readiness for walking, gait analysis, and the effectiveness of walking once it is achieved. Effective treatment is based on the therapist's ability to define problems of movement, stability, balance, and alignment in relation to functional ambulation. Evaluation of changes in ambulation assists in determining the efficacy of treatment as well as projecting realistic expectations for children's mobility.

In the following case studies, specific assessment, goal setting, treatment planning, and treatment techniques for children of different ages and with different developmental disabilities are described.

CASE STUDIES

CASE NO. 1 — JASON
Cerebral Palsy, Right Hemiparesis, 18 Months

Jason is an eighteen month old with a right hemiparesis who has the following strengths and weaknesses related to ambulation. Jason has adequate muscle strength, joint ROM, postural reactions, and muscle tone to get into and maintain independent standing. However, Jason always initiates getting into a standing position with his left side. He moves through half-kneeling bringing his right leg forward every time because he is unable to balance with the right hip in extension and is unable to keep his pelvis rotated forward for weight bearing.

In standing, Jason's posture is characterized by weight bearing primarily on the left with the pelvis rotated back on the right, the right hip externally rotated, and the right foot in valgus. This position widens his base of support. His equilibrium is adequate to balance within his base of support, but if he falls, he cannot extend his right arm to protect against the fall.

Jason began ambulating independently at fifteen months, well within normal expectations for a child with hemiplegia. [14,70] Jason's gait is characterized by both a short stance and swing phase on the right when compared to the left. The pelvis is rotated back on the right throughout swing and stance. On initial contact, the right pelvis is retracted with the hip in external rotation. Spasticity is present in the gastroc-soleus group and Jason is unable to obtain adequate dorsiflexion. The entire foot contacts the floor with weight more on the medial side, placing the foot in equinovalgus. On midstance, the weight transfer is across the medial side of the foot, the ankle is in plantar flexion, the knee hyperextends, and the hip remains in flexion. During pre-swing the heel leaves the floor rapidly so the period of full foot contact is minimal and out of phase. On initial swing, the knee does not flex enough to allow the foot to clear the floor. Jason compensates by keeping the pelvis rotated back, hip externally rotated and abducted, and foot in valgus to make the limb shorter during swing. Stride length on the right is short due to the backward rotation of the pelvis and inability to use momentum to bring the right leg forward. Step length and forward momentum are produced by forces acting on the left leg during left swing and stance. This adds to the asymmetry of his gait so that with continued walking the left side leads the entire body and orientation through space.

By the time Jason is 2 to 2 1/2 years of age, his lower extremity pattern will change. While still having backward rotation of the pelvis on the right side, the femur will internally rotate and the foot will be in a position of equinovarus. Equinus which develops in children with hemiplegia is multifactorial. It may result from shortened muscles, foot-drop, tonic spasticity, rigidity, compensation for a short limb, fixed contracture at the hip, secondary to chronic toe-walking, or abnormalities in the visco-elastic properties of a muscle. [70] Because this position results in his right lower extremity being longer in comparison to the left, he compensates in standing with knee flexion. This is the typical pattern of the older child with hemiplegia. It is important to identify the developmental progression of the hemiplegic gait as it changes in relation to normal developmental changes and the underlying neuromuscular disorder.

Jason can initiate walking at will. He can control stopping and starting. The pattern of walking deteriorates with speed since he cannot rapidly change from extension to flexion during swing and stance. The pattern described is more exaggerated with speed. He cannot vary stride length and changes directions only by pivoting on the left foot. He walks backwards and sideways slowly and deliberately. Because he must control ascent and descent with the non-hemiplegic leg, he climbs stairs with a railing by leading up with the left leg and down with the right leg.

General Treatment Goals:

1. increase control of forward rotation of the pelvis on the right side.
2. improve ability to shift weight and maintain weight bearing on the right side, freeing up the left side for functional movement.
3. decrease gastroc-soleus stiffness.
4. increase control of selective reciprocal movement of the right knee.

Short-Term Objectives:

Following treatment, Jason will:

1. come to a standing position from a low bench with feet and legs parallel, three of five times.
2. sit on a small bench and place his left foot on the bench to assist in putting on his shoe and sock, each time attempted.
3. stand with neutral alignment of hips and knees and with both feet flat on the floor for 30 seconds.
4. not hyperextend the knee in the stance phase when walking a distance of 10 feet.

The following activities might be included, in this sequence, in a single session to meet the objectives:

Sitting astride a small bolster so that weight is evenly distributed across the hips, Jason leans forward to play at a low bench. This position encourages weight shift in both sagittal and frontal planes across the hips and feet. In this position Jason may come to a partial standing position, varying the amount of hip and knee flexion,

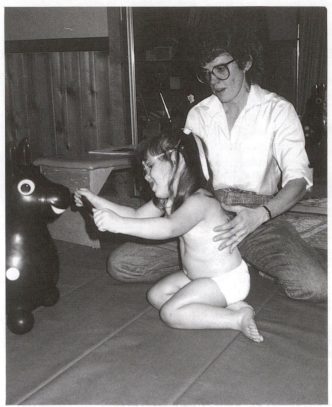

FIGURE 12. *Side sitting on the right, this child prepares to "feed the horse a carrot stick." A stick is used to keep the right arm forward and engage the right hand.*

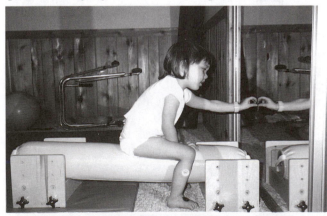

FIGURE 11. *Astride a bolster to encourage lateral weight shifts, this child takes weight on her right hand and places stickers on a mirror, a variation on the activity described in the text.*

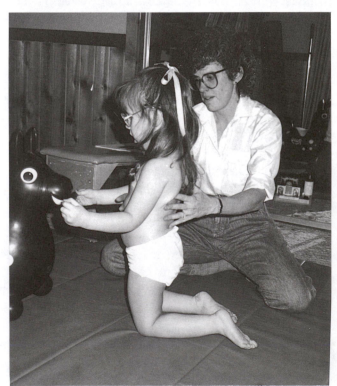

FIGURE 13. *From side-sitting the child moves to kneeling, maintaining alignment of trunk and pelvis with hip extension.*

which requires control of hip and knee flexion with ankle dorsiflexion (Figure 11).

Jason can then lean down to floor, first over the left side then to the right, to retrieve a toy and place it on the bench. This activity adds full weight bearing onto either lower extremity. This same sequence could be modified so that Jason begins straddling a small bolster between parallel standing poles and ends the sequence with hip, knee, and trunk extension as he stands.

Jason moves from side sitting on the right to kneeling while the therapist maintains weight bearing on the right (Figures 12 & 13). From kneeling, an equilibrium response is facilitated so the left leg moves forward for half-kneel and weight is maintained on the right with the hip extended.

From half-kneel, Jason can come to stand to play. The therapist can facilitate small weight shifts from side to side without allowing him to change the width of the base of support.

Once in standing, the therapist can place Jason's left leg forward on a small bolster, then shift his weight from the extended right leg to the left leg with knee flexion. The same sequence should be repeated with the right leg forward since Jason needs to be able to shift the body forward over the right dorsiflexed ankle without hyperextending the knee, as well as take weight with right knee flexion, which is needed during stance. [6]

To prevent hyperextension of the knee in stance, the therapist will facilitate external rotation at heel-strike to prevent him from locking the knee. This will be done by facilitating a diagonal weight shift onto the right side either through the pelvis or right shoulder.

CASE NO. 2 — JILL
Cerebral Palsy, Spastic Quadriparesis, Mental Retardation, 7 Years

Jill is a seven year old with severe spastic quadriplegia and mental retardation. Because of increased muscle tone, limited active and passive ROM, persistent tonic reflexes imposing asymmetries of the head and trunk, and lack of selective movement responses and balance reactions, she has no potential for ambulation.

While Jill has no potential for walking and actively moves very little, she is at risk for developing contractures of the hip and knee flexors. She has a mild scoliosis which may progress since she has a strong ATNR to the left and very little ability to change her posture.

To prevent increased deformity while increasing social and educational opportunities, Jill needs to be positioned in sitting and standing to encourage symmetry and midline orientation. An adapted wheelchair would be appropriate for positioning for activities, social interactions, meals in the classroom and at home, and for transportation on the school bus. [71-73] A stander in the classroom would provide an alternative to sitting,

allowing trunk, hip, and knee extension while maintaining symmetry and positioning of the upper extremities. [74-76]

Both the wheelchair and stander would need specific adaptations to meet Jill's needs. For example, in the wheelchair a firm back is needed to support a vertical pelvic position. A firm seat elevated 10 degrees will assist with equal weight bearing across the pelvis and decrease the pull of the hamstrings. Adjustable footrests, lateral pelvic supports, lateral trunk supports, and an adductor wedge also may be necessary. A removable lap board would assist posture of the thoracic spine and shoulders by supporting the elbows and forearms and provide a surface for feeding, educational activities, and communication.

An adjustable height stander would allow Jill to stand near the floor for peer interaction. Adjustable anterior leg supports, adaptable foot supports, a pelvic belt, and an adjustable, attachable tray would all be appropriate for Jill (See Chapter 12).

CASE NO. 3 — TAYLOR
Myelomeningocele, Repaired L 1-2, 4 Years

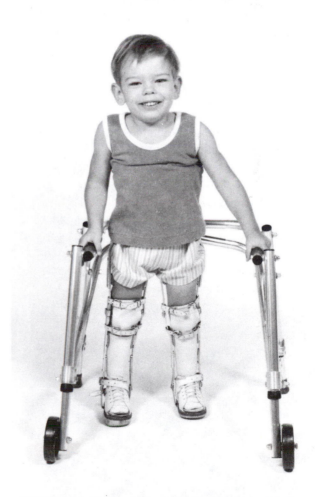

FIGURE 14. *Even without standing balance, this four-year-old boy can use the Posture Control Walker to develop appropriate body alignment, exploration, and mobility.*

Taylor is a four year old with L 1-2 level myelo-meningocele. He has the following strengths and weaknesses related to ambulation. Taylor lacks strength in his lower trunk, hips, legs, and feet to get into a standing position without the support of his braces. He is able to get into a sitting position and into a hands and knees position, although he cannot walk. He attempts to pull up to kneeling at a low table or bench but must take most of his weight on his abdomen since hip strength and balance prevent him from kneeling upright.

Upper extremity strength, interest in mobility, and a sense of security in his parapodium indicate that he is ready for assisted ambulation.[77]

Taylor recently received long leg braces with a pelvic band and is currently using a Posture Control walker to provide external balance and alignment with trunk and hip extension.[13] (Figure 14) The LSU reciprocation brace was considered to take advantage of Taylor's active hip flexors and allow reciprocal movements of the lower extremities.[12, 78] However, it was decided that Taylor might progress faster with ambulation and achieve better alignment in spite of contractures if long leg braces with a pelvic band were used. As Taylor achieves greater confidence and independence, the LSU reciprocation brace could be considered. In his braces and walker, Taylor uses a swing-to gait. In this fashion he is able to walk around his home and preschool classroom.

Taylor is not able to get into a standing position or lock his braces without assistance. He is unable to negotiate ramps, slopes, stairs, or rough terrains and therefore cannot ambulate outside without assistance. He can change directions by pivoting with his walker. He walks slowly and fatigues easily due to lack of strength in his arms and shoulders.[79]

General Treatment Goals:
1. increase strength in the upper extremities and trunk.
2. increase ability to initiate walking with weight shift and hip flexion.
3. improve balance and security in the upright position.
4. increase independence in use of the braces.

Short-Term Objectives:
Following treatment, Taylor will:
1. walk 10-20 feet with the hip joints unlocked using his walker.
2. stand with loftstrand crutches and take 10 steps with assistance.
3. walk to his car along the sidewalk and across his lawn with his braces and walker.
4. lock and unlock his braces and get into and out of his wheelchair independently, 3 of 5 times.

The following activities might be included, in the following sequence, in a single treatment session to achieve the treatment objectives. Beginning without braces, the therapist holds Taylor around his trunk while he is prone and his trunk is horizontal. He supports himself on his hands on a small bench. In this position Taylor reaches forward taking all his weight on one arm then the other.

The therapist then takes Taylor on her lap while she sits on a ball. Taylor places his hands behind him on a bench. This position requires a great deal of strength in the scapular adductors and depressors as well as in muscles controlling the shoulders, elbows, and wrists (Figure 15).

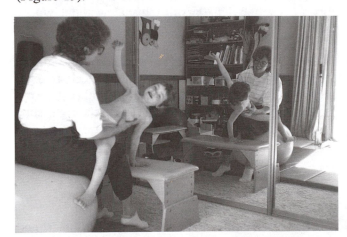

FIGURE 16. *Rotation of trunk over weight bearing shoulder.*

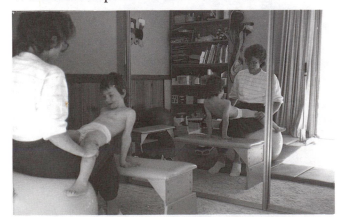

FIGURE 15. *Weight bearing in this position requires head and trunk strength as well as upper extremity and scapular strength.*

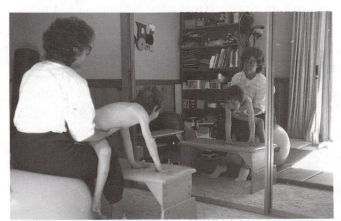

FIGURE 17. *This activity requires all muscles of the upper trunk and shoulder girdle and arms to move and stabilize as the child changes positions.*

From this position the therapist rotates Taylor's trunk so that all the weight is on one hand and Taylor reaches into the air. Taylor continues to rotate over his shoulder until he supports himself prone on hands on the bench (Figure 16 & 17).

Now Taylor sits on the floor, pushes down on his hands, and scoots backward across the floor. To scoot forward, the therapist may need to support Taylor's legs to remove the resistance against the floor.

With his braces on, Taylor is placed prone and pushes up onto his hands. The therapist supports his legs and Taylor wheelbarrow walks across the room.

In his braces, Taylor stands leaning onto a bench. Taylor supports his weight on one hand and reaches down to unlock one hip then the other. Taylor then pivots around to sit on the bench. Once in sitting, he unlocks his knee joints.

CASE NO. 4 — ASHLEY
Down Syndrome, 15 Months

Ashley is a 15 month old with Down syndrome. She has the following strengths and problem areas related to her ambulation potential. Ashley is sitting independently and can get into sitting from prone by spreading her legs 180 degrees and using her hands to push to a sitting position, ending with hips widely abducted moving in the sagittal plane. This is a typical pattern for a child with Down syndrome.[80] She can pull to stand and stand at a small table or bench. However, she pulls to stand primarily by pulling up with her arms and supporting with her abdomen on the table. She stands with weight against her abdomen, the hips flexed, and the knees hyperextended. She cannot adjust her feet under her to provide a stable base of support. At the table, she can extend her arms when standing, but to reach out to play she drops back to supporting on elbows since she does not have the shoulder and trunk stability to permit weight shift necessary for reaching.

Ashley is unable to walk alone. She will take steps with her hands held. She stands and steps with a broad base and does not flex her knees during swing phase. The hips are abducted and facilitate foot clearance. During stance her knees are hyperextended. Both during swing and stance the hips are flexed and she cannot align her trunk and pelvis over the lower extremities. Her swing phase is short as is her step length. She does not yet have any rotation around the body axis. She has limited balance reactions for standing or walking. Ashley is receiving physical therapy along with her early intervention program with the goal to improve those components of movement which are currently interfering with her motor performance.[81,82]

General Treatment Goals:
1. increase ability to shift the center of gravity outside the base of support.
2. improve trunk stability in standing.
3. increase hip extension in rising to stand and standing.
4. decrease base of support in standing.

Short-Term Objectives:
Following treatment, Ashley will:
1. move from kneeling to side sitting with assistance from the therapist, each time requested.
2. maintain support on extended arms at a small table without leaning on her abdomen for 30 seconds.
3. rise to stand from a small bench by pushing up with her legs, 2 of 3 times.
4. accept weight transfer while cruising along a bench, 5 feet in each direction.

The following activities might be included in a single treatment session to achieve these objectives:

Therapy begins with Ashley sitting on a small bench. Blocks are placed on the bench to her left and a container is placed on a bench or table in front of her. The therapist shifts Ashley's weight to the left so that weight is supported on the left hand while she picks up a block with her right. Caution must be taken that Ashley does not move her feet in an attempt to widen her base of support, but actually shifts her trunk over her feet and pelvis thereby shifting her center of gravity over her base of support. Support is given around her trunk so that Ashley can come back to a sitting position and drop the block into the container.

Ashley then is encouraged to place her hands on the bench in front of her and rise to stand. The therapist assists Ashley at the trunk to rise to stand, and once standing, pressure is placed down through Ashley's shoulders and hips to facilitate cocontraction of her trunk muscles.

Now the bench is removed and Ashley remains in standing. The therapist continues to provide support to Ashley's trunk and encourages her to lean on a wall, mirror, or easel. She can lean on one hand to play with magnetic pieces or stickers. The therapist shifts Ashley's weight to the right, adducting the left leg, and then shifts her weight back to the left, adducting the right leg to narrow her base of support.

Side stepping along the mirror or wall can be facilitated as she moves along the mirror to reach for stickers. This will encourage weight transfer from one leg to another over a narrow base of support (Figure 8).

Standing is fatiguing, so Ashley is brought down into side sitting. Toys are placed so that she has to move into a hands and knees position to reach them. Then she has to move back to side sitting to play. The therapist assists these movement transitions and Ashley's stability in these positions. ❏

References

1. Beck RJ, Andriacchi TP, Kuo KN, et al: Changes in the gait patterns of growing children. J Bone Jt Surg 63A: 1452-1457, 1981

2. Burnett C, Johnson EW: Development of gait in childhood: Part II. Dev Med Child Neurol 13:207-215, 1971

3. Norlin R, Odenrick P, Sandlund B: Development of gait in the normal child. J Ped Ortho 1: 261-266, 1981

4. Okamoto T, Kumamota M: Electromyographic study of the learning process of walking in infants. Electromyography 12: 149-158, 1972

5. Statham L, Murray MP: Early walking patterns of normal children. Clin Ortho Related Res 79: 8-24, 1971

6. Perry J: Cerebral palsy gait. In Samuelson RL (ed): Orthopedic Aspects of Cerebral Palsy. Clinics in Dev Med Nos 52/53: Philadelphia, PA, JB Lippincott, 1975, pp 71-97

7. Mann R: Biomechanics in cerebral palsy. Foot and Ankle 4: 114-119, 1983

8. Pope K, Wigglesworth JS: Haemorrhage, Ischaemia and the Perinatal Brain. Clinics in Dev Med Nos 69/70, Philadelphia, PA, JB Lippincott, 1979

9. Woods BT, Teuber HL: Early onset of complementary specialization of cerebral hemispheres in man. Trans Am Neurol Assoc 98: 113-117, 1973

10. Campbell S: Central nervous system dysfunction in children. In Campbell S (ed): Pediatric Neurologic Physical Therapy, New York, NY, Churchill Livingstone, 1984, pp 1-12

11. Bobath B, Bobath K: Motor Development in the Different Types of Cerebral Palsy. London, William Heinemann, 1975

12. Badell-Ribera A: Myelodysplasia. In Molnar G (ed): Pediatric Rehabilitation, Baltimore, MD, Williams and Wilkins, 1985, pp 176-206

13. Ryan KD, Plaski C, Emans JB: Myelodysplasia-the musculoskeletal problem: Habilitation from infancy to adulthood. Phys Ther 71: 935-946, 1991

14. Hoffer MM, Fiewell E, Perry J, et al: Functional ambulation in patients with myelomeningocele. J Bone Jt Surg 55A: 137-148, 1973

15. DeSouza MB, Carroll N: Ambulation of the braced myelomeningocele patient. J Bone Jt Surg 58A: 1112-1118, 1976

16. Capute AJ, Shapiro BK, Palmer TB: Spectrum of developmental disabilities: Continuum of motor dysfunction. Ortho Clin N Am 12: 3-22, 1981

17. Cratty B: Motor Activities in the Education of Retardates, ed 2. Philadelphia, PA, Lea and Febiger, 1974

18. Shapiro B, Accardo P, Capute A: Factors affecting walking in a profoundly retarded population. Dev Med Child Neurol 21: 369-373, 1979

19. Donoghue E, Kuman B, Bullmore GH: Some factors affecting age of walking in a mentally retarded population. Dev Med Child Neurol 12: 781-792, 1970

20. Melyn M, White D: Mental and developmental milestones of noninstitutionalized Down syndrome children. Ped 52: 542-545, 1973

21. Holt KS: Review: The assessment of walking in children with particular reference to cerebral palsy. Child Care, Health and Dev 7: 281-297, 1981

22. Campbell SK, Wilhelm IJ: Developmental sequence in infants at high risk for central nervous system dysfunction: The recovery process in the first year of life. In Stack J (ed): The Special Infant: An Interdisciplinary Approach to the Optimal Development of Infants. New York, NY, Human Sciences Press, 1982

23. Molnar GE, Gordon SU: Cerebral palsy: Predictive value of selected signs for early prognostication of motor function. Arch Phys Med Rehabil 57: 153-158, 1976

24. Badell-Ribera A: Cerebral palsy: Postural-locomotor prognosis in spastic diplegia. Arch Phy Med Rehabil 66: 614-619, 1985

25. Largo RH, Molenari L, Weber M, et al: Early development of locomotion: Significances of prematurity, cerebral palsy and sex. Dev Med Child Neurol 27: 183-191, 1985

26. Molnar GE: Cerebral palsy: prognosis and how to judge it. Pediatric Annals 8: 596-604. 1979

27. Molnar GE: Cerebral Palsy. In Molnar GE (ed): Pediatric Rehabilitation. Baltimore, MD, Williams and Wilkins, 1985, pp 420-467

28. Bleck EE: Locomotor prognosis in cerebral palsy. Dev Med Child Neurol 17: 18-25, 1975

29. Scherzer A, Tschamuter I: Early Diagnosis and Therapy in Cerebral Palsy. Pediatric Habilitation Vol. 3, New York, NY, Marcel Dekker, 1982

30. Sparling JW: The transdisciplinary approach with the developmentally delayed child. Phys Occup Ther Pediatr 1: 3-15, 1980

31. Harris SR: Transdisciplinary therapy model for the infant with Down syndrome. Phys Ther 60: 420-423, 1980

32. Saturen P: Skeletal Disorders in Children. In Molnar GE (ed): Pediatric Rehabilitation. Baltimore, MD, Williams and Wilkins, 1985, pp 390-419

33. Staheli LT: Medial femoral torsion. Orthop Clin North Am 11: 39-50, 1980

34. Cusick BD: Progressive Casting and Splinting for Lower Extremity Deformities in Children with Neuromotor Dysfunction. Tucson, AZ, Therapy Skill Builders, 1990

35. Bleck EE: Orthopedics Management in Cerebral Palsy. Philadelphia, PA, JB Lippincott, 1987

36. Berger W, Quintern J, Dietz V: Pathophysiology of gait in children with cerebral palsy. Electroenceph and Clin Neurophysio 53: 538-548, 1982

37. Csongrada J, Bleck EE, Ford WF: Gait electromyography in normal and spastic children, with special reference to quadriceps femoris and hamstring muscles. Dev Med Child Neurol 21: 738-748, 1979

38. Gueth V, Steinhausen D, Abbink F: The investigation of walking of patients with cerebral palsy by the electromyogram using surface electrodes. Electromyogr Clin Neurophysiol 24: 225-240, 1984

39. Lee EH, Nather A, Goh J, et al: Gait analysis in cerebral palsy. Annals Acad Medicine, 14: 37-43, 1985

40. Skrotzky K: Gait analysis in cerebral palsied and nonhandicapped children. Arch Phys Med Rehabil 64: 291-295, 1985

41. Simon SR, Deutoch SD, Nuzzo RM, et al: Genu recurvatum in spastic cerebral palsy. J Bone Jt Surg. 60A: 882-894, 1985

42. Sutherland D: Gait analysis in cerebral palsy. Dev Med Child Neurol 20: 807-813, 1978

43. Chong KC, Vojnic DC, Quanbury AO, et al: The assessment of the internal rotation gait in cerebral palsy. Clin Ortho and Related Res 132: 145-150, 1978

44. Sutherland D, Cooper L: The pathomechanics of progressive crouch gait in spastic diplegia. Orth Clinics North Am 9: 143-154, 1978

45. Woltering H, Guth V, Abbink F: Electromyographic investigation of gait in cerebral palsied children. Electromyogr Clin Neurophysiol 19: 519-533, 1979

46. Wong MA, Simon S, Olshen RA: Statistical analysis of gait patterns of persons with cerebral palsy. Stat in Medicine, 2: 245-354, 1983

47. Gage JR, Fabia D, Hicks R, et al: Pre and post operative gait analysis in patients with spastic diplegia: A preliminary report. J Ped Ortho 4: 715-725, 1984

48. Hoffer MM, Perry J, Melkonian GJ: Dynamic electromyography and decision making for surgery in the upper extremity of patients with cerebral palsy. J Hand Surg 4: 424-431, 1979

49. Perry J, Hoffer M M, Antonelli MS, et al: Electromyography before and after surgery for hip deformity in children with cerebral palsy. J Bone Jt Surg 58A: 201-208, 1976

50. Perry J, Hoffer MM: Preoperative and post operative dynamic electromyography as an aid in planning tendon transfers in children with cerebral palsy. J Bone Jt Surg 59A: 531-537, 1977

51. Palisano RJ: Investigation of Electromyographic Gait Analysis as a Method of Evaluating the Effects of Neurodevelopmental Treatment in a Child with Cerebral Palsy. Master's Thesis, Division of Phys Ther, School of Med, U. of N Carolina at Chapel Hill, 1981

52. Watabe S, Otabe T, Kii K, et al: Improving the walking of a spastic diplegic child. Totline 7: 14, 1981

53. Leonard CT, Hirschfeld H, Forssberg H: The development of independent walking in children with cerebral palsy. Dev Med Child Neurol 33:567-577, 1991

54. Rose J, Medeiros J, Parker R: Energy cost index as an estimate of energy expenditure of cerebral-palsied children during assisted ambulation. Dev Med Child Neurol 27: 485-490, 1985

55. Stallard J, Rose GK, Tart J, et al: Assessment of orthoses by means of speed and heart rate. J Med Engineering Tech 2: 22-24, 1978

56. Bard G, Ralston HJ: Measurement of energy expenditures during ambulation with special references to evaluation of assistive devices. Arch Phy Med and Rehabil 40: 415-420, 1959

57. Campbell J, Ball J: Energetics of walking in cerebral palsy. Ortho Clinics of North Am 9: 374-376, 1978

58. Dahlback GO, Norton R: The effects of corrective surgery on energy expenditure during ambulation in children with cerebral palsy. Europ J of Applied Physio 54: 67-70, 1985

59. Manning J: Facilitation of movement - the Bobath approach. Physio 58: 403-407, 1972

60. Harryman SE: Lower-extremity surgery for children with cerebral palsy: Physical therapy management. Phys Ther 72:16-24, 1992

61. Logan L, Byers-Hinkley K, Ciccone CD: Anterior versus posterior walkers: A gait analysis study. Dev Med Child Neurol 32: 1044-1048, 1990

62. Levangie PK, Chemira M, Johnston M, et al: The effects of posterior rolling walkers vs the standard rolling walker in gait characteristics of children with spastic cerebral palsy. Phys Occup Ther Pediatr 9: 1-17, 1989

63. Wilson JM, Park TS, Ortman M: Changes in ambulation in children with spastic diplegia following selective dorsal rhizotomy. Paper presented at Physical Therapy Management of the Cerebral Palsy Child Undergoing Selective Dorsal Rhizotomy. St. Louis, Nov 1991

64. Storrs BB, McLane DG: Selective posterior rhizotomy in the treatment of spasticity associated with myelomeningocele. In Marlin AE (ed): Concepts Pediatric Neurosurg, Basel Kargen 9:173-177, 1989

65. Thomas SE, Mazur JM, Child ME, Supan TJ: Quantitative evaluation of AFO use with myelomeningocele children. Z Kindrichir 44:38-40, 1989

66. Bertoti DB: Effect of short leg casting on ambulation in children with cerebral palsy. Phys Ther 66: 1522-1529, 1986

67. Watt J, Sims D, Harckham F, et al: A prospective study of inhibitive casting as an adjunct to physiotherapy for cerebral palsied children. Dev Med Child Neurol 28: 480-487, 1986

68. Cahan LD, Adams JM, Perry J, et al: Instrumental gait analysis after selective posterior rhizotomy. Dev Med Child Neurol 32:1037-1043, 1990

69. Montgomery PC: A clinical report of long term outcomes following selective posterior rhizotomy: implications for selection, follow-up, and research. Phys Occup Ther Pediatr, 12:69-88, 1992

70. Brown JK, Rodda J. Walsh EG, Wright GW: Neurophysiology of lower limb function in hemiplegic children. Dev Med Child Neurol 33, 1037-1047, 1991

71. Bergen AF, Presperin J, Tallman T: Positioning for Function; Wheelchairs and Other Assistive Technologies. Valhalla, NY, Valhalla Rehab Pub, 1990

72. Matlock WJ: Seating and positioning for the physically impaired. Orth Prost 31: 11-21, 1977

73. Alexander MA: Orthotics, adapted seating, and assistive devices. In Molnar G (ed): Pediatric Rehabilitation. Baltimore, MD, Williams and Wilkins, 1985, pp 158-175

74. Finnie N: Handling the Young Cerebral Palsied Child at Home, ed 2. New York, NY, E.P. Dutton, 1975

75. Shephard RF: Physiotherapy in Paediatrics, ed 2. London, William Heinemann, 1980

76. Trefler E (ed): Seating for Children with Cerebral Palsy. Memphis, TN, U of TN Rehab Engineering Dept, 1984

77. Matlock WJ: The parapodium: An orthotic device for neuromuscular disorders. Artificial Limbs 15: 36-47, 1971

78. Douglas R, Larson PF, D'Ambrosia R, et al: The LSU reciprocation-gait orthosis. Orthopedics 6: 834-839, 1983

79. Wallace S: The effect of upper-limb function on mobility of children with myelomeningocele. Dev Med Child Neurol 15 (Supp. 29): 84-91, 1973

80. Lydic J: Assessment of the quality of sitting and gait patterns in children with Down syndrome. Phys Ther 59: 1489-1494, 1979

81. Piper MC, Pless IB: Early intervention for infants with Down syndrome: A controlled trial. Pediatrics 65: 463-469, 1980

82. Harris SR, Shea AM: Down Syndrome. In Campbell SK. (ed): Pediatric Neurologic Physical Therapy, ed 2. New York, NY, Churchill Livingstone, 1991

CHAPTER 11

DEVELOPING HAND FUNCTION

Regi Boehme, OTR

◆

The shoulder girdle is one of the most complicated kinesiological systems in the human body. Structurally, it consists of the scapulas, clavicles, and sternum. When looking at functional performance, however, the humerus, rib cage, and spine are considered integral parts of the shoulder girdle (Figures 1 & 2) and provide attachments for the muscles of the shoulder girdle. When there is a lack of proper joint alignment or a lack of adequate joint mobility in any of these structures, the shoulder girdle cannot function dynamically to support the control of the arm. Dynamic function of the shoulder girdle has several important roles in upper extremity control. Enough proximal stability is needed for the arms to accept part of the body weight during transitional movements. For example, proximal stability of the shoulder girdle is evident when the scapulas maintain their active connection with the rib cage as the body weight is shifted over the arms in any position. When the scapulas and rib cage separate, scapular winging is evident medially and inferiorly. Scapular winging is not, in and of itself, abnormal or atypical. Normal children and adults may exhibit scapular-rib cage separation during portions of upper extremity weight shifting. This scapular winging is created by changes in the center of gravity. The scapulas and rib cage may separate briefly, but they are also able to hold together during at least part of the movement pattern. When scapular instability on the rib cage is a problem, the child will compensate in a variety of ways. For example, in quadruped, the child may markedly internally or externally rotate the upper arms to achieve mechanical stability or hip flexion may be used to keep most of the body weight on the legs instead of the arms. The child may move quickly between positions using momentum rather than postural control to shift weight. The child may "fixate" muscles on one side of his body for stability, and direct his movements asymmetrically, always moving one favorite side. The child may not feel secure enough, proximally, to attempt transitional movements, thereby limiting his own ability to move and explore the world. Scapular instability is a problem only when it interferes with the child's ability to develop gross motor movement patterns. The scapula must be dynamically stable on the rib cage, and it also must be mobile. Movement of the humerus in space depends on movement of both the scapula and clavicle. When shoulder girdle movement is blocked for any reason, the humerus cannot move through its potential range. The head of the humerus is large in comparison to the glenoid fossa of the scapula. As the humerus moves in space during reach, the scapula has to move

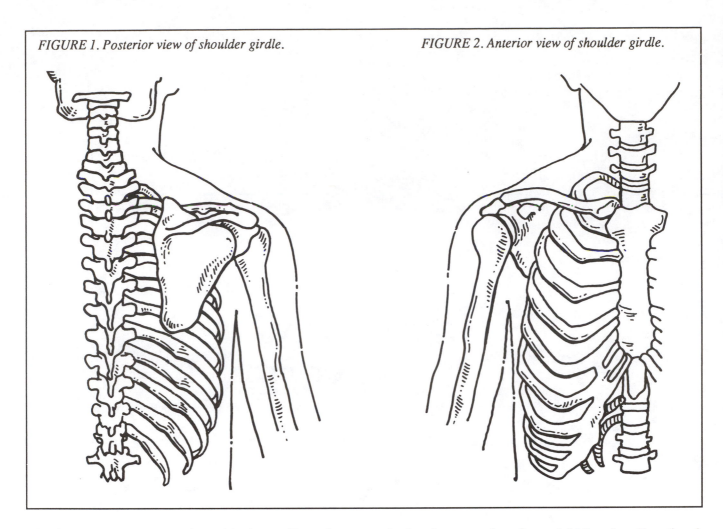

FIGURE 1. Posterior view of shoulder girdle.

FIGURE 2. Anterior view of shoulder girdle.

with it to avoid a bone on bone blockage. Since the scapula's only boney attachment to the body is at the acromio-clavicular joint, the clavicles also must be mobile during reach. Scapular movement then, is dependent upon clavicular mobility.

The scapula and humerus act together during reach. As the humerus adducts horizontally toward and beyond midline, the scapula must abduct or move away from the spine. Active horizontal ranges of the humerus are those movements expressed at 90 degrees. As the humerus horizontally abducts, the scapula must adduct or move toward the spine. As the humerus moves into extension, the scapula moves into downward rotation and the inferior border moves closer to the spine. As the humerus moves above 90 degrees in either forward flexion, abduction or adduction, the scapula must upwardly rotate and its inferior border moves away from the spine and under the axilla. When scapular upward rotation is blocked, as is often seen with cerebral palsy, the child will not be able to raise the arm above 90 degrees.

THE FUNCTIONAL ROLE OF THE HUMERUS

The upper arm is used primarily for reaching. Specifically, its job is to project the hand in a wide and varied range of space, to direct the hand to an object, or to place the hand on a surface for weight bearing. Functional humeral control means that the upper arm can reach, hold the reaching posture in mid-space, and correct or change the direction of reach during movement. As larger muscles move the humerus, smaller rotator cuff muscles hold the humeral head in the glenoid fossa and depress it slightly. These small rotator cuff muscles also alter the rotational component of the humerus during reach, making it possible for the large humeral head to clear the joint easily and comfortably.

The humerus needs stability and freedom in the glenoid fossa for controlled movement. When the joint capsule is not malleable and when the humeral head is poorly positioned in the joint, humeral range is restricted. Joint capsule tightness thus can result from a lack of active movement on the part of the child. A poorly aligned humeral head also may be due to an imbalance of muscle activity around the glenohumeral joint. When small rotator cuff muscles (Figure 3) are shortened or tight, humeral range again is restricted. As the child attempts to reach, the humerus may pull the scapula away from the rib cage, creating lateral winging. This is described commonly as scapulohumeral tightness, but is often a combined problem of both shortened musculature and scapular-rib cage instability.

Therapeutic Exercise In Developmental Disabilities

The Functional Role Of The Elbow

The elbow brings the hand to and from the body. It can make the arm shorter or longer during reach and transitional movement patterns. Dynamic elbow control means that the elbow can move through its maximum range slowly, can stop and hold in midrange, and is strong enough to make the arm longer or shorter as it is loaded with partial body weight. A child may be able to quickly flex or extend the elbow during reach, but lack the ability to make slow graded movement.

Generalized movement disorders that interfere with the experience of developmental transitional movements result in weak triceps. A child may be able to use the elbow for reaching out in space, but may not be able to use the elbow once the arm is loaded with body weight. Triceps weakness inevitably will interfere with gross motor treatment and the child's ability to use ambulation aids. The development of elbow control depends on both glenohumeral activity and adequate hand placement for effective loading on extended arms. When positioned on extended arms, the child may compensate for lack of stability by locking the elbows into extension, which then interferes with dynamic weight shift. The child may fist the hands tightly to increase the stability in the arms in lieu of elbow control, but this compensation will interfere with weight shift.

The Functional Role Of The Forearm And Wrist

The forearm and wrist orient the hand in space during reach and in preparation for weight bearing or weight shifting. Forearm rotation is critical for function and develops as a result of controlled humeral rotation, balanced elbow flexion and extension, and prone weight shifting experiences. Prone play experiences allow the child to isolate forearm movements while the humeral movements are restricted through the weight bearing posture. When any of these components are at risk, the development of forearm rotation may be blocked or functionally restricted. Limited freedom of forearm movement in either pronation or supination has a greater negative impact on hand function than it does on weight shifting. The capability for wrist control depends on a balance of long finger flexion and extension across the wrist joint. When children lack range in wrist movement, hand placement is limited both in space and weight bearing. As the child attempts to load the hand with body weight, compensations are evident. The child may bear weight on the knuckles or back of the hand when wrist extension is limited (Figures 4 & 5). When joint range is limited in either direction, the child will bear weight on the extreme radial or ulnar side of the hand. These compensations will impact the quality of

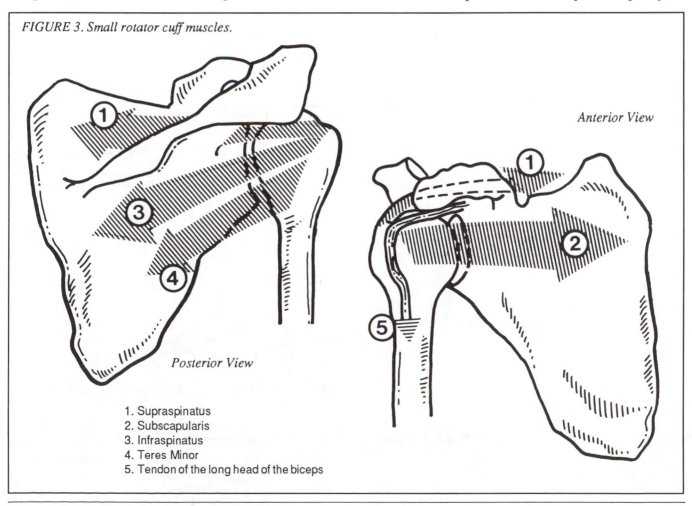

FIGURE 3. Small rotator cuff muscles.

Anterior View

Posterior View

1. Supraspinatus
2. Subscapularis
3. Infraspinatus
4. Teres Minor
5. Tendon of the long head of the biceps

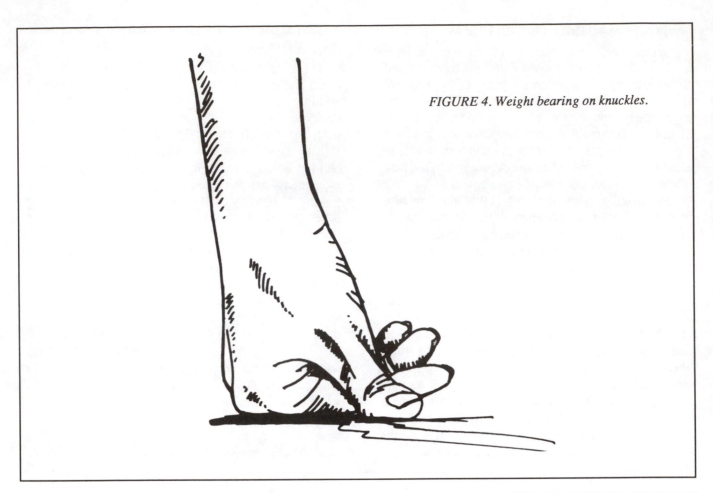

FIGURE 4. Weight bearing on knuckles.

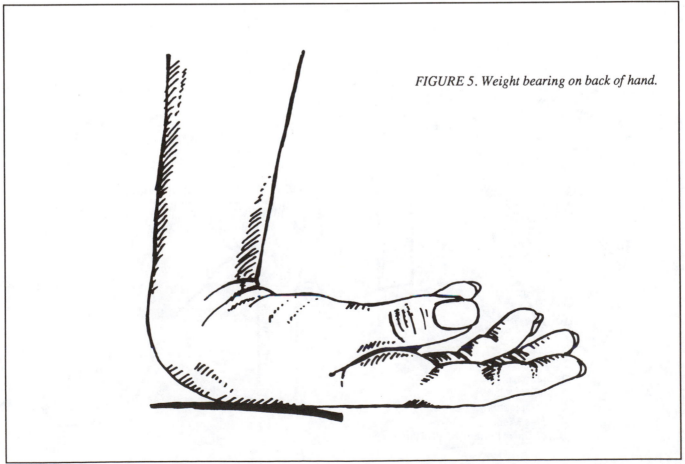

FIGURE 5. Weight bearing on back of hand.

Therapeutic Exercise In Developmental Disabilities

weight shifting, but should not completely prevent movement transitions.

When wrist range is adequate, but muscle co-activation around the circumference of the wrist is poor, the child may feel unstable in weight bearing. Wrist instability creates the need for other compensations. The child may take weight on the palmar surface of the metacarpal heads, forming a modified tripod effect (Figure 6). This virtually locks the wrist joint so that it feels stable, but inevitably stretches out the metacarpal-phalangeal (MP) tendons. Other children with wrist instability will opt to flex the fingers and adduct the thumb in an effort to gain distal stability in lieu of wrist control during weight shifting.

THE FUNCTIONAL ROLE OF THE HAND

The hand has many functional and critical roles. Generally, it shapes itself around an object and accommodates its own shape to the shape to be held or the shape and contour of the weight bearing surface. In order to do this, it must be expandable enough to flatten out for weight bearing. It must also be malleable enough to shape itself around both large and small objects. The hand at times needs to be powerful and at other times delicate in its approach to grasp and manipulation. The ability of the hand to be functional in all of these situations depends on a variety of arching systems in the palm. The capability for arch development in the hand relies on balance of activity between the long finger flexors and extensors, the capability for neutral alignment between wrist and hand, mobility of the carpal and metacarpal bones, and activity of the intrinsics.

Ongoing sensory-motor experiences prepare the hand for its long term development of both simple and complex patterns of movement. The young child's hand-to-hand, hand-to-knee, and hand-to-foot play help the hand to experience its accommodating potential. Ungraded pressure with the child's first attempts to grasp helps make the arches malleable. Early weight shifting experiences on extended arms help to expand the hand and develop balance reactions from the arches. The young child does not actually develop a controlled grasp until the hand is used in a neutral position at the wrist. Once this basic hand pattern is established the fingers are able to develop more distal control for more refined function.

TASK ANALYSIS

Therapists share a common goal in treatment. We make every attempt to guide children toward a life of independent function. The ability to tend to one's own needs is basic to our belief that we have some control over our lives and ultimately our destinies. As we make

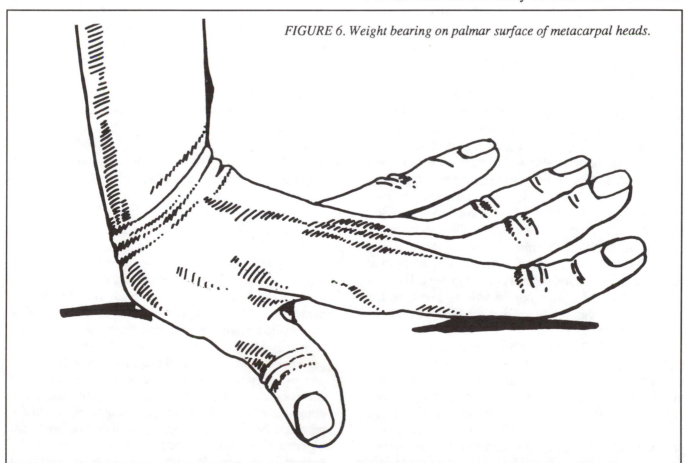

FIGURE 6. Weight bearing on palmar surface of metacarpal heads.

commitments to specific functional goals for the children, we need to understand what we are asking them to do. We can achieve the same functional outcomes in different ways. For example, there are a variety of methods for putting on a pair of shoes or a T-shirt. To determine the basic motor prerequisites for these tasks, move through the tasks yourself. An erroneous assumption is made if you think you understand the motor components, just because you do them automatically. Move through a task in slow motion and ask yourself what parts of your body are moving? What points of stability are you using to make your body move? Where do you feel yourself "holding" your position against gravity? What's preventing you from falling? Normal children may have developed many of the necessary motor prerequisites for movement and self-care by the age of two years. Yet, it takes many more years of practice to become graceful and controlled with movement and adept at dressing and other self-care skills. Independent functional skills develop long after the motor components are available. Developing independence requires motor planning and sequencing, focused attention on the task, and goal-oriented behavior.

ASSESSMENT

Identify the child's functional skills. Can he use the upper extremities to help with movement in and out of positions? Can the child dress, use the toilet, self-feed, use the hands for classroom learning, and use the hands to explore and play with objects in the environment? Can the child use his arms and hands for mobility aids or transfers?

How does the child function? Does he move the arms normally during activity? Is there an increase in muscle tone, abnormal patterns, or compensations? Identify those skills that the child is unable to perform. What consistent problems seem to interfere with function? Problems with functional independence may be due to a lack of mobility. The child may not have enough joint range to accomplish the functional task. It could be due to poor joint alignment. For example, the child may not be able to position the hips adequately to obtain a functional base of support for sitting. The child may have a lack of postural control against gravity. If this is the case, the child may not be able to maintain his balance during the weight shifting needed for a particular functional task.

If there is a lack of muscle activity, the child may not be able to organize his body and plan his movements. Confusion about sensory input may also interfere with the child's motor abilities (see Chapter 6). Sensory organization contributes to the child's ability to plan his movements and interact with his world. The inability to organize oneself and process sensory information may make learning frustrating. When describing the child's

use of arms and hands, use functional descriptions. For example, the upper arm can be described in terms of range of reach, holding the reaching posture against gravity, correcting the reach during movement, accepting weight on forearms, weight shifting on forearms, moving in and out of prone propping, demonstrating asymmetrical arm and hand use, demonstrating a bilateral approach, and demonstrating unilateral control. Functional descriptors for the elbow may include bringing the hand to the body, face, or foot, accepting weight on extended arms, and moving in and out of extended arm weight bearing postures. In the area of forearm and wrist control, does the child demonstrate the ability to orient the lower arm and hand appropriately in space in preparation for grasp, use a variety of forearm positions, or hold an object while moving the forearm and wrist? Evaluation of hand function may address the child's ability to bear weight on the hand, weight shift over an opened hand, grasp or immobilize an object in the hand, manipulate an object between two hands, manipulate an object inside one hand, or release an object without having to fling it or flex the wrist to let it drop out. The information gathered during assessment needs to be analyzed from a functional perspective. Why does the child move as he does? What motor components are present and which ones are missing? What abnormal movements is the child using? How does he compensate for the limitations of his body? Do the compensations help or hinder the child's attempt at function? Can the child do a part of the functional task? Does he have the cognitive/perceptual skills for the functional task? Is this a skill that the child is motivated to do? It's easier to reach a functional goal that the child, the professional, and the parent discuss and choose together. The child does not have to approach the task in the usual or "culturally acceptable" way. Allow him to try his own way. For example, a child may be able to undress himself while lying on the floor, but could not even begin to do the same task while sitting on a bench or chair.

TREATMENT

Many functional skills are learned cognitively and rely on voluntary movement rather than the automatic movements used in balance reactions. Voluntary movements require effort and this may increase the atypical or less desirable muscle tone and poor postural control seen in the child with cerebral palsy. Preparing the child before practicing a skill will make the task less effortful and will help the child to develop some of the motor components that he may be missing. Achieving scapulo-humeral mobility, for example, will give the child the potential for increased range of reach during functional movement. The normal baby acquires freedom of the humeri in the scapulo-humeral joints with movement from supine to sidelying and from supine through rolling to prone. As the weight of the trunk is loaded onto the upper arm in these transitional movement patterns, elongation of the musculature between humeri and scapula and between humeri and rib cage will give the child the freedom to initiate upper arm movements in a greater range. Reaching in prone then stimulates the child to use this new range. Scapulo-humeral mobility develops in the normal baby between three to six months of age.

Facilitating scapular-thoracic activity will give the child the stability needed for controlling reach in midranges. Active thoracic extension is the prerequisite for medial scapular stability because it prevents excessive scapular winging. The normal baby develops active thoracic extension initially in prone play where he can work from the stability provided by the weight bearing surface. Appropriate prone play requires that the body weight be transferred off the shoulders and onto the abdomen and thighs. With the weight shifted posteriorly, the child can begin to push up on forearms and the spine extends smoothly. With volitional or accidental weight shifting, the scapula begins to hold onto the rib cage. As the child develops endurance in spinal extension, reach can be added. Control of reach in space depends on scapular-rib cage stability, which begins to develop as early as two months in the normal baby. Increasing shoulder girdle and elbow strength is an important aspect of the child's ability to use the arms for transitional movements, functional transfers, and use of mobility aids. Facilitation of slow graded movements where the child uses the arms to push from one position to another is the way the normal baby develops strength and endurance in the shoulders and elbows. This developmental play begins with the five-month-old's experience with prone on extended arms. But the quality of this control depends on the child moving from propping on his side up to sitting, sitting to quadruped, and creeping in quadruped. Developing isolated elbow movements is critical for self-care skills. Hand to body play emerges in supine in the three-month-old, with hand-to-chest along with hand-to-mouth play, and is used functionally throughout life. The child continues to develop isolated elbow movements in prone play at five months of age by shifting weight from the forearms, back to the elbows where the lower arm is freed for elbow flexion/extension and the humeral movements are inhibited by the weight bearing position. The child then generalizes this sensory motor experience in other positions, using the elbow movement to activate or explore a toy. The elbow movements are used again as the child attempts to hold his bottle at six to seven months of age, and again in finger feeding at eight to nine months of age. Without these experiences in treatment, the child will be dominated by either excessive elbow flexion or extension. The child may be able to move the elbow throughout the range, but will have difficulty grading it and using it in functional movement patterns. Prone on elbow play at five months of age also helps the child to gain isolated forearm and wrist control. He actually develops the mobility for forearm rotation at four months of age by weight shifting prone on forearms. He then shifts his weight back to the elbows and plays with movements of the forearm and wrist. The child generalizes the movement of the forearm in supine and sitting by first holding the upper arm against the rib cage for stability. Active forearm rotation, however, is not used functionally until about eight to nine months of age. An important developmental experience that prepares the wrist for eventual control is active weight shifting on extended arms. This play elongates the muscles around the wrist. The child generalizes the isolated wrist control during self-feeding and play at eight to nine months of age. For example, the child places a bread stick or toy in the mouth, stabilizes it with the jaw, and then plays with wrist movement. These varied experiences can be used in therapy to help the child use the forearm and wrist to orient the hand during functional movement.

Facilitating hand function requires a combination of many therapeutic experiences. Weight shifting on extended arms in quadruped and in transitional movement patterns helps to expand the hand so that it will be malleable enough to actively arch during grasp and manipulation. Ongoing hand to body play provides the hand with a sensation of accommodation, where the hand shapes itself around the object. Helping the child to grasp with the hand held in a neutral position at the wrist will facilitate an appropriate balance between flexion and extension over the wrist, through the palm, and over the metacarpal joints. The palm of the hand is the proximal point of control for the fingers. Digit activity is merely a reflection of palmar activity. The development of release is based on the child first learning to work long finger extensors from a point of stability. Experience with release begins with simple hand-to-hand play. The child then works on transferring objects from one hand to another, working from the stability provided by the first grasping hand. Children then let go of objects on a surface, the surface being the stable point. They also release objects to an adult who stabilizes the object. This process is generalized at eight to nine months of age, when the child has enough internal stability to release an object in space.

Simulating the skill through play helps the child to use the movements and plan the sequence without the stress of the actual task. For example, pushing a large toy or therapy ball will give the child experience with elbow extension for crutch walking. Placing hoops on the feet will prepare the child for putting on socks, orthotic devices, and shoes.

PRACTICING THE SKILL

Children learn to develop skills through successive approximation with much repetition. Repetition brings the skill from a voluntary to a more automatic level. Preparing the child will not in itself create a functional skill. The skill must be practiced and the handlers need to help the child cope with any problems that exist. Functional skills are learned in small parts. If the child is not having success in the development of independence, the task may need to be broken down into smaller steps (refer to Chapter 3 regarding motor learning issues). Many verbal cues are needed. The child can be coached as he practices in therapy and at home. He may not always know when he is moving well and when his movements are less desirable. He does not necessarily recognize normal or better movement. Temporary adaptations are appropriate during the training program. Seating devices, for example, help the child to work on the upper extremity movements required in a task without demanding that he control his whole body at the same time. Temporary adaptations should be reevaluated frequently.

CARRY-OVER

Carry-over is a critical concept. It allows the child valuable sensory repetition, which creates independence. Children with disabilities need even more repetition, because they have developed many nonfunctional habits. Carry-over should be based on reasonable expectations that take into account individual and environmental factors. Expecting parents to work with their child on dressing in the morning when the child has to go to school may not be reasonable. It is reasonable to ask parents to work on dressing and undressing in the evening at bath time or in the family room after school when the child can practice in a leisurely manner. It may not be reasonable to ask a teacher to work on independent spoon feeding during school lunch, when time is limited and many children need to be fed. It is reasonable, however, to ask a teacher to work with a child during snack time.

CASE STUDIES

CASE NO. 1 — JASON
Cerebral Palsy, Right Hemiplegia, 18 Months

Jason exhibits sensory disregard on the right side. Sensory deficits in children with hemiparesis are related directly to a lack of weight bearing and weight shifting experiences on the involved side. Jason's inability to tolerate or interpret light touch and his hypersensitive palmar grasp response also are consistent with a lack of weight bearing. Loading the arm and hand with weight provides sensory information into the joints, tendons, and muscles, as well as the skin.

Inactivity of the right shoulder girdle complex is consistent with hemiparesis and puts the entire upper extremity development at risk. This inactivity prevents Jason from developing full symmetrical flexion and extension in the trunk for optimal anterior/posterior righting responses. This further blocks lateral righting and diagonal control. The response of Jason's less involved shoulder is to increase activity to compensate for the hemiplegic side.

Inadequate shoulder girdle stability on the rib cage is a consequence of Jason's basic problem of inactivity. The most obvious instability is seen in scapular winging. Other subtle areas of instability are found in the gleno-humeral joint, the clavicle, and the right side of the rib cage. Instability interferes with Jason's ability to support his weight through the right arm during transitional movements.

Atypical posturing of the right arm in humeral extension, adduction, internal rotation, and elbow flexion, along with his associated reactions during effort are his way of attempting to control posture and movement without the proximal prerequisites. His posturing may be considered an adaptive balance reaction. To define the problem as simply increased muscle tone will not tell us how to correct the problem.

As a consequence of his scapular/rib cage instability, Jason's reach is limited to 90 degrees of humeral abduction with internal rotation. There is poor scapulo-humeral rhythm with his attempts at movement. Because the scapula pulls away from the ribs, rather than upwardly rotating as he reaches, the humerus mechanically cannot move above 90 degrees.

Weakness in elbow extension is due to several factors. Elbow flexion is used as a point of stability in lieu of proximal control, creating a situation where flexion dominates the posture of the arm. He can extend his elbow in space, but does not have the strength and endurance to extend his elbow when it is loaded with partial body weight.

Jason's lack of isolated forearm and wrist movements is a consequence of his lack of symmetrical prone play experiences in combination with the hypertonus in the hand that has developed with his efforts at movement against gravity.

Jason's hand function is limited to a gross grasp with an uncontrolled release. He lacks the hand expansion normally developed during extended arm weight bearing. He also lacks the hand to body play so important for shaping the hand.

General Treatment Goals:
1. improve sensory awareness in right arm and hand.
2. increase symmetrical activity in shoulder girdle.
3. increase range and variety of reaching patterns.
4. decrease muscle stiffness and associated reactions

which dominate the posture of the right upper extremity.

5. increase active forearm rotation and wrist extension.
6. increase functional hand use.

Short Term Objectives:

Following treatment, Jason will:

1. reach for a 12 inch diameter ball with two hands, 2 of 5 times.
2. reach overhead with elbow fully extended, 3 of 3 times.
3. reach to midline, 2 of 6 times.
4. grasp a dowel shaped toy with the right hand without abnormal posturing of the arm, 3 of 6 times.

Sample Activities:

Weight shifting over forearms and extended arms will improve sensory awareness. It also will increase shoulder girdle stability, elbow extension strength, and endurance. Symmetrical flexion and extension can be facilitated through assisted sitting on a therapy ball. Playing in prone over a roll can facilitate increased range of reach of the right arm and, at the same time, inhibit non-functional posturing.

Playing with weight taken on the elbows can help free up the forearm and wrist for functional skills.

Finger feeding with the right hand will stimulate functional use of the right hand, using the mouth as an intermediate point of stability. Sticker play will facilitate simultaneous use of two hands, especially when the sticker is placed first on the right hand.

CASE NO. 2 — JILL
Cerebral Palsy, Spastic Quadriparesis, Mental Retardation, 7 Years

Jill's use of head and neck hyperextension with tongue retraction virtually locks the neck and upper body together. She responds to the head and neck hyperextension by pulling the shoulders forward. This is her way of correcting her center of gravity. She also is using shoulder elevation to support her head.

Jill's eye tracking is inadequate in that she cannot visually scan her environment. Her lack of downward gaze is consistent with neck hyperextension. Her eyes and head attempt to move together, but her head control is too poor to allow coordinated eye-head coordination.

Shoulder girdle immobility limits her reach to 60 degrees of humeral abduction. Limited spine and rib cage mobility result in a poor base of support for dynamic shoulder girdle function. Scapulo-humeral and humeral-rib cage immobility limit her arm movements to humeral extension, adduction, and internal rotation. This prevents free and varied reach for play and environmental interaction.

Jill makes attempts to grasp, but her hand closes involuntarily prior to obtaining objects. This indicates that she has not yet developed any voluntary control of the hands. Without a basic palmar grasp pattern, the development of release and manipulation is blocked.

General Treatment Goals:

1. decrease muscle rigidity and increase mobility of spine, rib cage, and shoulder girdle.
2. increase thoracic extension and shoulder girdle activity to support a greater range of reach.
3. develop eye tracking with emphasis on downward gaze; free head and neck from shoulder girdle to support visual tracking.
4. develop basic palmar grasp and release.

Short Term Objectives:

Following treatment, Jill will:

1. reach above 60 degrees, 3 of 5 attempts, in supported sitting.
2. visually follow moving objects without moving her head, 50% of the time.
3. grasp an object 6 of 10 attempts in supine and 4 of 10 attempts in supported sitting.
4. release an object that is stabilized by a therapist, 5 of 5 attempts in any position.

Sample Activities:

Slow, passive trunk rotation will increase spinal and rib cage mobility and will help normalize muscle tone. Slow oscillating movement of each gleno-humeral joint will facilitate relaxation and increase her potential range and variety of reach. Movement in and out of sidelying will improve mobility between the scapula and humerus. These treatment strategies will be followed by the facilitation of active reaching. Expansion of the hand, along with pressure of her hand onto her knee and other body parts, will be followed by the facilitation of active grasp and assisted release.

CASE NO. 3 — TAYLOR
Myelomeningocele, Repaired L 1-2, 4 Years

Taylor has developed basic grip, manipulation, and release. Visual-motor integration delays are present that interfere with school skills. Spatial perceptual problems seem directly related to limitations in movement experience. Taylor lacks upper extremity muscle strength and endurance necessary for prolonged ambulation with aids. He is unable to accomplish lower body dressing independently.

General Treatment Goals:

1. improve visual-motor integration.
2. improve upper extremity muscle strength and endurance.
3. develop independence in lower body dressing.

Short Term Objectives:

Following treatment, Taylor will:

1. maneuver through an obstacle course while using the arms to push a scooter board.
2. accomplish 10 straight arm pushups from sitting.
3. accomplish 15 prone pushups.

4. don and remove lower body clothing with minimal assistance.

Sample Activities:

Negotiation of scooter board obstacle courses will improve visual-motor integration, spatial perception, and coordinated use of the arms for planned movements. Straight arm pushups from sitting will increase arm strength and endurance in preparation for assisted ambulation. Time will be spent on direct practice of adapted dressing techniques on the floor, bench, toilet, and mat table.

CASE NO. 4 — ASHLEY
Down Syndrome, 15 Months

Low muscle tone is present and Ashley demonstrates a poor base of support for movement. Ashley has a basic palmar grasp, but cannot release with control. She flings objects to dispose of them. She cannot pick up pellet-sized objects. She has not yet developed goal-directed play but does enjoy playing randomly with objects. Ashley uses her arms to help with movement transitions, but locks her elbows into extension and externally rotates her humerus to compensate for poor scapulo-thoracic stability. This limits her to the use of anterior and posterior movement transitions. She is unable to control movement patterns that require rotation of body weight over either arm.

General Treatment Goals:

1. improve muscle coactivation around major joints with emphasis on shoulder girdles.
2. develop release and pinch.
3. develop goal directed play.

Short Term Objectives:

Following treatment, Ashley will:
1. move in and out of positions without locking elbows in 3 of 6 transitional movement patterns.
2. release an object, without flinging, 5 of 10 times.
3. pick up a small pellet-sized object, without raking, 3 of 10 times.
4. participate successfully in a goal directed activity during each treatment session.

Sample Activities:

Assisted bouncing on extended arms on a small trampoline, therapy mat, or therapy ball will help increase muscle coactivation around the joints. This will be followed by facilitation of diagonal movement patterns in quadruped. Play with weighted, resistive toys will improve hand strength, improve sensory proprioception, and upgrade prehension patterns. Sticker play and finger feeding, with facilitation of palmar arches, will help develop pinch. Goal directed play will be used during therapy to facilitate functional cognitive learning. ❏

SUGGESTED READINGS

1. Bly L: The Components of normal movement during the first year of life and abnormal motor development. Chicago, IL, Neuro Developmental Treatment Association, 1983
2. Bobath B, Bobath K: Motor Development in the Different Types of Cerebral Palsy. New York, NY, Heinemann, 1975
3. Bobath K: A Neurophysiological basis for the treatment of cerebral palsy. Clinics in Developmental Medicine No. 75, Philadelphia, PA, J.B. Lippincott, 1980
4. Boehme R: Developing Mid-Range Control and Function in Children with Fluctuating Muscle Tone. Tucson, AZ, Therapy Skill Builders, 1990
5. Boehme R: The Hypotonic Child. Tucson, AZ, Therapy Skill Builders, 1990
6. Boehme R: Improving Upper Body Control: An Approach to Assessment and Treatment of Tonal Dysfunction. Tucson, AZ, Therapy Skill Builders, 1988
7. Cailliet R: The shoulder in hemiplegia. Philadelphia, PA, F.A. Davis Co, 1980
8. Connor F, Williamson G, Siepp J: Program Guidelines for Infants and Toddlers with Neuromotor and Other Developmental Disabilities. New York, NY, Teachers College, 1978
9. Erhardt RP: Developmental Hand Dysfunction: Theory, Assessment, Treatment. Laurel, MD, Ramsco, 1982
10. Erhardt R: Developmental Visual Dysfunction Models for Assessment and Management. Tucson, AZ, Therapy Skill Builders, 1990
11. Finnie N: Handling The Young Cerebral Palsied Child At Home. New York, NY, E.P. Dutton, 1975
12. Kapandji IA: The Physiology of the Joints: Upper Limb, Vol I, ed 3, New York, NY, Churchill Livingstone, 1982
13. Richer P: Artistic Anatomy. New York, NY, Watson-Guptill, 1971
14. Scherzer A, Tscharnuter I: Early Diagnosis and Therapy in Cerebral Palsy. New York, NY, Marcel Dekker, Inc, 1982
15. Turbiana R: Examination of the Hand and Upper Limb. Philadelphia, PA, W.B. Saunders Company, 1984

CHAPTER 12

SELECTION AND USE OF ADAPTIVE EQUIPMENT

Janet M. Wilson, M.A.C.T., PT

◆

Over the past 15 years, the use of adaptive equipment for positioning and mobility has become an integral part of the therapeutic management of children with developmental disabilities. Establishing goals and rationale for intervention are the first steps in the process of providing a child with adaptive equipment. The rationale and treatment philosophy described in this chapter can be stated simply. Children with movement problems resulting from central nervous system (CNS) dysfunction need to initiate movement from a good postural base to improve the quality of movement and maximize functional skills. Posture is viewed as a dynamic base for movement and ultimately function. In this context, the amount of external support given through adaptive equipment enhances posture and movement, but does not limit or restrict the child's initiation of goal directed, purposeful movement.

GOALS

The following goals encompass the current concepts and popular practices that many therapists believe can be achieved by using adaptive equipment. [1-5]

Goal #1: Gain or Reinforce Normal Movement

Adaptive equipment is used to reinforce or gain normal movement components by providing the opportunity for appropriate skeletal alignment, weight shifts, and postural adjustments during functional movements. Adaptive equipment supports the body in good alignment, with the necessary stability to allow the child to repeat movements with ease and control from a variety of postures. Adapted seating and standing eliminate excessive effort which can produce abnormal posture and tone and unequal muscle pull on the joints. The movements the child makes produce a more normal sensorimotor base for learning and reinforce functional movement patterns.

Several investigators have evaluated the relationship between seating and upper extremity functions in children with cerebral palsy. Nwaobi et al. reported that the angle of hip flexion had a positive effect on timed upper extremity movement. [6] McCleneghan and colleagues investigated the effects of seat surface inclination on both postural stability and functional use of the upper extremities in children with cerebral palsy. [7] They concluded that a slight posterior tilt to the seat improved active upper extremity function. Seeger et al., however, did not find that an increase in hip flexion improved hand function [8] and McPhearson found no significant differences in hand function attributable to seat position. [9] O'Brien and Tsurumi evaluated the effect of two body positions on head righting in severely disabled individuals with cerebral palsy and found no differences in duration or frequency of head righting when the child was seated in an adapted wheelchair or a prone positioner.[10] Hulme and colleagues reported significant improvement in sitting posture, head control, and grasp in children with multiple handicaps when fitted with adaptive seating devices.[11] The conflicting results of these studies suggest that therapists must evaluate carefully the effect seating has on each child.

Goal #2: Achieve Normal Postural Alignment

Adaptive equipment provides the support to maintain the integrity of the joints, symmetry of body parts, and alignment of the body relative to the base of support and the effect of gravity. Adaptive equipment allows the child to experience support to the appropriate body parts that will free the child's head, arms, and legs for purposeful use.

Several studies suggest that the manipulation of the seat surface aids postural alignment. Nwaobi et al. in a study of tonic myoelectric activity of the low back extensors of children with spastic cerebral palsy changed in response to seat inclination, reported less electric activity when the seat elevation was 0 degrees and backrest at 90 degrees.[12] Bablich and colleagues found that an anteriorly tipped seat facilitated extension of the spine and decreased deviation from midline.[13] Miedaner found that sitting on an anteriorly tipped seat facilitated trunk extension.[14] However Dilger, et al. found that the kyphotic sitting posture of children with developmental delays improved by using a posteriorly inclined wedge.[15] Cristarella compared the sitting posture of a child with cerebral palsy when seated on a child's chair and when seated on a bolster seat.[16] She found a more vertical pelvis and hip and knee flexion of 90 degrees when the child straddled a bolster. Posture and spinal curves approximated a normal child's posture.

Goal #3: Prevent Contractures and Deformities

Adaptive equipment can decrease liklihood of contractures and deformities in two ways. First, adaptive equipment can place a child in positions that he otherwise cannot assume or maintain. These positions can counteract the deforming forces of his disability, such as persistent asymmetry, skeletal deformities (scoliosis or kyphosis), abnormal joint positions (hip adduction or internal rotation), or habitual patterns (always uses one side for movement).

Second, adaptive equipment can counteract the inadequate support from everyday furniture which contributes to existing deformities, such as the kyphotic posture commonly seen in children who sit in chairs with inappropriate seat depth. Another example is the neck extension, lordotic thoracic spine, and scapular retraction related to the stress of maintaining trunk extension because the chair is too high and the child's feet cannot

be supported on the floor to assist balance and aid the base of support.

Gibson and associates found that incorporating lumbar extension and lateral supports in the wheelchairs of children with Duchenne muscular dystrophy decreased the frequency and severity of scoliosis in these children.[17] Myhr et al. demonstrated a decrease in asymmetrical tonic neck postures in children with severe spastic quadriplegic cerebral palsy when placed in a forward tipped seat with firm back, arms supported on a table, and feet behind the knees.[18]

Goal #4: Increase Opportunity to Participate in Social or Educational Programs

Adaptive equipment provides seating, standing, and mobility systems so that a child can establish interactions with the world outside his immediate family. This allows the child to choose and access various environments with participation within the limits of his disability, but at his mental, emotional, and social level. Appropriate equipment permits the child to direct his energies toward participation in educational or social programs, rather than maintaining posture and gaining mobility.

Burt-DuPont described the use of adaptive equipment as a key element in allowing children with developmental disabilities to participate in developmental dance programs with greater independence.[19] Butler evaluated the changes in frequency of self-initiated interactions with objects, spatial exploration, and communications with the care giver and found that if children with cerebral palsy had independent powered mobility, they improved in all three behaviors.[20]

Goal #5: Provide Mobility and Encourage Exploration

Mobility and exploration are often the goals for providing adapted standard or powered wheelchairs for children who have no means of mobility or whose movements are so slow that the effort is not worth the goal. Orthotics and walkers often are provided for young children with spina bifida to begin ambulation at an early age. Ambulation aids provide support for children with cerebral palsy before they develop independent balance for walking.

Hulme and colleagues assessed the benefits of adaptive equipment in homes of non-ambulatory, multiple handicapped children.[21] They found that adaptive chairs were the most consistently used equipment. There was significant improvement in the number of times the client left the home and an increase in places visited by the client in the community if adaptive equipment was available.

Several studies have evaluated the impact of walker design on the mobility of children with cerebral palsy. LeVangie and colleagues[22] and Logan et al.[23] compared ambulation abilities for children with cerebral palsy using standard forward walkers and reverse posture control walkers. Both studies reported improvements in various parameters of gait and in upright posture using posture control wheeled walkers.

Goal #6: Increase Independence in Activities of Daily Living and Self Help Skills

If properly positioned, a child may feel secure and motivated to practice new skills, such as feeding, toileting, grooming, or other self-help skills. Appropriate support frees the hands for manipulation, the head and mouth for speaking, and the eyes for social interaction.

Wolf and colleagues evaluated four different powered wheelchairs and determined which chair provided the greatest mobility for indoor activities.[24] They stated that powered wheelchairs with different designs have different strengths and weaknesses. In a separate single case study, Deitz and associates found an increase in indoor functional activities on level surfaces, rough terrain, and negotiating curbs using a specific powered wheelchair.[25] Hulme et al. reported a change in self help skills and activities of daily living and a significant increase in eating and drinking along with a decrease in time needed to eat a meal.[21]

Goal #7: Assist in Improving Physiological Functions

Adaptive equipment can have a positive effect on respiratory and cardiac efficiency, digestive processes, skin integrity, and skeletal alignment. Proper positioning can decrease the fatigue caused by the struggle to maintain a seated position, propel a chair, or the necessity to prop with the upper extremities. The risk of infections and deformities which are secondary to the developmental disabilities will be decreased.

Nwaobi and Smith examined changes in pulmonary function in children with cerebral palsy when seated in a sling-type wheelchair versus an adaptive seating system.[26] Improved vital capacity and forced expiratory volume were found when the children were properly seated and positioned. The authors hypothesized this was related to improved alignment of the neck, thorax, and abdomen while in the adapted seating system. Stallard and colleagues reported that heart rate decreased and speed of ambulation increased when children with spina bifida used orthoses.[27] Bard and Ralston evaluated gait in children with cerebral palsy using ambulation aids and found that the closer the gait pattern was to normal gait, the less energy expended.[28]

Goal #8: Increase Comfort

Being comfortable is important for any child who is dependent on equipment for sitting, standing, and mobility. Comfortable positioning may need to accommodate for structural deformities which interfere with normal alignment and movement. Children who are uncomfortable often are irritable and unhappy which produces negative interactions with caregivers and peers and rejection of the positioning methods. Positioning for comfort may require a compromise between improving function and supporting the biomechanical and physical properties of the child's growing body. Hulme et al. showed a significant decrease in the time spent in the bedroom when the client could be comfortably positioned in an adaptive chair.[21]

METHODS OF POSITIONING

Ward described three methods of positioning to enhance a child's program.[4] The first is using an adult's body to position the child. This method is used by therapists, teachers, and parents and has the advantage of being a dynamic system which changes instantaneously to the child's need for support and control of movement depending on the functional goal. The disadvantage is that it requires the presence of an adult and limits both the child's and adult's independence from one another.

The second method is positioning through standard furniture. Many of the ideas for commercially available products have originated this way. For very young children who change rapidly, this may be an acceptable alternative to purchasing or constructing special seating. The advantage is immediate access to positioning in any environment. The limitation is the non-specific nature of household furniture so that it may not be modified to meet individual needs.

The third method is constructing or purchasing a specialized product. Adaptive equipment is available and responsive to the needs of children. The advantage of purchasing commercially available products is that they adapt to the developing needs of the child and may be funded by medical insurance. The disadvantage may be the inability to respond to specific deformities, unusual postures, or abnormal movements. The advantage of individually constructed products is that they can be tailored to the unique requirement of a child, but often in doing so, cannot accommodate growth or change. The primary disadvantages are the labor intensive construction and cost.

Whichever method is used, adaptive equipment must meet the needs of the child as he grows, gains better control of his posture and movement, and develops educational and daily living skills. Appropriately selected, adaptive equipment allows movement and encourages the child to make postural adaptations necessary in any given situation. Adaptive equipment should not restrict the child's movement, but rather increase the child's possibilities to practice and use developing movement. Adaptive equipment limits the parameters of the environment to the extent that movement is possible without the stress which may produce abnormal tone and movement patterns. Adaptive equipment must be designed to adapt to the changing needs of the child, caregivers, and the environment if it is to become an integral part of the total management of the child.

ASSESSMENT

PART I - THE NEEDS OF THE CHILD

Physical Abilities and Limitations

The therapist first must assess the child's present motor abilities, need for movement, and potential functional independence. A child should be given the opportunity to use whatever abilities he has, thereby allowing him to control and adjust his posture by himself whenever possible. Adaptive equipment should be restricted to the minimum amount of support necessary to provide maximum function with minimal pathology. [2]

It also is important to assess the child's range of motion and joint mobility as these factors may determine whether the appropriate base of support is available for sitting or standing. Fitting a child with a chair or a stander begins with the base of support. If full range is not available at the hips and pelvis for sitting or ankles and feet for standing, it may be necessary to contour the seat to accommodate the available range. If skeletal deformities or contractures are fixed, then the base of support may need to be customized for the child.

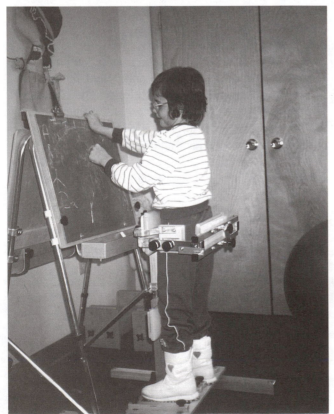

FIGURE 1. This 7 year old girl with spastic diplegia has no standing balance. The vertical stander provides balance and alignment while allowing her to use her hands for writing skills.

Evaluating strength will help determine how much external control is needed. For example, if the child has the strength to gain and maintain an upright posture in sitting, it is not necessary to use an anterior chest harness. If the child cannot regain an upright position if he falls to the sides, then lateral supports will be an integral part of the chair or stander.

Balance is another important component. A child may lack balance in various positions and while he can achieve the posture, he cannot maintain it without holding on with hands. This may suggest the need for additional support at the pelvis, a seat belt, or pommel, or other supports until the trunk is stable without depending on the arms and hands.

Finally, the therapist must evaluate the child's need to function in different environments, such as school or home. The need for posture and movement may be quite different in various environments. For example, if a child can pull to stand, but cannot free his hands in a standing position, he may need to be supported on a prone or vertical stander at school so that his hands are free for school work. At home, the child's parents may be available to provide the support needed to use his hands in a standing position and adaptive equipment is not needed. (Figure 1)

Communication

The therapist must evaluate the effects of position on the ability to communicate. Children with cerebral palsy may need to be upright for adequate breath support for speech. Children who use direct selection communication systems will need very carefully selected trunk and head supports in order to use their motor function for expression. Prone standers, corner chairs, individually adapted wheelchairs, or other modified chairs may be used to provide the support needed to promote communication skills. The therapist may find that children need more external control during communication than during times which are less stressful or less demanding on posture. The supports can be removed during less stressful times so that developing postural control is used.

Daily Living Skills

The therapist must evaluate the effect of posture on the degree of independence in activities of daily living. Many children with cerebral palsy are ready for self feeding or toilet training or can assist in dressing and grooming if properly supported (Figure 2). Activities of daily living provide functional goals for movement and are motivating as an opportunity to practice newly learned movements. In addition, being able to care for oneself is important in building self esteem and a positive self image; all efforts to allow children to participate in these activities should be encouraged. Special potty chairs, benches, adapted high-chairs, or childrens' chairs can be used to promote this important aspect of development.

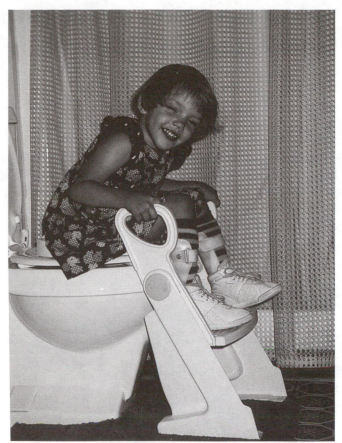

FIGURE 2. This 4 year old girl sits independently on the toilet when she uses a potty seat with hand grips and foot supports.

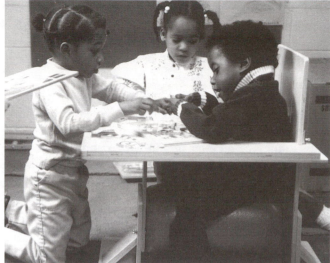

FIGURE 3. Seated on a bolster chair places this child at a level to interact with his peers while providing appropriate pelvic and spinal alignment along with hip and knee flexion.

Social Interaction

The effect position has on social interaction should be evaluated. Good positioning which reduces unusual appearing postures makes the child more approachable and more acceptable in social settings. A young child with a disability carried in his mother's arms looks like a baby and there is no expectation for age appropriate behavior. The same child sitting well and looking attentive in an adapted stroller or wheelchair is expected to demonstrate a higher level of independence, emotional control, and social interaction. Attractive equipment can help make a child with developmental disabilities appear more like other children and be accepted more easily by persons who do not understand about the effects disabilities have on posture and movement. (Figure 3)

Education

Evaluation of the effect posture and movement have on the child's educational experience is important. To participate in group activities, the child often must have some means of mobility through walkers, scooters, wheelchairs, or strollers. This allows the child to move or be moved by the teacher to different areas in the classroom, to the library, lunch room, or recess. Often with appropriate adaptive equipment a child can func-

tion in a regular classroom setting having greater options for educational programs and age appropriate social interactions. Powered wheelchairs make it possible for the child to move quickly and easily within the school, leaving energy and attention for learning and

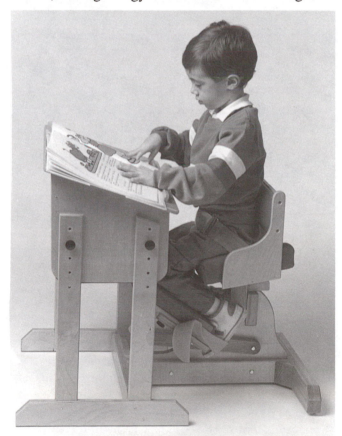

FIGURE 4. In a classroom, this 6 year old boy with spastic diplegia uses a chair with forward tipped seat and leg support to aid back extension and lumbar lordosis.

interaction. Attractive adaptive equipment can help to focus on the similarities between a child with developmental disabilities and his normal age mates rather than the differences (Figure 4).

Mobility

Mobility should be assessed. Some children who use their hands to propel a wheelchair become much stiffer in the lower extremities with this effort. An adaptive tricycle may be a better option, when appropriate, for these children (Figure 5). Children with athetosis usually have better control of the lower extremities and can use walkers when they are unable to propel a wheelchair. The decision to use electric wheelchairs often depends not only on the mental and motor capabilities of the child, but also the needs of the environment. Certainly children should have the opportunity to move around if at all possible, even if this means only one method of mobility which will not meet all the normal experiences of going under, over, in, and out as normal children do. The ability to follow through when children are motivated to change settings or go after a toy or a favorite person should be a prime consideration in providing mobility equipment.

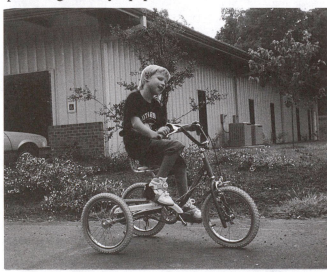

FIGURE 5. *This 9 year old boy with spastic diplegia has good reciprocal movement and strength, but cannot balance on a bicycle. This adapted tricycle allows him some independence in his neighborhood.*

Growth and Development

The therapist must evaluate the child's age, size, and extent of disability to determine which needs can best be met through adaptive equipment. Equipment that is appropriate at one age is not necessarily appropriate at another. A young child can be pushed in an adapted stroller since the needs to be independent from a caregiver are not very great. Once the child enters school, he may need to be more independent and wheelchairs, trikes, walkers, and scooters become more important. A severely involved child, however, can be maintained in a stroller for a much longer time, since this child cannot get himself in or out of his chair or function independently once his destination has been reached.

Physiological Needs

A child with myelodysplasia may need to move from a walker to crutches to increase his mobility in elementary school, but the demands on respiration and energy may be so great that this decision will limit use to inside the classroom, using the walker only for long distances (Figure 6). Transitions from one type of equipment to another or to less support often need to be gradual in order to work within the physiological parameters associated with the developmental disability.

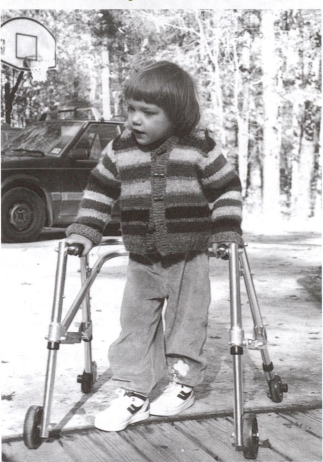

FIGURE 6. *The posture walker allows independent exploration and rapid mobility when the transition to crutch walking is still slow and energy consuming.*

Psychological Needs

Therapists should be sensitive to the psychological and emotional needs of the child regarding the impact of adaptive equipment. Whenever possible, depending on age and ability to understand and make decisions, the child should be included in the decision to purchase equipment. If other features are equal between two products, perhaps the child can pick color or style, or help determine when and where the product will be used. Children wish to be like their peers, to be included in family activities, educational programs, and social events. It can be extremely revealing to ask the child what is important to him and whether equipment will make him more like his peers or different from them. Therapists and parents must be realistic and, if only one product will produce the desired result, not frustrate the child by asking for his input.

Needs of the Caregiver

In addition to evaluating the needs of the child, the therapist must evaluate the needs of the caregivers regarding the use of adaptive equipment. Equipment must be provided which is convenient to use and meets the needs of the caregivers if it is to be incorporated into the therapeutic program. First, the therapist must know who are the primary caregivers responsible for using the adaptive equipment. They might include parents, teachers, ward personnel, babysitters, grandparents, or volunteers. The therapist then must evaluate the caregiver's understanding of the child's disability and acceptance of adaptive equipment to meet some of the child's needs. The caregiver must understand why adaptive equipment is being used. If not, she may believe that if the equipment changes the child's habitual posture it makes the child uncomfortable, and therefore will not use it.

The therapist must consider the caregiver's physical ability to handle the child and equipment. A mother with arthritis may find it particularly difficult to maneuver a child in a travel type chair into a car. A grandparent may not be able to place a child on a prone stander or a pregnant teacher may be unable to lift a child from his wheelchair. Physical limitations, temporary or permanent, must be considered in providing equipment.

In addition, the therapist must consider the caregiver's understanding of the use of the equipment and changes in its use as the child grows and abilities change. Adaptive equipment will need adjustment over time to assure good alignment and maximal movement of the child. Furthermore, the same piece of equipment may need to be adjusted differently for different activities in a single day. For example, for a child beginning to develop head control, head supports may be necessary when additional axial control is needed, such as during self-feeding. This complex skill requires coordination of eyes, hands, mouth, head, and trunk which may be very demanding for a young child. Yet it may be important to remove the head supports during activities which are less demanding on the child's posture so that the child has an opportunity to use head control which is developing. (Figure 7)

The therapist must assess the caregiver's needs in managing the child, including transportation, positioning for feeding, toileting, bathing, or positioning for educational or play activities. The life style and pace of the family are important if adaptive equipment is to be used during family functions. Some families are very active and make every attempt to include the child in the community (Figure 8). Strollers and wheelchairs become a necessity. Other families are more inclined to leave a young child at home with a family member when shopping or keeping appointments. Equipment to be used in home management then takes on greater importance. As often as possible, adaptive equipment should respond to the life style of the family making care more

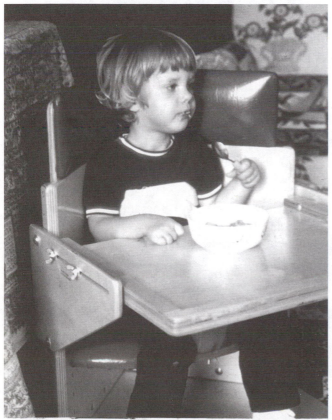

FIGURE 7. This 3 1/2 year old girl with athethosis needs additional axial support provided by head supports on her corner chair during self feeding.

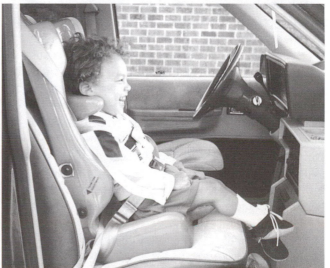

FIGURE 8. This 4 year old boy needs maximal head, neck and trunk support for transportation. He can sit well and attend to his environment and family if comfortably and securely positioned.

Therapeutic Exercise In Developmental Disabilities

convenient, while responding to what the family wants for the child. Therapists must understand that families represent various subcultures with their own sets of priorities, values, interests, and ethics, and that these differences will be reflected in the family's need for and interest in adaptive equipment.

The Needs of the Environment

The environment in which the equipment will be used must be evaluated. This includes the physical space, size of rooms, width of doors, lighting, types of floor coverings, width and length of hallways, and other equipment and furniture in the environment. Equipment must meet the physical constraints of the environment in order to be effective in that setting. Tile floors may make it easier for a child to move a scooter, but may not offer enough resistance to control a walker.

The therapist must consider the presence and activity level of children and adults in the environment. Equipment used in schools often must meet quite different standards of safety and durability than equipment used in the home.

Consider the need to move the equipment within the environment. If two classrooms share a stander or special chair, it must be possible to move the equipment quickly and easily. The equipment must fit through doorways and hallways. If the room is small, it is important to be able to move the equipment out of the way when it is not in use.

Finally, family members may be sensitive to an abundance of equipment in the home, either because of social stigma or limited space. If the family cannot deal with this problem directly, they may store equipment in an inaccessible place, making its use most inconvenient.

While adaptive equipment often can assist in meeting the many needs of a child with a developmental disability, there are limitations. The provision of equipment necessarily limits some sensory feedback. Because of the nature of posturing, some parts of the body may be maintained in a static posture with constant pressure and relative joint immobility, limiting tactile and kinesthetic feedback. To minimize this effect, all efforts should be made to provide equipment that controls but does not entirely limit the amount or direction of movement. Whenever possible, feet should be placed on a footrest but not secured. Lapboards and trays should support the arms and hands but not stop the child from leaning forward or to each side. Above all, a child should not be positioned in any piece of equipment no matter how good he looks, to the exclusion of other movement experiences. Good position in adaptive equipment does not substitute for initiation of active movement or the subtle controls of movement achieved through a therapist's hands.

Criteria for Selection of Specific Equipment

Once it has been decided that adaptive equipment can increase the child's function and make management more convenient, then the therapist, along with the caregivers, must decide what adaptive equipment is most appropriate. The final selection of equipment for use in home and schools requires close attention to therapeutic and educational goals and family expectations. The process of selecting appropriate equipment requires consideration of the following criteria.

Availability

Is the equipment available for rent or purchase? Is it available from a commercial source? If so, how quickly can it be obtained? Is there a source to build the equipment: parent, friend, high school shop class, or social club? If it is built, will the source be available for repairs or adjustments in the future?

Cost

What is the initial purchase or rental price? What will be the cost per year? How long will the child use the equipment before he outgrows it, before his functional needs change, or before it becomes medically obsolescent? What other things must the family or program do without if money is spent on equipment? If the item is custom built, does this increase or decrease the cost? Based on cost per time of use, is it better to rent or buy? Is the product under warranty? How costly and frequent are repairs?

Source of Funding

Does the family have the financial resources to rent or buy commercial or custom built products? Do they have medical insurance which pays for equipment? Are they funded through a state Crippled Children's Program? Medicaid? Muscular Dystrophy Association? March of Dimes? United Cerebral Palsy? Lions Club? Easter Seals? Will a parent group, church, or social club provide equipment? If purchased for a program, does the program have an equipment budget? What methods for payment are available? If a program buys equipment for a specific child, to whom does it belong? Will new equipment need to be purchased if the child leaves the program?

Portability

Will the equipment be used in a variety of places? Does it have to be transported from home to school? Daily? Does it have to be moved from place to place within a room or program? Does the equipment have provisions for transporting? Does it collapse or have wheels or casters? Is it lightweight? Can it easily be carried? Will it fit in the trunk of a car? If it is lightweight enough to be moved easily, does this compromise the stability? Will a vehicle need special adaptations for transporting, such as lifts in van or tie downs on bus?

Stability

Is the equipment stable enough to let the child and caregiver feel safe and secure? Is it stable enough so that other children cannot tip it over? Can it be attached to the floor or table or other permanent objects in the room? Does the stability make it difficult to move?

Ease of Adjustment

Is the equipment designed for a single child or are a variety of children going to use the same piece of equipment? How often during the day does the equipment need to be adjusted? How long does it take to make the adjustments? Do the adjustments require a variety of tools? Can the adjustments be made while the child is using the equipment? How much time can be allowed to adjust the equipment? Do the adjustments accommodate growth and development or new motor skills? Can supports be removed when no longer needed or will new equipment be necessary?

Ease of Modifications

Can the equipment be modified for a specific child's problem? Can it be modified with growth or development of a specific motor pattern? How complicated are modifications? Does it take simple or complex tools? Can a therapist, teacher, or parent make the modifications or will special resources for welding or carpentry be required? Does the manufacturer or supplier make modifications?

Construction

What are the basic materials used in the equipment: wood, metal, plastic, foam, vinyl? What is the type of finish? What advantages do the different materials have? What are the limits of the construction or materials? Will the materials last with continual use over time? Can the equipment easily be cleaned? Repaired? Reupholstered? What is the preference of the child and caregiver concerning different materials? Is it important to "match" the adaptive equipment to other furniture in the environment? What kind of warranty does the manufacturer or custom maker offer on construction and materials?

To help the therapist make knowledgeable decisions about selecting adaptive equipment, the appendix provides a list of manufacturers and distributors of adaptive equipment. While this list is not all inclusive, it includes the majority of products available on the commercial market. In addition to sources for commercial products, the references include books on planning, designing, and building adaptive equipment[26-30]. By assessing the needs of the child, the caregivers and the environment and by becoming familiar with the possibilities for obtaining and building adaptive equipment, therapists should be better able to make decisions whether or not to use adaptive equipment to help meet the needs of children with disabilities.

CASE STUDIES

The assessment process and treatment principles as applied in selecting and using adaptive equipment in management of children will be illustrated through the following four case studies.

CASE NO. 1 - JASON
Cerebral Palsy, Right Hemiparesis, 18 Months

Jason is an 18 month old boy with right hemiplegia. He walks independently. His right hand function is limited and he receives home-based physical therapy twice a week.

Goals for Adaptive Equipment:
1. reinforce normal movement through symmetrical weight bearing in sitting and normal postural adjustment during functional activities.
2. provide normal postural alignment in sitting.
3. increase independence in daily living.

Short Term Objectives:
1. sit with hips and knees flexed 90 degrees and feet flat on the floor to place sticker on mirror in front of him.
2. in sitting, shift weight, pick up right or left foot to assist with shoes and socks, each time attempted.
3. in sitting, will exhibit equal weight bearing on hips while reaching up with both hands to pull shirt on or off.

At 18 months, Jason is showing interest in dressing and undressing, as well as other grooming and self-help skills. The therapist, working in Jason's home, is able to help his parents position him on a small bench to encourage him to sit with equal weight bearing across his hips and feet flat on the floor. From this position, Jason is encouraged to pick up his foot to assist with shoe and sock (Figure 9). This develops weight shifting from side to side during a functional activity. Since Jason's floor sitting is very asymmetrical, the parents wanted a

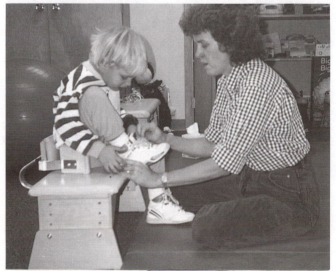

FIGURE 9. This 2 1/2 year old boy with hemiplegia uses an adjustable bench with pelvic support as he assists with shoes and socks, incorporating weight shift and equilibrium with a functional skill.

bench that would get him up off the floor and position his feet in front of him. For this reason, an adjustable height bench was purchased for use throughout his pre-school years. Jason uses his bench for all dressing activities and with a small table to sit and play with toys.

Since Jason is seen by the speech pathologist in his home, this bench can be used during speech therapy to provide good postural alignment during speech production.

In addition, Jason's family bought a small barrel chair at the local Toys-R-Us. This chair, because of its rounded back, forces Jason to sit flat on his bottom with feet in front (Figure 10). This plastic chair is light enough for Jason to carry and use when watching Sesame Street. Jason can stand up from this chair easily, but to do so must lean forward and shift his weight onto his feet.

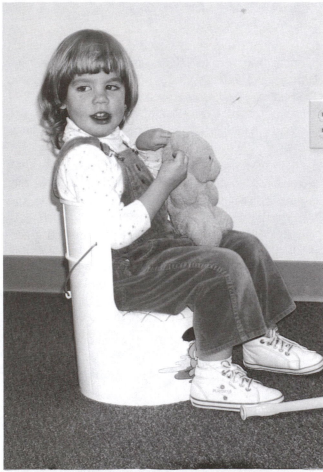

FIGURE 10. *This 3 year old girl with hemiplegia sits in a barrel chair, which encourages symmetrical weight bearing across the hips and neutral rotation of the femurs.*

CASE NO. 2 - JILL
Cerebral Palsy, Spastic Quadriparesis, Mental Retardation, 7 Years

Jill is a 7 year old with severe spastic quadriplegia and mental retardation. Increased tone or stiffness interferes with both active and passive range of motion. Persistent

tonic reflexes produce asymmetries of the head, trunk, and upper extremities. She moves very little, but enjoys assisted movement and social interaction. She attends an all day special education classroom which is open and spacious.

The following goals can be met with adaptive equipment:
1. achieve postural alignment.
2. decrease contractures and deformities.
3. increase opportunity to participate in social and educational programs.
4. assist in improving physiologic functions.
5. increase comfort.

Short Term Objectives:
1. Jill will stand in a vertical stander for 20 minutes while playing with a classmate to maintain range at hips, knees, and ankles.
2. Jill will stand in her prone stander during story reading and listening games and during classroom meals.
3. Jill will lie on her side during a 1/2 hour rest period while listening to tapes.

Using adaptive equipment is an important part of Jill's school day since she has no ability to change her own position. Jill lives with her mother, grandmother, and two younger brothers in a double-wide trailer. There is no room for equipment, other than her wheelchair. Her mother takes her out of the chair to lie on the floor after dinner. She admits she simply doesn't have the time or energy to do more for her daughter at home. Jill is transported to and from school in her wheelchair on a special school bus with a wheelchair tie-down system (Figure 11).

It is important to properly position Jill to maximize her eye contact, attention, and interest, as well as to

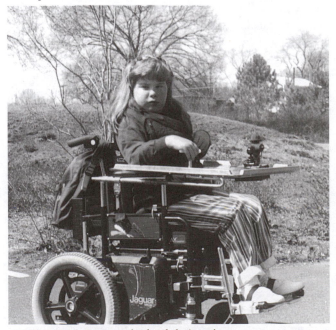

FIGURE 11. *Powered wheelchairs give access to many environments to children who otherwise would have no mobility.*

Therapeutic Exercise In Developmental Disabilities

promote active upper extremity reaching and passive range of motion and to prevent further progression of her scoliosis. Since Jill has no adaptive equipment in her home, the school purchased a prone stander, vertical stander (supine stander), and positioning pillow to allow a variety of positions other than sitting.

Initially, Jill used her wheelchair and prone stander in the classroom. The prone stander allowed partial weight bearing through her lower extremities with hips and knees extended (Figure 12). Since her stander has a tray, she can be positioned with her arms forward and weight on forearms and hands. This inhibits some of her upper extremity asymmetry and aids head lifting and neck extension.

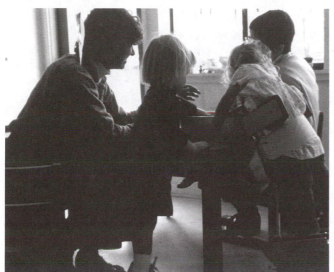

FIGURE 12. This 3 1/2 year old girl uses her pre-school prone stander to position her with her school mates for interaction and education.

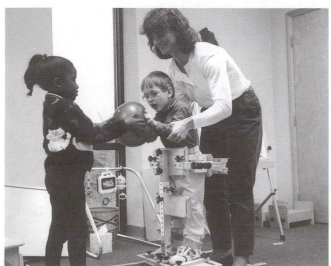

FIGURE 13. This 6 year old boy with spastic quadriplegia uses a vertical stander to achieve full weight bearing in appropriate alignment for assisted play and peer interaction.

This year, the school also purchased a vertical stander which positions Jill with both hips and knees extended, but places her fully on her feet. This stander requires her to extend her trunk and control her head. In this stander she can be assisted to reach with both hands and use her arms in play. Jill loves interaction with other students and this position makes her easily approachable by classmates (Figure 13).

In the past, Jill used a side-lyer during rest periods and when she listened to tapes and operated her tape recorder. She now is able to maintain side lying with less support and uses a positioning pillow for this purpose. This is less restrictive than the side-lyer and can be used at home, either on the floor or on her bed. Her physical therapist has shown her mother how to use this pillow to position her in sidelying with top arm and leg flexed, pelvis rotated forward, and head supported in midline. Jill's mother seems to be accepting of this and Medicaid will purchase this item for therapeutic positioning.

CASE NO. 3 - TAYLOR
Myelomeningocele Repaired L 1-2, 4 Years

Taylor is involved currently in a special education pre-school. This placement has allowed him to become comfortable using his wheelchair both outside and inside the classroom. He can propel his chair from the bus to the classroom, as well as within the smaller space of the classroom. The plan is to place Taylor in a regular kindergarten class next year. While his school is wheelchair accessible, his classroom will have limited space for his chair and he will need precise maneuverability. In addition, Taylor is ambulating currently with a posture walker and long braces. It is hoped that by next year he will use loftstrand crutches for increased mobility.

General goals for adaptive equipment:
1. increase opportunity to participate in social or educational programs.
2. increase independence in activities of self-help and daily living.
3. provide mobility and encourage exploration.
4. achieve appropriate postural alignment.

Short Term Objectives:
1. Taylor will propel his wheelchair from the school bus to the classroom each day.
2. Taylor will walk from the classroom to the lunch room and bathroom with braces and walker each day.
3. Taylor will use his wheelchair outside in the play area daily.
4. Taylor will transfer from wheelchair to walker and back 100% of the time.

These goals for Taylor are to prepare him for a regular classroom setting. The physical therapist is working on upper extremity strengthening which is a prerequisite for propelling his chair, using his walker, and eventually using crutches. The teachers and his aide will ensure that Taylor propels himself from the bus to his class. His classmates are very helpful and are eager to push him. It will be necessary to structure the setting so the other children can help by carrying his lunch box and walking beside his wheelchair.

While Taylor needs bathroom assistance, he will walk to the bathroom with his aide to increase his independence in toileting. Taylor's day can be structured to incorporate the goals for using his equipment as a natural part of the day. This may require that Taylor be given extra time if he is walking or even if he must propel his chair for long distances.

As the therapist introduces crutches, time will be made to allow him to ambulate with his crutches with assistance (Figure 14). It is important to give him other opportunities to walk independently with his walker to encourage independent exploration as he makes this transition.

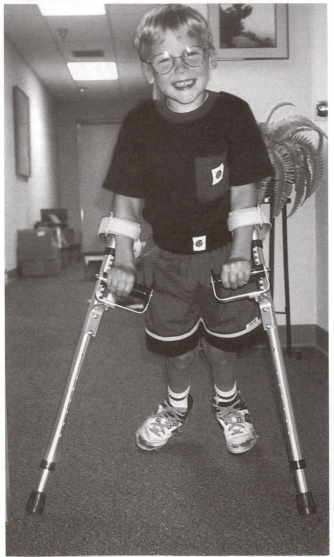

FIGURE 14. These developmental crutches have adjustable hand grips to accommodate the forearm pronation which many young children still have. As the upper extremity posture changes, the grip can be rotated so that hands move in the sagittal plane.

CASE NO. 4 - ASHLEY
Down Syndrome, 15 Months

Although Ashley attends a mother-infant early intervention program, which includes PT, OT, and speech, much of her program is carried out by her parents at home. Ashley is an only child and her parents had difficulty accepting the diagnosis and any intervention. After Ashley's first birthday, her mother began to recognize her developmental delays. Attending the mother-infant program and meeting other families has helped her to identify Ashley's strengths and weaknesses. Ashley's father enjoys playing with her, but still denies any need for direct therapeutic management. For this reason, in the home "adaptive equipment" means using the household furnishings to support her posture and increase mobility. Any "special" equipment is introduced only at the intervention program and the mother is instructed as to how she can modify materials or furniture in her home to carry over the goals and activities demonstrated.

General goals of adaptive equipment:
1. gain normal movement.
2. achieve appropriate postural alignment.
3. provide mobility and exploration.
4. increase independence in activities of daily living.

Short Term Objectives:
1. Ashley will sit on a bench with appropriate spinal alignment and feet on the floor during songtime and finger games.
2. Ashley will push a walker-wagon to the playground each day.
3. Ashley will sit in a chair for snacks and self feeding.

Ashley sits on a modified bench that has pelvic and lateral hip supports. The bench is adjusted so her feet are on the floor and the support at her pelvis assists in developing better trunk alignment since she sits with her

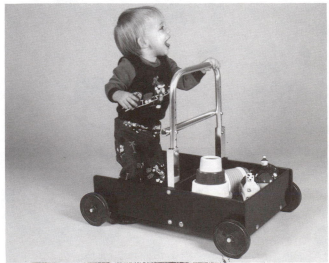

FIGURE 15. A walker wagon is an appropriate support for children who lack balance for walking but need to develop independence in exploration.

Therapeutic Exercise In Developmental Disabilities

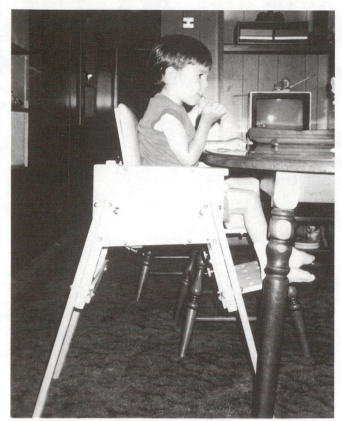

FIGURE 16. This 3 year old boy sits well in a Kinder highchair which supports his hips, knees and ankles at 90 degrees. Back and side supports assist spinal alignment in both sagittal and frontal planes.

flex to 90 degrees, a straight back, arm rests to prevent arm propping, and a foot rest to stabilize her lower extremities, she can use her hands to begin cup drinking and finger feeding (Figure 16). Her mother observes how much more capable Ashley is if she has proper support at the table. Ashley's mother hopes to have the father build a chair for Ashley to use at home. He is a talented carpenter and she believes if he can "do something" to help Ashley, he will be more aware of her difficulties and more tolerant of her needs. ❑

trunk rounded (Figure 9). In this posture, her mother can work in front of her to encourage eye contact and focus her attention for singing/clapping and finger play. This is the beginning of following directions and attending to responding to verbal cues. Since her mother does not need to hold her, Ashley can begin to feel independent of family members and develop responsibility for her posture.

Ashley is beginning to pull to stand and cruise. She does this with a broad base of support. Walking behind a wagon will help her develop stride, yet provide the security and stability she needs (Figure 15). Ashley's mother is encouraged to take this "toy" home for similar support. While most of the push toys use light weight plastic and are not stable enough for Ashley, her mother can request the father to stabilize an existing toy.

Mealtime is frustrating for Ashley and her parents. Her highchair seat depth is too great and she slides and sits with a rounded back. The footrest is too shallow to support her feet and they dangle. Her mother constantly is repositioning her in the chair. Ashley becomes agitated and uncomfortable and feeding is messy. Her mother has been asked to bring in the highchair for modification of the footrest and seat depth so that Ashley is more stable at the table at home. When Ashley is positioned with a seat depth that allows her knees to

MANUFACTURERS & SUPPLIERS OF ADAPTIVE EQUIPMENT
FOR CHILDREN WITH DEVELOPMENTAL DISABILITIES

Product Key:

WC	—	Wheelchairs, (power, manual)
S	—	Strollers
CS	—	Car Seats
SC	—	Special Chairs (seats, accessories)
SA	—	Standing Aids
SH	—	Self Help and Daily Living Aids
T	—	Tricycles
TP	—	Therapy Products
WA	—	Walkers, Crutches and Canes
SE	—	Sports Equipment

*Product Categories**

Achievement Products, Inc.
1621 Warner Avenue S.E.
P.O. Box 9033
Canton, Ohio 44121
(216) 453-2122
FAX (216) 453-0222
WC, S, CS, SC, SA, SH, T, WA

Amigo Mobility International, Inc.
6693 Dixie Highway
Bridgeport, Michigan 48722
(517) 777-8184
WC

Anthony Brothers Manufacturing
1945 S. Rancho Santa Fe Road
San Marcos, California 92069
(619) 744-4763
T

Aquatic Therapy
123 Haymac
Kalamazoo, Michigan 49004
(616) 349-9049
SE

Ball Dynamics International
1616 Glenarm Place, Suite 1900
Denver, Colorado 80202
(800) 752-2255
FAX (303) 893-0524
TP

Cleo Rehabilitation
3957 Mayfield Road
Cleveland, Ohio 44121
(216) 382-9700
(800) 321-0595
WC, S, SC, SA, SH, TP, WA

Consumer Care Products
Box 684
Sheboygan, Wisconsin 53082
(414) 489-8353
SC, SA, SH, WA, TP, T

Columbia Medical Manufacturing
P.O. Box 633
Pacific Palisades, California 90272
(213) 454-6612
CS, SH

Convaid Products
Box 2458
Ranchos Palos Verdes, California 90274
(213) 539-6814
SA, SC, S

Danmar Products, Inc.
221 Jackson Industrial Drive
Ann Arbor, Michigan 48103
(313) 761-1990
SE, SC

Equipment Shop
P. O. Box 33
Bedford, Maine 01730
(617) 275-7681
FAX (617) 275-4094
SC, SA, SH, T, TP

Everest and Jennings
3233 E. Mission Oaks Blvd.
Camarillo, California 90310
(805) 987-6911
(800) 235-4661
WC

Flaghouse, Inc.
150 N. MacQuesten Parkway
Suite 92726
Mt. Vernon, New York 10550
S, SC, SA, SH, T, WA, SE

Fred Sammons, Inc.
145 Tower Drive
Burr Ridge, Illinois 60521
(800) 323-5547
FAX (708) 323-4602
S, SC, SA, SH, TP, WA

Freedom Designs, Inc
2241 Madera Road
Simi Valley, California 93065
(800) 331-8551
WC

Guardian Products, Inc.
12800 Wentworth Street
Box C
Arleta, California 91331-4522
(818) 504-2820
WA

Gunnell, Inc.   WC, S, CS, SC
8440 State
Millington, Michigan 48746
(800) 551-0055
FAX (517) 871-4563

Invacare Corp.   WC, S
20 Kilmar Road
Edison, New Jersey 08817
(201) 572-6100

Jesana, Inc   C, S, SE, WA, T, SA
P.O. Box 17
Irvington, New York 10533
(800) 443-4728
FAX (914) 591-4320

Jay Medical, Ltd.   SC
P. O. Box 18656
Boulder, Colorado 80308-8656
(800) 648-8282

Kaye Products, Inc.   SC, SA, SH, TP, WA
535 Dimmocks Mill Road
Hillsborough, North Carolina 27278
(919) 732-6444
FAX (919) 732-1444

Kid-Kart/Kid Care   S
126 Rosebud, #1
Belgrade, Montana 59714
(800) 388-5278

Life Enhancement Products, Ltd. S
1916 Main Street
Acton, Maine 01720
(508) 263-9088
FAX (508) 263-5230

Marshall Electronics, Inc.   S
600 Barclay Boulevard
Lincolnshire Illinois 60069
(800) 323-1482
(312) 634-6300

Mulholland   WC, S, CS, SC, SA
P. O. Box 391
Santa Paula, California 93060
(805) 525-7165
FAX (805) 933-1082

Ortho-Kinetics   S, CS, SA, SC
P.O. Box 1647
Waukesha, Wisconsin 53187
(800) 824-1068

J.A. Preston   WC, S, SC, SA, SH
P.O. Box 3697
Grand Rapids, Michigan 49501-3697
(800) 631-7277

Quickie Designs, Inc.   WC
2842 Business Park Avenue
Fresno, California 93727-1328
(209) 292-2171

Rifton   S, SC, SA, SH, TP
P. O. Box 901
Rifton, New York 12471
(800) 374-3866
FAX 914-658-8065

Snug Seat, Inc.   S, CS
P. O. Box 1739
Matthews, North Carolina 28106
(800) 336-7684

TherAdapt Products, Inc.   SC, SA, WA, TP
17W163 Oak Lane
Bensenville, Illinois 60106
(708) 834-2471
FAX (708) 834-2478

Tramble Company   TP, SC
894 St. Andrews Way
Frankfort, Illinois 60423
(815) 469-2938
FAX (815) 726-9118

Triaid   T
P. O. Box 1364
Cumberland, Maryland 21502
(800) 868-5856
(301) 759-3525

Tumble Forms   TP, S, CS, SC
P. O. Box 3697
Department 1151
Grand Rapids, Michigan 49501
(800) 631-7277

ADDITIONAL SOURCES OF PRODUCTS

Annual Mobility Guide
Exceptional Parent Magazine
1170 Commonwealth Avenue, 3rd Floor
Boston, Massachusetts 02134

The Illustrated Directory of Handicapped Products
Trio Publishing, Inc.
3600 W. Timber Court
Lawrence, Kansas 66049

Physical Therapy Resource and Buyers Guide
Annual Supplement to Physical Therapy
1111 N. Fairfax Street
Alexandria, Virginia 22314-1488

Medical Equipment Distributors, Inc.
3223 South Loop 289, #150
Lubbock, Texas 79423

The Wheelchair
Annual Supplement to Home CareMagazine
Post Office Box 16448
North Hollywood, California 91615-6448

REFERENCES

1. Alexander MA: Orthotics, adapted seating and assistive devices. In Molner G (ed): Pediatric Rehabilitation. Baltimore, MD, Williams and Wilkins, 1985, pp 158-175

2. Bergen AF, Presperin J, Tallman T: Positioning for Function: Wheelchairs and Other Assistive Technologies. Valhalla Rehab Pub, Valhalla, NY, 1990

3. Trefler E (ed): Seating for Children with Cerebral Palsy: A Resource Manual. Memphis, TN, U of TN Rehab Engineering Dept, 1984

4. Ward D: Positioning the Handicapped Child for Function: ed 2. Chicago, IL, Phoenix Press, 1984

5. Wilson J: Cerebral Palsy. In Campbell S (ed): Pediatric Neurologic Physical Therapy: ed 2. New York, NY, Churchill Livingstone, 1991, pp 301-360

6. Nwaobi OM, Hobson DA, Trefler E: Hip angle and upper extremity movement time of children with cerebral palsy. Dev Med Child Neurol, 28: 24, 1986

7. McClenaghan BA, Thombs L, Milner M: Effects of seat surface inclination on postural stability and function of the upper extremities of children with cerebral palsy. Dev Med Child Neurol, 34: 40-48, 1992

8. Seeger BA, Caudrey DJ, O'Mara NA: Hand function in cerebral palsy: the effect of hip flexion angle. Dev Med Child Neurol, 26: 601-606, 1984

9. McPhearson JJ, Schild R, Barsamian, et al: Quantitative analysis of the quality of upper extremity movement: A comparison of individuals with cerebral palsy and without cerebral palsy in four sitting positions. AJOT, 45: 123-129, 1991

10. O'Brien M, Tsurumi K: The effect of two body positions on head righting in severely disabled individuals with cerebral palsy. AJOT, 37: 673-680, 1983

11. Hulme JB, Gallacher K, Walsh J, et al: Behavioral and postural changes observed with use of adaptive seating by clients with multiple handicaps. Phys Ther, 67: 1060-1066, 1987

12. Nwaobi OM, Brubaker CE, Cusick B, Sussman M: Electromyographic investigation of extensor activity in cerebral palsied children in different seating positions. Dev Med Child Neurol, 25: 175-183, 1983

13. Bablich K, Sochaniwskyj A, Koheil R: Positional and electromyographic investigation of sitting posture of children with cerebral palsy. Dev Med Child Neurol, 28: 25, 1986

14. Miedaner JA: The effects of sitting positions on trunk extension for children with motor impairment. Ped Phys Ther 2: 11-14, 1990

15. Dilger NJ, Ling W: The influence of inclined wedge sitting on infantile postural kyphosis: Dev Med Child Neurol, 28: 23, 1986

16. Cristaralla M: Comparison of straddling and sitting apparatus for the spastic cerebral palsied child. AJOT, 29: 273-276, 1975

17. Gibson DA, Koreska J, Robertson D, et al:: The management of spinal deformities in Duchenne muscular dystrophy. Orthop Clin North Am, 9: 437-450, 1978

18. Myhr U, Von Wendt L: Improvement of functional sitting position for children with cerebral palsy. Dev Med Child Neurol, 33: 246-256, 1991

19. Burt-DuPont B: Developmental dance therapy. Clinical Management, 5: 20-25, 1985

20. Butler C: Effects of powered mobility on self-initiated behaviors of very young children with locomotor disability. Dev Med Child Neurol, 28: 325-332, 1986

21. Hulme JB, Poor R, Schillein M, et al: Perceived behavioral changes observed with adaptive seating devices and training programs for multihandicapped developmentally disabled individuals. Phys Ther, 63: 204-208, 1983

22. Levangie P, Chimera M, Johnston M, et al: Effects of posture control walker versus standard rolling walker on gait characteristics of children with spastic cerebral palsy. Phys Occup Ther Pediat, 9: 1-18, 1989

23. Logan L, Byers-Hinkley K, Ciccone C: Anterior versus posterior walkers for children with cerebral palsy: A gait analysis study. Dev Med Child Neurol, 32: 1044-1048, 1990

24. Wolf LS, Massagli TL, Jaffe KM, Dietz J: Functional assessment of the Joncare Hi-Low Master Power Wheelchair for children: Phy Occup Ther Pediat, 11: 57-72, 1991

25. Deitz J, Jaffe KM, Wolf LS, et al: Pediatric power wheelchairs: Evaluation of function in the home and school environments. Assistive Technology (in press)

26. Nwaobi OM, Smith P: Effect of adaptive seating on pulmonary function of children with cerebral palsy. Dev Med Child Neurol, 28: 24-25, 1986

27. Stallard J, Rose GK, Tart J, et al: Assessment of orthoses by means of speed and heart rate. J Med Engineering and Tech, 2:22-24, 1978

28. Bard G, Ralston HJ: Measurement of energy expenditures during ambulation with special references to evaluation of assistive devices. Arch Phy Med and Rehabil, 40: 415-420, 1959

29. Hofmann R: How to Build Special Furniture and Equipment for Handicapped Children. Springfield, IL, Charles C. Thomas, 1970

30. Lowman E, Klinger J: Aids to Independent living. New York, NY, McGraw Hill, 1969

31. Macey P: Mobilizing Multiply Handicapped Children: A Manual for the Design and Construction of Modified Wheelchairs. Lawrence, KS, Univ Kansas, 1974

32. Robinault I (ed): Functional Aids for the Multiply Handicapped. Hagerstown, PA, Harper and Row, 1973

33. Tri-Wall (R) Pattern Portfolio. Tucson, AZ, Skill Therapy Builders, 1991

CHAPTER 13

PHYSICAL THERAPY IN THE EDUCATIONAL ENVIRONMENT

Wendy L. Tada, Ph.D., PT

Susan R. Harris, Ph.D., PT, FAPTA

Joanell A. Bohmert, M.S., PT

◆

Enactment of Public Law 94-142, (PL 94-142) the Education for all Handicapped Children Act, (EHA) in 1975, significantly increased the demand for physical therapists in the public schools.[1] By mandating a free and appropriate public school education for all school aged children with disabilities, PL 94-142 opened schools' doors to children with severe disabilities who had not been served previously. This influx of students with severe orthopedic, neurologic, and gross motor impairments into the public schools brought immediate attention to the importance of physical therapy services within educational settings.

In 1986, enactment of Public Law 99-457, (PL 99-457) the EHA Amendments, significantly changed services for infants and young children.[2] Part B extended mandated services to children between three and five years of age. Additionally, Part H provided financial incentives for "states to plan, develop, and implement a comprehensive, statewide, interagency system of early intervention services" for infants and toddlers.[2]

The purpose of this chapter is to discuss the role of the physical therapist in the educational environment. Aspects of PL 94-142 and PL 99-457 most pertinent to the school physical therapist will be highlighted. Types of physical therapy services in the educational environment and the roles and functions of the school physical therapist will be discussed. Special emphasis will be placed on the relevance of physical therapy services to educational goals. The chapter will conclude by addressing the physical therapy needs of the case study children in a school settings.

EDUCATIONAL LAWS

Educational laws are the bases for provision of services for children with disabilities in public schools. To understand the role and function of the physical therapist in an educational setting, we must understand the contents and implications of the laws. We also must understand the history of educational law and understand the interaction between federal and state laws. EHA, passed in 1975, was the first Federal law to define special education and related services. In 1986, PL 99-457 was passed to provide amendments to EHA. It contained two principle parts: Part B which applies to children ages 3 through 5 years, and Part H which applies to infants and toddlers from birth through 2 years of age. In 1991, Congress reauthorized Part H and the Amendments to Part B of the EHA and renamed the Act, Individuals with Disabilities Education Act (IDEA).[3]

Federal law defines how children should be served, what the States are mandated to provide, and what is permissive. States must write legislation to define how they will provide these services. Therapists need to be familiar with their state's educational rules, and regulations so their practice reflects the state's legal guidelines. Therapists also need to be familiar with their state's physical therapy practice act and how that impacts practice in an educational setting.

PUBLIC LAW 94-142

Purpose

As stated by Congress, the purposes of PL 94-142 are "1) to insure that all handicapped children have available to them a free and appropriate public education, 2) to assure that the rights of handicapped children and their parents are protected, 3) to assist states and localities to provide for the education of all handicapped children, and 4) to assess and insure the effectiveness of all efforts to educate such children." [3]

Definitions

The definition of "handicapped children" in the law virtually is unprecedented in its inclusiveness. Children with handicaps are defined as children who are "mentally retarded, hard of hearing, deaf, speech impaired, visually handicapped, seriously emotionally disturbed, orthopedically impaired, other health impaired, deaf-blind, multi-handicapped, or as having specific learning disabilities who because of those impairments need special education and related services." [1] The law established priorities, first, to children with disabilities who currently are not served, and second, to children who are served inadequately due to severely disabling conditions.

The broad scope of the law can be appreciated by examining the extent to which it specifically defines key phrases. "Special education" is defined as "specifically designed instructions" provided at no cost to parents or guardians to meet the individual needs of each handicapped child. [1] Instruction includes "classroom instruction, instruction in physical education, and instruction in hospitals and institutions. [1] This also includes the provision of "related services" to assist the child to benefit from special education. Physical therapy is listed specifically as one such related service along with occupational therapy, psychological services, speech-language pathology and audiology, school health services, and transportation. The provision for these related services expands the traditional definition of special education to include a complex of mandated services that traditionally have been the responsibility of noneducation agencies. [4]

The law requires documentation of due process and the plan for special education. Due process consists of procedural safeguards to assure that the rights of parents and children with disabilities are maintained in the educational setting. Due process includes informed consent; confidentiality; timelines for assessment, placement, and service; and procedures for the resolution of conflicts. A separate "individualized education program" or "IEP" must be written for each child that qualifies for special education. The child's parent(s) must be involved in the development of the program. Components of the IEP include:

- a statement of the child's present levels of educational performance;
- a statement of annual goals, including short-term objectives;
- a statement of specific special education and related services to be provided to the child and the extent to which the child will be able to participate in regular education programs;
- the projected date for initiation of services and the anticipated duration of such services; and
- appropriate objective criteria and evaluation procedures and schedules for determining, on at least an annual basis, whether instructional objectives are being achieved. [5]

In addition, the law requires that children with disabilities are educated in the least restrictive environment with children without disabilities. The separation of children with disabilities from the regular education environment "occurs only when the nature or severity of the handicap is such that education in regular classes with the use of supplementary aids and services cannot be achieved satisfactorily." [1]

PUBLIC LAW 99-457

Purpose

Congress amended the EHA in 1986 stating there was an urgent and substantial need "(1) to enhance the development of handicapped infants and toddlers and to minimize their potential for developmental delay, (2) to reduce the educational costs to our society, including our Nation's schools, by minimizing the need for special education and related services after handicapped infants and toddlers reach school age, (3) to minimize the likelihood of institutionalization of handicapped individuals and maximize the potential for their independent living in society, and (4) to enhance the capacity of families to meet the special needs of their infants and toddlers with handicaps." [2]

As a result, Congress established a policy to financially assist states "(1) to develop and implement a statewide, comprehensive, coordinated, multi-disciplinary, interagency program of early intervention services for handicapped infants and toddlers and their families, (2) to facilitate the coordination of payment for early intervention services from Federal, State, local, and private sources (including public and private insurance coverage), and (3) to enhance its capacity to provide quality early intervention services and expand and improve existing early intervention services being provided to handicapped infants and toddlers and their families."[2]

Definitions

The definition of handicapped was expanded in PL 99-457 to include infants and toddlers "from birth to age 2, inclusive, who need early intervention services because they (A) are experiencing developmental delays, as measured by appropriate diagnostic instruments and procedures in one or more of the following areas: cognitive development, physical development, communication development, social or emotional development, or adaptive development, or (B) have a diagnosed physical or mental condition which has a high probability of resulting in developmental delay."[2] Individual states may include definitions of individuals who may be at risk. While the law defines the term "handicapped infants and toddlers", it allows the states to define the term " developmental delay". This allows the states to define their target population and establish criteria for service.

Early intervention services are defined as developmental services and may include family training, counseling, and home visits; special instruction; occupational therapy; physical therapy; speech and language therapy; psychological services; medical services for diagnostic or evaluation purposes; health services; case management services; and early identification, screening, and assessment services.

PL 99-457 does not define related services, but instead identifies related service providers as primary providers. The infant or toddler may receive physical therapy singularly as the early intervention program according to federal law. However, the states may define this differently so that physical therapy can be provided only if the child receives service from a teacher or speech and language clinician.

Instead of the IEP, PL 99-457 requires an Individual Family Service Plan (IFSP). Prior to development of the IFSP the law requires a "multidisciplinary assessment of the unique strengths and needs of the infant or toddler and the identification of services appropriate to meet such needs."[3] The IFSP must contain:

"a statement of the infant's or toddler's present levels of physical development, cognitive development, communication development, social or emotional development, and adaptive development,
- a statement of the family's resources, priorities, and concerns,
- a statement of the major outcomes expected to be achieved for the infant and toddler and the family,
- a statement of specific early intervention services,
- a statement of the natural environments in which early intervention services shall appropriately be provided,

- the projected dates for initiation of services and the anticipated duration of such services,
- the name of the service coordinator, and
- the steps to be taken to support the transition of the infant and toddler to services provided under part B" (3 to 5 year old program).[2]

Family Focus

A significant change in Part H is the move from child-focused service to family-focused service. Family-focused means the assessment and present level of performance and needs must address not only the child but also the family. The parents, while being part of the focus, are also a part of the team. Parents need, and want, to be involved in the entire process, especially before decisions are made.[6,7] The focus on the family is needed as the parents are the child's primary care-givers and as such the child's primary teachers.[8] To empower the parents, to recognize the knowledge they have regarding their child, and to acknowledge their ability to become the child's "teachers" are important aspects of intervention.[9]

When working with families, therapists need to recognize and acknowledge that each family is different. Each family has a different value system which may be different from that of the therapist.[8,10,11] Cultural differences need to be addressed in the assessment, identification of expected outcomes, and in materials and techniques used in intervention. The family's level of acceptance of the child and assistance from outsiders will impact their ability to participate in the IFSP process. There are a variety of models for assessing family needs and in planning programs.[12,13] The responsibility of the team is to determine which model and tools will address the individual family's needs appropriately.

In the development of the IFSP the family's priorities and needs should be addressed before establishing expected outcomes or goals and objectives.[8,10] Once the goals and objectives are established they should not be considered static, but rather changing and evolving.[6,14]

Collaboration of Services

The law recognizes the complex and varied needs of families of children with disabilities. It also recognizes that one agency cannot meet all these needs. To meet the needs of families, collaboration of services is required from multiple agencies.

Another unique requirement of PL 99-457 is the establishment of a State Interagency Coordinating Council. The designated agency for services for children ages 3 through 21 years is education, however, each state must designate a lead agency (education or other) to manage the implementation of PL 99-457.

Services to meet the needs of infants and toddlers with disabilities and their families should be provided in natural environments as much as possible with children

The key differences between Part B and Part H are:

	Part B	Part H
Age Level Served:	School-aged children	Infants and toddlers
Program Focus:	Program focuses on child	Program focuses on family
Services Providers:	Services provided by single agency	Program provided by multiple agencies
Role of PT:	PT is a related service	PT is a primary service
Service Site:	Site is generally classroom	Site is generally child's home
Individual Plan:	IEP	IFSP
Outcome Measures:	Goals and objectives	Expected outcomes

without disabilities. For most infants and toddlers this would be their home, however, it also may include day-care or preschool settings.

Part B and Part H of IDEA (formerly EHA) are similar in the requirements for providing appropriate educational services for children, however, there are several key differences which are listed in Figure 1.

ROLES AND FUNCTIONS OF PHYSICAL THERAPISTS IN THE SCHOOLS

The purpose of physical therapy is the promotion of optimal function. The emphasis of therapy will depend on the program in which the child is participating. The role of the physical therapist in the educational setting is to assist the child to benefit from special education. The primary focus for the physical therapist in the educational setting is to assist the child in the development of functional mobility and to assist the child to access the educational environment.

The patterns of practice in an educational setting are unlike those in the typical medical setting where direct one-to-one services are provided to each patient. Physical therapists in the schools need to adjust and redefine their treatment programs and treatment objectives to assist the child to benefit from special education. Physical therapists are considered a part of the child's IEP or IFSP team whose members jointly identify needs and develop goals and objectives.

Teaming

A critical aspect of working in an educational setting is the ability to function effectively on a team. Teaming is required by law for assessment and the development of the child's IEP or IFSP. Two primary reasons for teaming are to provide better programming and to improve the use of available resources. Teaming is considered a dynamic process which requires teams to go through stages of development before becoming effective. Having an effective team requires work and commitment from the team members as well as from the school administration.

The four types of teams physical therapists could participate on are described in Figure 2. Teaming concepts have progressed from multidisciplinary to interdisciplinary and transdisciplinary. The use of inter-disciplinary and transdisciplinary teams in educational settings has become increasingly popular for the provision of service to children with disabilities. The advantage of the interdisciplinary model is increased communication and coordination of services with more disciplines directly involved with the child. The transdisciplinary model requires even more communication and interaction among team members as there are fewer disciplines involved directly with the child. This is seen as an advantage for infants, toddlers,[15] and children with severe and multiple disabilities.[16,17]

Transdisciplinary teaming requires members of the team to teach others aspects of their own discipline and to learn aspects of the other team members' disciplines. While this is defined as role release, many believe they are "giving away their profession" and are threatened by this process. York, Rainforth, and Giangreco attempted to clarify some of the misconceptions of transdisciplinary teamwork and integrated therapy.[18] They stated that loss of direct student contact is not a result of released professional skills but is a cooperation among team members to enhance the child's ability to function in natural settings. An important aspect of working in an educational setting is teaching others how to set up the environment and practicing skills in the environment in which the child needs to use them. Traditionally the special education teacher has been the primary interventionist, but with Part H the therapist can be the primary interventionist with the parent viewed as the child's primary teacher and care-giver.[19]

Caution must be used so that the concept of the transdisciplinary approach is not used to limit the availability of or access to any discipline. For effective teaming, adequate time must be committed to and provided on a regular basis by the administration and team members.

Basic components for an effective team include: defined purpose for the team; clearly established team goals; high communication among team members; high commitment from team members; understanding of own and other professional's roles; respect and value for each others profession; equal participation, power, and influence; participation by all members; defined decision-making and conflict resolution process; and encouragement of differing opinions. There are numerous references that further describe the process of effective teaming and factors which can interfere with it.[20-24]

Reimbursement of Therapy Services

When EHA was first enacted, states were required to provide students with disabilities the same resources as students without disabilities. To assure equal treatment, Congress specifically stated that all children with disabilities are to receive a "free appropriate education which includes special education and related services."[25] It was not the intention that education assume all of the health costs incurred by these children but that other agencies would continue providing health and/or medical services. There has been confusion as to the extent the schools are responsible for providing health-related services. In an attempt to clarify this issue, Congress amended Section 612(6) of the EHA by adding "This paragraph shall not be construed to limit the responsibility of agencies other than educational agencies in a State from providing or paying for some or all of the costs of a free appropriate public education to be provided handicapped children in the State."[2] The law also states that education is the payor of last resort if funding from private or public sources would have paid for the same service.

FIGURE 2.   Models of Teaming

	Assessment	Goal Setting	Intervention	Communication
Uni-disciplinary	by discipline	by discipline	by discipline	none
Multi-disciplinary	by discipline	by discipline	by discipline	minimal
Inter-disciplinary	by discipline	by team	by discipline	intermittent to regular for program planning and coordination of services
Trans-disciplinary	by discipline by team (arena)	by parent/ caregiver and team	most appropriate profession(s)	regular/high level required training of other team members

Part H incorporated the idea of sharing in the costs of services for infants and toddlers by requiring interagency cooperation with a family focus. The IFSP can be used as a document that describes all the services (educational, health, medical) the child needs and clearly states who (school district, county, insurance) is responsible for payment. Unfortunately, it is not this clear for children 3 through 21 years of age because the IEP does not require inclusion of outside services nor does it address payment.

In 1988, Congress passed the Medicare Catastrophic Coverage Act, PL 100-360. Section 411 (k) (13) specifically states that states cannot deny payment for Medicaid services "...because such services are included in the child's individual education program established pursuant to Part B or the Education of the Handicapped Act or furnished to a handicapped infant or toddler because such services are included in the child's individualized family service plan adopted pursuant to part H of such Act."[26] Because this amendment was a technical amendment to Medicaid law, it has no impact on Medicare or third party insurers unless they are involved in the state Medicaid program. However, many states and individual school districts interpreted this as allowing them to seek reimbursement for therapy services from Medicaid and third party payers. As Roybal stated "...the amendment gives states the flexibility to claim federal Medicaid funds for health-related services provided through the public school system, but does not require any state to take advantage of this option."[27]

Confusion and concern continue regarding the implications of public schools seeking reimbursement for health-related services.[28,29] Rogers discussed "dangers to the family" that exist when schools access their private insurance. These include "depletion of available lifetime coverage; depletion of annual or service charge; loss of future insurability; premium increase; or discontinuation of coverage."[29] She suggested that families evaluate their situation carefully and to "just say no" as schools must have the parent's permission before seeking reimbursement. The impact to school therapists may include additional documentation to meet the standards of the insurer, pre-authorization, and denial with possible appeal. The services the child receives, however, cannot be dependent on whether reimbursement will be sought and/or received. The child must receive the services required to meet identified educational needs immediately and the services cannot be delayed nor denied due to reimbursement issues. The physical therapist may be able to assist the educational agency in the pros and cons of seeking reimbursement and its cost effectiveness.

Medical vs Educational Services

Physical therapists usually are considered medical professionals, rather than educational professionals, because they are trained and most frequently provide service in a medical setting. As a result, the service of physical therapy is usually considered a medical service. Ottenbacher addressed the conflicts that may arise between "professional belief systems" when therapists trained in a medical model assume roles in an educational model.[30] As he explained, the logic of the medical model is to discover the underlying cause of problems. Therapists following this model may direct their treatment toward remediating the underlying disorder. This medical approach may run counter to a more educationally and behaviorally oriented approach of task analysis and remediation through compensatory strategies. While this latter approach often is criticized as teaching "splinter skills," it often is more functionally-oriented, including specific, educationally-relevant objectives.

Defining or identifying what is "medical" or what is "educational" physical therapy is becoming more difficult. Education used to be what happened in the classroom. With the changes in laws, however, education now encompasses teaching children in a variety of settings which include the home, classroom, playground, lunchroom, bus, community, and work sites. At the same time, the medical model has changed from the hospital setting to the home, community, and work site. As a result, there is potential overlap between medical and educational services. Medical and educational services both address function. Both are concerned with the "whole child" and both are concerned with the quality of the child's life.

One major difference between medical and educational services is the process for accessing the service. In the medical model, any child can receive physical therapy services. In the educational model, the child must meet a minimum of two conditions before physical therapy services can even be considered. First, the child must be identified as handicapped, as defined in federal and state statutes, and second, must be determined to be in need of special education. For children ages 3 through 21 years, only when these first two conditions are met can physical therapy be considered to assist in meeting the child's identified special education needs. Infants and toddlers also must be identified as handicapped and in need of special education, however physical therapy, by federal law, can be the special education.

The question now becomes, what is a medical service and what is an educational service for children who receive special education? Many believe it is critical to define the difference since education is responsible to pay only for educational services and many private insurers will pay only for medical services. In 1988 Congress passed PL 100-360, Section 411 (k) (13) which allows education to seek reimbursement for "medically necessary" health-related services provided as part of a child's special educational program. This has added to the confusion because "medical" services can now be provided and reimbursed by Medicaid in educational settings.

It is not easy to define the difference between medical and educational therapy because the therapist uses the same base of knowledge and techniques to provide "physical therapy". Physical therapy is physical therapy. Perhaps the difference lies in the primary purpose for which the therapy is to be provided. For example, the primary purpose of physical therapy in a medical role for using a positioning program is to prevent contractures, maintain muscle length, and prevent loss of bone density while the primary purpose of physical therapy in an educational model is to attain functional abilities needed in the educational setting, such as sitting on the floor during class, sitting at a lunch table, or attending to class instruction. It is important, however, that a continuum of physical therapy services be available both in medical and educational settings.

Questions to consider when determining if the service to be provided fits the medical or educational model include:

- Is the child functionally independent in the educational setting?
- Is therapy necessary for the student to function in the educational setting?
- Is it a life-long need or an educational need?
- Is the child functionally independent in the non-educational setting?
- Did a medical intervention change the child's special education needs or just the need for therapy services?
- Is it an acute situation requiring frequent intervention?
- Does it require the expertise of a PT or could it be done by staff/parent(s)?
- Is it necessary to enhance a medical procedure i.e., before/after surgery?

Deciding whether therapy services are medical or educational is up to the individual states, school districts, and the IEP team. The law requires that physical therapy must be provided that is necessary to "assist the child to benefit from special education." [3] IEP and IFSP teams which include physical therapists must determine what is educationally necessary.

These are complex and difficult issues which need to be answered and which may cause hesitation or resistance by some physical therapists to a more educationally oriented model. The need to address these issues as well as the changing role of the physical therapist in school settings has been the subject of a number of recent articles in professional therapy journals. [30-35]

SERVICE DELIVERY

Types of Physical Therapy Services

Physical therapists in the schools provide a variety of services in many different settings. Listed below are the services that may be provided by physical therapists in the schools as adapted from the American Physical Therapy Association (APTA). [36]

Screening — Identification of students with previously undetected problems, for example scoliosis and gross motor delays.

Evaluation — Identification of a student's present level of function and special education needs.

Program Planning — Development of IEP or IFSP goals and objectives in collaboration with the educational staff based on the student's identified special education needs.

Treatment — Provision of direct or indirect services to students whose evaluations indicate a need for the expertise of a physical therapist.

Consultation — Interaction with teachers, administrators, parents, and other professionals regarding educational programming and long range planning for children with disabilities within the educational and vocational environments.

Administration — Coordination and implementation of services in a manner consistent with district, state, and federal regulations.

Education — Provision of information to personnel in the educational environment through formal and informal inservice programs.

TREATMENT

Physical therapy services may be direct or indirect. The assumption should not be made that one type is better or worse than the other. The service the child receives will depend on the individual child's identified needs.

Direct service consists of service provided directly to the student. Direct service includes individual and group therapy. Individual therapy allows the therapist to continually monitor and alter the therapy program to meet the changing needs of the student. Small group therapy allows the physical therapist to serve a larger number of students and provides an opportunity for peer interaction and socialization which may be more motivating and enjoyable for some students.

Indirect service consists of service provided to other staff, parents, and the child when appropriate. Service may include direct contact with the child for the purpose of training, progress review, and reevaluation. Other activities include review of records, consultation, inservice training, monitoring, program planning and review, ongoing communication with staff and parents, and the modification and/or adaptation of the child's educational environment.

Indirect physical therapy services may be provided through consultation and in-services to teachers, aides, parents, and other professionals and the child when appropriate. These are considered indirect services, since program suggestions and therapy-related activities are carried out by someone other than the physical therapist. Educational goals and objectives which require the physical therapist's expertise should be included in the IEP or IFSP.

Physical therapy consultation may be provided for a child or group of children and may include recommendations for proper positioning, use of adaptive equipment, functional mobility, gross motor programs, evacuation plans, accessing playground equipment, modifications or adaptations of academic materials, and pre-vocational and vocational planning. Physical therapy consultation may be particularly important in facilitating a child's adaptation to a regular classroom, especially if the teacher is not familiar with the special equipment and educational needs of children with disabilities.

The physical therapist also may consult with a child's physician, private physical therapist, or other public and private agencies concerned with the child. This consultation is important to ensure that services are coordinated and that classroom and therapy programs are consistent with the child's overall needs.

EDUCATION

Information to teachers, parents, administrators, and other professionals can be provided through in-service training. General information applicable to children with disabilities, such as medical terminology, body mechanics for lifting and transferring students, general handling and positioning principles, and other topics that would complement the teacher-directed educational program should be provided. Physical therapists also can provide information regarding removal of architectural barriers, transportation needs, evacuation plans, special equipment needs, transition planning, pre-vocational and vocational planning, and long-range planning for the student.

SERVICE DELIVERY MODELS

School physical therapists work in a variety of settings which vary among school districts. Therapists may be center-based, serving a large number of students in one setting, or itinerant, traveling between several schools to provide services. Whether the therapist works in one school or travels from school to school is a decision based on the structure of the special education system within that district. One choice which may reside with the therapist is the decision to use an isolated or integrated therapy model.[37]

The isolated therapy model is more traditional and reflects the strong influence of the medical model. In this model, the student is removed from the classroom and treated in a separate therapy room. The treatment is carried out for the prescribed amount of time, and the student is transported back to the classroom. The advantages of this model are the ready accessibility to any special equipment and the elimination of distractions.[38] The disadvantages of this model are that the child is practicing skills in an artificial environment which may have little carry over into the natural environment,[39] and that the staff is unaware of the activities performed with the therapist thus decreasing the chance for integration of activities into the child's daily routine.

In the integrated therapy model, the physical therapist brings needed equipment into the home, classroom, or worksite and provides therapy within that setting. This allows the physical therapist more contact with the parent or teacher and facilitates the use of therapy for the achievement of educationally-appropriate goals. When in the classroom setting, the student does not lose valuable class time or opportunities for peer interaction and is spared the stigmatization of removal from the classroom. The integrated therapy model also provides an ideal opportunity for the therapist to model appropriate handling and positioning activities to the parent or teacher.[38] This therapy model seems especially appropriate for the child with multiple handicaps who may require the services of a number of different support service personnel. Removal from the classroom for each of these special services would mean the loss of a great deal of class time and continued interruptions for the teacher and remaining students in the classroom.

In a study of in-class vs out-of-class therapy, Cole et al found that there was no significant difference in performance of children with developmental delays but that teaching staff preferred the in-class model.[40] Houck and Radonovich described an expanded continuum of motor options for students with disabilities in preschool and kindergarten from services in their least restrictive setting (classroom) to most restrictive (home based/or noncenterbased).[41] A major benefit of providing integrated services is that the teaching staff and/or parents become more aware of, and assume more responsibility for, motor programming.[40,41]

MAKING SERVICE DELIVERY DECISIONS

Decisions regarding the type of physical therapy service to be provided are based on the child's identified educational needs and goals and objectives. The level of expertise needed for the person to assist the child is determined for each of the child's goals. Not every child who has an identified goal for increased functional mobility will be appropriate for physical therapy services. For example, one child may be limited only because of lack of experience and another because of musculoskeletal limitations. The first child can be taught by the teacher, whereas the second child requires the expertise of the physical therapist. In addition, therapy should not be thought of as a life-long need, but as a service which is on a continuum and will change as the child's needs change. It is very appropriate for a child to move back and forth between direct and indirect services as skills change. It also is appropriate to discontinue therapy service and initiate an evaluation years later as the child moves into a different educational setting which requires different skills, such as vocational experiences. The duration of service must be stated on the IEP and IFSP and by law can be no longer than one year from the date of the IEP or IFSP. Thus, reevaluation must be done on an annual basis. Therapists need to change from providing automatic continuation of services to informing the parents and staff of the need to reevaluate children yearly. The child and family should not assume that the level of physical therapy services will remain the same throughout the child's academic career.

Once it has been determined that the expertise of a physical therapist is needed, the team must decide if the service will be direct or indirect. Decisions regarding the selection of students for direct or indirect therapy services and the frequency, intensity, and duration of such therapy are based on a number of variables. Zimmerman described several factors that are used in the Occupational/Physical Therapy Profile which include "chronological age, expected outcome, extent of previous therapy, extent to which needs are met in other programs, priority of direct therapy in relation to educational program, and immediacy of need." [42] In addition, the child's desire or motivation to move must be considered as well as the priorities of the family and the child.

No definitive research has been offered which suggests what amount of therapy is most beneficial for a particular diagnosis at a specific age. Therapists must, however, make definitive statements on the IEP and IFSP about the number of therapy sessions per week, their duration, and the types of services to be provided. Parents and therapists may assume that "more is better" and "direct is better than indirect" and fail to consider the infringement that multiple therapy sessions or direct intervention may have on other academic and social needs of the child. The focus may be inappropriately placed on the specific amount and type of service rather than the more important issues of yearly goal attainment and incorporation of activities that address the child's needs into the daily program.

How long should direct therapy aimed at changing motor performance be continued? In a study by Beals, walking performance of children with spastic diplegia generally improved until the age of 7 years. [43] In reviewing this study, Bleck concluded that physical therapy to improve walking patterns beyond age 7 was unlikely to be worth the time and effort expended, and he stressed that other areas of function should take precedence. [44] Based on clinical experience, Ellis concurred that by age

7 or 8 years, emphasis should change to more functional goals using equipment and adaptive devices to allow the child to be as functional and active as possible. [45] This viewpoint is controversial and reflects a move from a disease-oriented to a function-oriented approach to children with cerebral palsy and other physical disabilities. [44]

Should the normal motor developmental sequence be used as a model for school therapy? Atwater questioned the use of a normal motor developmental sequence as a theoretical model in pediatric physical therapy. [46] This hierarchical model requires motor skills to build on each other in a specific sequence. VanSant stated "the extent to which early tasks lay the foundation for later skills is a matter of conjecture." [47] Current theories in movement science suggest that development is a dynamic process dependent on many factors or variables. The child and task interaction results in organization of movement to a preferred form (dynamical systems approach). [48-50] With this in mind, the goal of intervention is to maximize function in the child's environment. Therapists need to teach functional abilities instead of motor milestones. [46,51] It has been suggested that the role of the physical therapist is to teach the individual the ability to develop movement solutions instead of imitating motor skills. [52,53]

Does the frequency of therapy make a difference? Jenkins and colleagues reported no significant differences in motor gains made by children with mild to moderate motor delays who received physical therapy three times a week compared with those who received therapy once a week. [54] Both groups of children, however, who received therapy made greater motor gains than a no-treatment control group. A similar study examining frequency of treatment was reported recently for children with spastic cerebral palsy. [55] Children who received almost three times as much neurodevelopmental therapy (intensive NDT group) did not do significantly better on measures of hand function or quality of movement when compared to children who received fewer treatments (regular NDT group).

Levine and Kliebhan suggested general guidelines for treatment time based on diagnosis, prognosis, and treatment possibilities. [56] Their recommendations range from less than one hour a month for a child on a maintenance program to two hours a week for an active therapy program. They recognized the need for more intensive therapy services for a limited amount of time (generally less than three months) for children following surgery, for children with no previous therapy, and for fabrication and ordering of equipment. Campbell and Finn suggested the need to determine the "best fit" of service for the child based on the child's individualized needs. [57] They discussed the need for the therapist to have an understanding of intervention approaches as they vary in theoretical framework, form, schedule of delivery, and the involvement of professionals in isolation or in collaboration with other professionals or parents. Therapists need to understand the central features and efficacy for the non-traditional and traditional therapy approaches. They emphasized that the service the child receives should be based on a match between the various treatment approaches and the specific characteristics of the child.

STAFFING CONSIDERATIONS

A needs assessment may be the first step in determining how best to provide physical therapy services. This information can facilitate cost-effective budgeting for staff, space, and equipment, and also can help in long-range planning. APTA guidelines on "Physical Therapy in Educational Environments" recommends a needs assessment with the following components:
• philosophy and models of service delivery,
• number and type of children with disabilities in the district who are eligible for physical therapy,
• location of the schools to be served,
• referral mechanisms,
• functional levels of referred children,
• facilities available for delivery of service,
• equipment needs of the children with disabilities,
• job descriptions,
• anticipated caseload,
• need for physical therapist assistants and secretarial support, and
• the orientation and staff development plan.[36]

Information from the needs assessment can assist in the determination of caseload numbers. Particular attention should be paid to the following factors when determining caseload numbers:
• the identified responsibilities of the therapist,
• the amount of travel time required,
• the range and severity of handicaps,
• the number and type of supportive personnel,
• the level of service (individual, group, consultation), and
• the experience and training of current staff members.[36,56]

Consideration also must be given for the time needed for administrative tasks, such as program planning, IEP or IFSP meetings, report writing, and in-service training.

Determination of caseload numbers is a difficult issue. Several surveys have reported ranges varying from 11 to 30 children served per week in a variety of service delivery models.[58-60] Attempts have been made to develop a method to determine appropriate caseloads, to establish the number of therapists required to serve a district, and to facilitate equal distribution of work among therapists. Both the Georgia Alliance of School Occupational and Physical Therapists[61] and the Washington State Special Education Advisory Council[62] have developed methods for determining maximum therapy caseloads. The latter group recommended the following therapist-to-student ratios according to degree of handicap: severe 1:8; moderate 1:12; mild 1:20.[62]

EMPLOYMENT OPTIONS

Physical therapists generally have two employment options, direct hire or contracting. In the direct hire option, the physical therapist is hired directly by a local education agency (LEA) or by a cooperative agency that serves several LEAs. Through this system, the therapist is placed on a teacher's contract and receives the same benefits as a teacher. The advantages of being an employee of the LEA are more direct contact with other staff, availability when needed, and more flexibility in scheduling. The disadvantages may include supervision by an educationally trained administrator, requirement to perform education-related duties such as bus supervision, and limited contact with other therapists.[36]

When contracting, the therapist does not receive any of the benefits of the LEA and must show proof of liability insurance. The advantages of contracting for the therapist may be in having to work only with a few students and deciding the maximum amount of time spent in the LEA. Generally, contracting is advantageous to the LEA, especially if there are few students that require service. Disadvantages include limited availability of the physical therapist for additional meetings and interactions with staff, and a fee-for-service arrangement which frequently results in the LEA only requesting therapist involvement for direct service and essential meetings.

Therapists should investigate both alternatives before deciding which option is best for them. Additional information is available in the APTA guidelines on "Physical Therapy Practice in Educational Environments".[36]

PERFORMANCE REVIEW OF PHYSICAL THERAPISTS IN EDUCATIONAL ENVIRONMENTS

Unlike most physical therapy practice settings, where the evaluating supervisor is a physical therapist, school physical therapists often are responsible to educational personnel, such as the school principal or the special education director. Several methods and types of evaluations which may be useful in the educational environment are:

Internal Peer Review: A method of review easily conducted within a physical therapy department is a periodic review of reports written by the therapy staff. Therapists critique reports written by other staff members to ensure the quality of reports. Exposure to different styles of report-writing also will enable therapists to improve their own report writing skills. Therapists may want to use the American Physical Therapy Association's

Standards of Practice[63] as a basis for minimum criteria for written documentation.

Evaluation of the quality of physical therapy services as it relates to the abilities of a therapist to perform specific therapy techniques is probably the most difficult assessment for educational personnel. Designation of a lead therapist or head therapist in school districts with large therapy staffs may assist educational administrators in this process.

External Peer Review: Special certification for physical therapists working in the public schools has been adopted by many states via external peer review. Such a method can assure attainment of competence by physical therapists in the areas of evaluation, program planning, and management of students within the educational system. Supervised experience in an educational setting often is required for initial certification with a more extensive peer review, including chart audits, required for continued certification.

Field Observation: While it may be difficult for educational administrators to evaluate the quality of therapy services, general performance standards applicable to all educational staff could be evaluated by on-site observations of the physical therapist in the classroom or therapy setting. Performance standards such as professionalism, communication skills, organizational abilities, and adaptability and flexibility in program planning could be adapted for use with physical therapists. Evaluations would be most appropriately conducted by those working closely with the therapist, such as the school principal or the special education teacher. Lindsey described a performance appraisal instrument for school physical therapists which can be used by non-therapist supervisors.[64] Specific educational agencies may have their own internal teacher performance review which they will use for physical therapists.

Chart Audit: An audit of physical therapy records could be conducted by educational administrators in much the same manner as chart audits are conducted in a medical setting. Prior to the institution of such a review process, the therapy staff and educational administrators would determine the items necessary for inclusion in each chart, such as records of therapy sessions scheduled and attended, data to document progress of IEP or IFSP objectives, and phone conversations with parents.

Individual Goals and Objectives: Another approach to the evaluation of school physical therapists would be to monitor the attainment of annual professional goals and objectives developed by the physical therapist with concurrent approval from the administrator. An important professional goal, for example, is enrollment in continuing education courses. Other goals might include completion of a certification process for a particular therapeutic procedure or development of a research project or paper pertinent to the practice of physical therapy in the schools.

CONCLUSION

Physical therapists play an important role in the educational environment. As integral members of a multidisciplinary or interdisciplinary team, physical therapists work to ensure the most appropriate education for children with disabilities. The physical therapist's unique skills in the management of physical disabilities assist teachers, parents, administrators, and other educational staff in assuring integration into the classroom. Educators, therapists, medical personnel, insurers, and parents need to understand that physical therapy provided in the educational setting only addresses educational needs and therefore should not be the only therapy available. Part H has begun to recognize this by requiring interagency collaboration with a family focus. This recognition of multiple agencies with multiple providers and payers needs to be carried over to meet the overall needs of children.

This chapter has presented an overview of the roles and functions of physical therapists in the educational environment, along with issues related to service delivery. These topics will now be addressed as they relate to the physical therapy needs in an educational setting for the case study children.

CASE STUDIES

CASE NO. 1 — JASON
Cerebral Palsy, Right Hemiparesis, 18 Months

Jason's IFSP was developed by an interagency team. The family's priorities are to improve Jason's feeding, right hand use, walking, and play skills. Additionally, the family would like more information on Jason's disability and are interested in a support group. At the IFSP meeting it was determined that the school district would be responsible for home-based occupational therapy once a week and a center-based family support and play group once every other week. The family's insurance is responsible for home-based, private physical therapy twice a week and speech therapy once a week. The home-based services allow the therapists to work closely with Jason's family members and to model appropriate handling techniques. Regular communication among the therapists was established.

The physical therapist consults with Jason's parents to ensure that he is properly positioned during feeding and play activities. A bench has been purchased for Jason which allows both feet to rest flat on the floor with hips and knees flexed to at least a 90 degree angle. This will facilitate a more symmetrical sitting posture and reduce the risk of eliciting the positive support reflex on his involved side. When seated at a table for play activities, it is recommended that Jason keep both arms on the table to encourage use of his involved extremity. These seating considerations are shared with the occupational therapist and speech pathologist who treat Jason in the home.

As many play activities take place on the floor, the therapist also provides Jason's parents with recommended floor sitting positions for him. Side-sitting on the right hip is recommended to increase weight-bearing on his involved side. It also is a good position to encourage weight-bearing on an extended arm and open hand. Another suggested position is ring sitting which will provide equal weight-bearing on both hips. Reverse tailor sitting ("W-sitting") is discouraged due to placement of the lower extremities in a total flexion pattern.

The physical therapist gives Jason's mother several general suggestions to be incorporated into play activities. She is reminded not to force Jason to use his involved arm and hand. Rather, activities are structured to encourage bilateral use of his extremities with his involved arm used as a "helper." For example, musical instruments such as cymbals or the triangle which require use of both hands should be encouraged. Tossing or rolling a large ball using both hands would be more beneficial for Jason than playing with a smaller ball which could be held with the uninvolved hand alone. A cup large enough circumferentially to require use of both hands also is recommended. Finally, Jason's mother is encouraged to provide sensory experiences to his involved extremities in activities such as finger-painting, water play, and sand play (see Chapter 6). Medically relevant goals and objectives are appropriate for Jason as described in Chapters 6-11.

CASE NO. 2 — JILL
Cerebral Palsy, Spastic Quadriparesis, Mental Retardation, 7 Years

Jill is enrolled in a full day special education classroom but is integrated with second graders for music and social studies. Since her enrollment in the public schools at the age of 4 years, Jill has received extensive direct physical therapy services. In addition, the physical therapist has worked closely with the parents, physician, and occupational therapist to adapt Jill's wheelchair so that she is positioned comfortably and in the best functional and therapeutic position possible. Jill's present level of performance for motor ability reveals a plateau in motor development. She requires adaptive equipment in order to access her educational environment and has no functional mobility. She can assist with a standing pivot transfer. Jill's special education motor needs include positioning and evaluation for functional mobility. The expertise of the physical therapist is needed on an indirect basis to establish a positioning program, pro-

vide adaptive equipment, train staff in transfer techniques, and evaluate Jill's potential for powered mobility. The therapist also will continue to provide regular in-services to the educational staff on such topics as wheelchair use, proper body mechanics for lifting and transferring students, and general handling and positioning principles.

The primary purpose for Jill's positioning program at school is so she can access different learning stations. A secondary reason for her positioning program is to maintain her flexibility for functional purposes as well as to maintain good hygiene, prevent skin breakdown, maintain range of motion, and minimize further progression of her scoliosis. Because Jill has limited ability to move independently, the therapist has recommended several positions for her to assume out of her wheelchair. These include positioning on a prone board to allow weight-bearing on the lower extremities, as well as to provide a means of maintaining Jill's range of motion following her heelcord and adductor releases. This position also can help maintain upper extremity range of motion by moving Jill's arms out of their typical pattern of adduction and flexion (Figure 3). This is an excellent position for classroom table top activities.

Use of a prone wedge will provide another opportunity to stretch out her lower extremities and to move her arms out of the flexed and adducted position (Figure 4). This is a good position for floor activities, especially reading books or playing board games.

A floor sitter will allow Jill to sit on the floor and be maintained in a comfortable and therapeutic position (Figure 5). The removable wedge can be adjusted to hold the seat in several reclining positions. This is another position for floor activities such as the opening classroom session, music, or when the teacher reads to the class.

A side-lying position will help stretch out or "lengthen" Jill's trunk muscles on the concave side of her scoliosis. A foam cut-out can be used to maintain her in this position. Commercially made side-lying positioners are available (Figure 6). This position allows Jill to use her top arm to manipulate objects, but puts her at a visual disadvantage.

The therapist works closely with the classroom teacher to develop a schedule for positioning which will be integrated with classroom activities. For example, Jill is placed on the prone board during a classroom activity which requires a table top. The therapist also ensures that all staff working with Jill understand how equipment is used and the importance of the positioning program to Jill's overall development and integration into the classroom. Diagrams and step-by-step procedures are outlined and given to the classroom teacher for easy reference.

Educationally-relevant goals and objectives for Jill include:

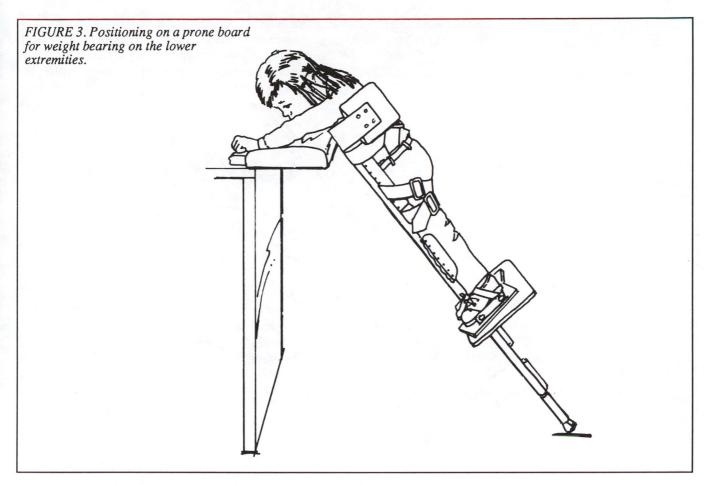

FIGURE 3. Positioning on a prone board for weight bearing on the lower extremities.

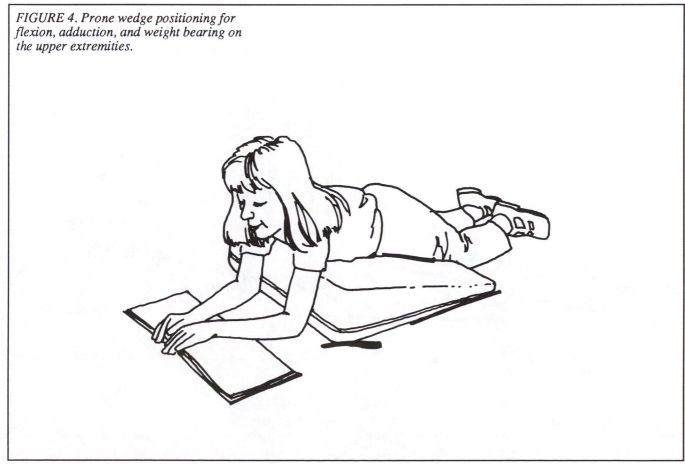

FIGURE 4. Prone wedge positioning for flexion, adduction, and weight bearing on the upper extremities.

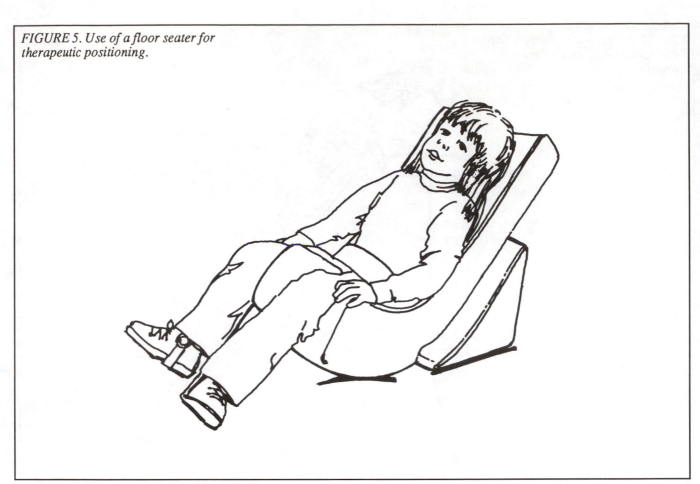

FIGURE 5. Use of a floor seater for therapeutic positioning.

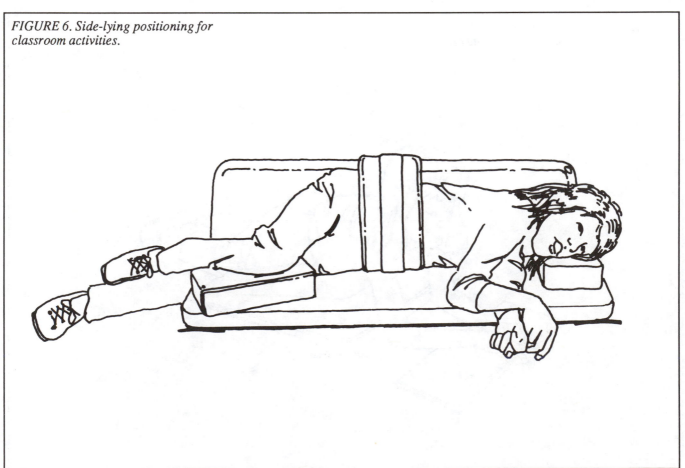

FIGURE 6. Side-lying positioning for classroom activities.

Annual Goal: Participate in activities in the classroom while in appropriate functional positions.

Short-term Objective: Jill will participate in the art activity while standing on the prone board for 30 minutes, twice a day, for 3 consecutive data days.

Annual Goal: Improve functional mobility skills.

Short-term Objectives:

1. Jill will complete a standing pivot transfer from her wheelchair to the toilet with decreasing physical assist, currently at moderate assistance, on 80% of the trials on 3 consecutive data days.

2. Jill will maneuver a powered wheelchair 100 feet in hallway, running into walls no more than 2 times on 3 consecutive data days.

Case No. 3 — Taylor
Myelomeningocele Repaired L 1-2, 4 Years

Taylor is completing his second year in a special education preschool. His parents, along with the multidisciplinary team, are considering placing Taylor in a regular education kindergarten next year. The physical therapist has been asked to determine what special assistance Taylor will need to be mainstreamed into a regular educational classroom given his physical limitations.

The physical therapist develops the following list for discussion at the next multidisciplinary staff meeting: wheelchair accessibility of the building, doors, locker/coat room, classroom, media area, music area, school health office, and the restrooms; set-up of classroom; mobility opportunities within the classroom; integration of positioning and mobility activities into class schedule; general classroom schedule; options for sitting at tables and on floor; playground accessibility and available equipment; classroom teacher's knowledge of myelomeningocele; Taylor's current medical status and projected needs including bowel and bladder training programs; and model for special education programming including integrated therapy.

Although some members of the team have recommended Taylor be assigned a full-time aide, the physical therapist recommends use of the school's health aide or other special education aide only for the toileting program. The therapist believes that Taylor must be given the opportunity to develop his independence by moving away from the constant one-to-one attention he has become accustomed to in the special education and therapy programs.

Taylor will continue to receive individual therapy services twice a week. He is a high priority for therapy at this time, because he is ready to begin ambulating with conventional orthoses and crutches. It is recommended that the sessions be a combination of in-class and out-of-

class depending on the specific activities the class is doing at the time of therapy. The therapist has consulted with Taylor's parents and physician regarding the orthoses and crutches Taylor will need. In order for the newly acquired skills to be carried over into the classroom and home, the therapist will remain in close communication with the teacher and parents regarding Taylor's progress and activities to incorporate into his day.

Educationally-relevant goals and objectives for Taylor include:

Annual Goal: Improve independent transfer skills.

Short-term Objective: Taylor will independently transfer from his wheelchair to his classroom chair and back, 100% of the time on 3 consecutive data days.

Annual Goal: Improve functional mobility.

Short-term Objectives:

1. Taylor will walk from his wheelchair to his classroom chair a distance of 10 feet using his orthoses and crutches, with stand-by assistance, on 3 consecutive data days.

2. Taylor will propel his wheelchair independently from the school entry to his classroom within 2 minutes, on 3 consecutive data days.

Case No. 4 — Ashley
Down Syndrome, 15 Months

Ashley attends an early intervention program for infants with disabilities twice a week. The program emphasizes parent training and provides one-to-one services to each family. The physical therapist works in the classroom with the teacher and parents for 45 minutes each week and provides them with appropriate motor activities to be incorporated at home and in the classroom.

The physical therapist suggested several activities for Ashley. Ashley should be encouraged to maintain her balance in a half-kneeling position (Figure 7), allowing her to use a bench for balance as needed. She should be encouraged to free her hands to reach for toys while maintaining her balance.

While standing using furniture for support, toys can be placed on the floor and Ashley can be encouraged to stoop down to pick them up and then return to standing. In all-fours, Ashley could be encouraged to reach out and push a large ball while maintaining balance on three extremities.

With Ashley seated on the adult's lap, her hips could be held and she could be tilted slowly to the right or left, with time given for her to bring her head back to midline. She also could be held at the hips and tilted back a short distance. She should be encouraged to keep her chin tucked during this activity.

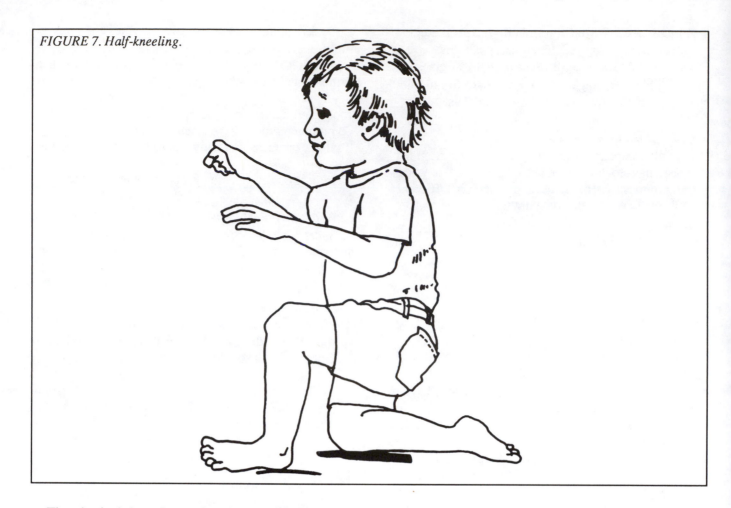

FIGURE 7. Half-kneeling.

The physical therapist works with the occupational therapist and speech clinician to coordinate Ashley's feeding program. In-service sessions also are provided periodically to the staff on such topics as normal and abnormal development and proper positioning and handling techniques.

Educationally-relevant goal and objectives for Ashley include:

Annual Goal: Improve functional mobility.

Short-term Objectives:

1. In 4 out of 5 trials, Ashley will creep up four 6" inch steps to attain a favorite toy.
2. In 3 out of 5 trials, Ashley will maintain independent standing for 5 seconds while playing with toys on a table. ❑

REFERENCES

1. Education for All Handicapped Children Act, Public Law 94-142. U.S. Congress, Senate, 94th Congress, first session, 1975

2. Education of the Handicapped Act Amendments of 1986, Public Law 99-457. U.S. Congress, Senate, 99th Congress, 1986

3. Individuals with Disabilities Education Act Amendments of 1991, Public Law 102-119. U.S. Congress, Senate, 102d Congress, 1991

4. Audette RH: Interagency collaboration. In Elder JO, Magrab PR (eds): Coordinating Services to Handicapped Children: A Handbook for Interagency Collaboration. Baltimore, MD, Paul Brooks, 1980, pp. 25-34

5. Ballard J, Zenel J: Public Law 94-142 and Section 504; What they say about rights and protections. Excep Child 44: 181, 1977

6. Able-Boone H, Sandall SR, Loughry A, et al: An informed, family-centered approach to Public Law 99-457: Parental views. Topics Early Childhood Spec Educ 10: 100-111, 1990

7. Cone J, Delawyer D, Wolf V: Assessing parent participation: The parent/family involvement index. Exceptional Children 51: 417-424, 1985

8. Bailey DB Jr, Simeonsson RJ: Critical issues underlying research and intervention with families of young handicapped children. J Division for Early Childhood 8:38-48, 1984

9. Dunst CJ, Trivette CM, Davis M, et al: Enabling and empowering families of children with health impairments. CHC 17: 71-81, 1988

10. Bailey DB: Collaborative goal-setting with families: Resolving differences in values and priorities for services. Topics Early Childhood Spec Educ 7: 59-71, 1987

11. Hanson M, Lynch E, Wayman K: Honoring the cultural diversity of families when gathering data. Topics Early Childhood Spec Educ 10: 112-131, 1990

12. Bailey DB Jr, Simeonsson RJ, Winton PJ, et al: Family-focused intervention: A functional model for planning, implementing, and evaluating individualized family services in early intervention. J Division for Early Childhood 10: 156-171, 1986

13. Bailey DB Jr, Simeonsson RJ: Assessing needs of families with handicapped infants. J Special Education 22: 117-127, 1988

14. Whitehead L, Deiner P, Toccafondi S: Family assessment: Parent and professional evaluation. Topics Early Childhood Spec Educ 10: 63-77, 1990

15. Spencer PE, Coye KW: Project BRIDGE: A team approach to decision-making for early services. Infants Young Children 1: 82-92, 1988

16. Campbell PH: The integrated programming team: An approach for coordinating professionals of various disciplines in programs for students with severe and multiple handicaps. J Assoc Severely Handicapped 12: 107-116, 1987

17. Sears CJ: The transdisciplinary approach: A process for compliance with Public Law 94-142. TASH J 6: 22-29, 1981

18. York J, Rainforth B, Giangreco MF: Transdisciplinary teamwork and integrated therapy: Clarifying the misconceptions. Ped Phys Ther 2: 73-79, 1990

19. Harris SR: Transdisciplinary therapy model for the infant with Down's syndrome. Phys Ther 60: 420-423, 1980

20. Abelson MA, Woodman RW: Review of research on team effectiveness: Implications for teams in schools. School Psychology Review 12: 125-136, 1983

21. Albano ML, Cox B, York J, et al: Educational teams for students with severe and multiple handicaps. In York R, Schofield D, Donder D, et al, (eds): Organizing and Implementing Services for Students with Severe and Multiple Handicaps. Springfield, IL: Illinois Board of Education, 1981, pp 23-34

22. Bailey DB Jr. A triaxial model of the interdisciplinary team and group process. Exceptional Children 51: 17-25, 1984

23. Lyon S, Lyon G: Team functioning and staff development: A role release approach to providing integrated educational services for severely handicapped students. J Assoc Severely Handicapped 5: 250-263,1980

24. Orelove FP, Sobsey D: Chapter 1: Designing transdisciplinary services. In Orelove FP, Sobsey D, (eds): Educating Children with Multiple Disabilities. Baltimore, MD: Paul H. Brookes, 1987, pp 1-24

25. Code of Federal Regulations 300.550(b) (1-2), July 1988

26. PL 100, cited in Roybal MR. Government affairs. Ped Phys Ther 1: 42, 1989

27. Roybal MR: Government affairs. Ped Phys Ther 1: 42, 1989

28. Long T: Editorial: School based physical therapy: Where are we headed? Ped Phys Ther 1: 47, 1989

29. Rogers, JJ: Schools, insurance, and your family's financial security. Exceptional Parent 76-78, 1991

30. Ottenbacher K: Transdisciplinary service delivery in school environments: Some limitations. Phys Occup Ther Pediatr 3: 9-16, 1983

31. Levangie PK: Public school physical therapists: Role definition and educational needs. Phys Ther 60: 774-779, 1980

32. McLaurin SE: Preparation of physical therapists for employment in public schools. Phys Ther 64: 674-677, 1984

33. Mullens J: New challenges for physical therapy practitioners in educational settings. Phys Ther 61: 496-502, 1981

34. Sellers JLS: Professional cooperation in public school physical therapy. Phys Ther 60: 1159-1161, 1980

35. Surburg PR: Implications of Public Law 94-142 for physical therapists. Phys Ther 61: 210-212, 1981

36. Physical Therapy Practice in Educational Environments: Policies, Guidelines. Alexandria, VA, American Physical Therapy Association, 1990

37. Sternat J, Messina R, Nietupski, et al: Occupational and physical therapy services for severely handicapped students: Toward a naturalized public school service delivery model. In Sontag E (ed): Educational Programming for the Severely and Profoundly Handicapped. Reston, VA, Council for Exceptional Children, 1977

38. Harris SR, Tada WL: Providing developmental therapy services. In Garwood SH, Fewell RR (eds): Educating Handicapped Infants: Issues in Development and Intervention. Rockville, MD, Aspen Systems Corporation, 1983, pp 343-368

39. Fetters L: Cerebral palsy: Contemporary treatment concepts. In Lister MJ (ed): Contemporary Management of Motor Control Problems: Proceedings of the II STEP Conference. Alexandria VA, Foundation for Physical Therapy, 1991, pp 219-224

40. Cole KN, Harris SR, Eland SF, et al: Comparison of two service delivery models: In-class and out-of-class therapy approaches. Ped Phys Ther 1: 49-54, 1989

41. Houck C, Radonovich S. Practice management: An expanded continuum of motor options for handicapped preschool and kindergarten students. Ped Phys Ther 1: 88-90, 1989

42. Zimmerman J: An OT/PT reporting system approach to school-based therapy. Totline, American Physical Therapy Association 12: 6-7, 1986

43. Beals R, cited in Bleck EE: Cerebral Palsy. In Bleck EE, Nagel DA (eds): Physically Handicapped Children: A Medical Atlas for Teachers, ed 2, New York, NY, Grune and Stratton. 1982, pp 59-132

44. Bleck EE: Cerebral Palsy. In Bleck EE, Nagel DA (eds): Physically Handicapped Children: A Medical Atlas for Teachers, ed 2, New York, NY, Grune and Stratton, 1982, pp 59-132

45. Ellis E: How long should therapy be continued? Dev Med Child Neurol 9: 47-49, 1967

46. Atwater SW: Should the normal motor developmental sequence be used as a theoretical model in pediatric physical therapy? In Lister MJ (ed): Contemporary Management of Motor Control Problems: Proceedings of the II STEP Conference. Alexandria VA, Foundation for Physical Therapy, 1991, pp 89-93

47. VanSant A: Motor control, motor learning, and motor development. In Montgomery PC, Connolly BH (eds): Motor Control and Physical Therapy: Theoretical Framework and Practical Applications. Hixson, TN, Chattanooga Group Inc, 1991, pp 13-28

48. Attermeier S: Should the normal motor developmental sequence be used as a theoretical model in patient treatment? In Lister MJ (ed): Contemporary Management of Motor Control Problems: Proceedings of the II STEP Conference. Alexandria VA, Foundation for Physical Therapy, 1991, pp 85-87

49. Kamm K, Thelen E, Jenson JL: A dynamical systems approach to motor development. Phys Ther 70: 763-775, 1990

50. VanSant AF: Life-span motor development. In Lister MJ (ed): Contemporary Management of Motor Control Problems: Proceedings of the II STEP Conference. Alexandria VA, Foundation for Physical Therapy, 1991, pp 77-83

51. Heriza C: Motor development: Traditional and contemporary theories. In Lister MJ (ed): Contemporary Management of Motor Control Problems: Proceedings of the II STEP Conference. Alexandria VA, Foundation for Physical Therapy, 1991, pp 99-126

52. Higgins S: Motor skill acquisition. Phys Ther 71: 123-129, 1991

53. Mulder T: A process-oriented model of human motor behavior; Toward a theory-based rehabilitation approach. Phys Ther 71: 157-164, 1991

54. Jenkins JR, Sells CJ, Brady D, et al: Effects of developmental therapy on motor impaired children. Phys Occup Ther Pediatr 2: 19-28, 1982

55. Law M, Cadman D, Rosenbaum P, et al: Neuro-developmental therapy and upper-extremity inhibitive casting for children with cerebral palsy. Dev Med Child Neurol 33:379-387, 1991

56. Levine MS, Kliebhan L: Communication between physician and physical and occupational therapists: A neuro-developmentally based prescription. Pediatrics 68: 208-214, 1981

57. Campbell PH, Finn DM: Programming to influence acquisition of motor abilities in infants and young children. Ped Phys Ther 3: 200-205, 1991

58. School Administrator's Guide to Physical Therapy and Occupational Therapy in California Public Schools, Fremont, CA, California Alliance of Pediatric Physical and Occupational Therapists, 1980

59. Gilfoyle EM, Hays C: Occupational therapy roles and functions in the education of school based handicapped students. AJOT 33: 565-576, 1979

60. Strategies for Implementing Occupational and Physical Therapy in Schools. Houston, TX, Harris County Department of Education, 1982

61. Effgen SK: Determining school therapy caseloads based upon severity of need for services. Totline, American Physical Therapy Association, 10: 16-17, 1984

62. Support Service Task Force Report, Washington, Washington State Special Education Advisory Support Services Task Force, 1976

63. Standards of Practice for Physical Therapy. American Physical Therapy Association, Alexandria, VA, 1991

64. Lindsey D: A model performance appraisal instrument for school physical therapists. Clinical Management Phys Ther 6: 20-26, 1986

CHAPTER 14

THE CHILDREN IN TREATMENT

Patricia C. Montgomery, Ph.D., PT
Barbara H. Connolly, Ed.D., PT

Children with developmental disabilities seldom have isolated problems, but rather multiple problems as identified in the preceding chapters. For teaching purposes, assessment and treatment of each problem area have been presented separately. However, in developmental therapy, we must deal with the whole child, not problems in isolation. The purpose of this chapter is to provide examples of several different, but comprehensive treatment sessions for the children used as case studies. In each of the cases, the long term goals are written for 12 months or for the duration of the school year. The short term objectives are appropriate for three months, or a quarter of the school year.

CASE NO. 1 — JASON
Cerebral Palsy, Right Hemiparesis, 18 Months

Goal: Increase sensory awareness of the right side of the body.

Objective: During play, spontaneously use the right upper extremity, 5 times in 3 minutes.

Objective: Remove all 5 stickers placed on the right arm within 1 minute.

Goal: Increase mobility of right side of the body, especially in the hips and thoracic spine, shoulder girdle, and forearm.

Objective: Rise from supine to sitting using a rotational pattern on request.

Objective: Lift an 8" ball 5" from the table with both hands, 2 of 3 times attempted.

Goal: Decrease tactile defensiveness.

Objective: Tolerate rubbing of the right upper extremity for one minute.

Objective: Spontaneously use right hand to "finger paint" with whipped cream on mirror.

Goal: Improve symmetrical activities in the upper and lower extremities.

Objective: Reach for a 12" ball with both hands equally, 2 of 3 trials.

Objective: Rise to standing from a small chair with equal weight on both feet.

Goal: Facilitate normal posture and movement.

Objective: Maintain neutral foot flat position on the floor in stance for one minute.

Objective: Grasp a dowel shaped toy and release into a container 5 times in 2 minutes.

Objective: Use the right hand for protection when falling to the right during walking, 2 of 3 times.

Goal: Increase active weight shifting to the right.

Objective: Maintain the quadruped position and point to the ceiling with the left hand on command without collapsing.

Objective: Rise to standing from a half kneeling position with the right leg forward, 50% of the time.

Goal: Increase symmetrical activity of the oral motor structures.

Objective: Maintain lip closure on the cup rim while drinking 50% of the time.

Objective: Produce a "b" and an "m" sound on command.

Goal: Improve coordination of respiration with oral motor activity.

Objective: Take 3-4 sips of liquid from a cup without pausing.

Objective: Blow bubbles through a wand for 3-5 seconds without interruption.

Treatment Session Goals

The following treatment session goals were set for a 45 minute home physical therapy visit. The mother was present to assist the therapist. Goals were to decrease tactile defensiveness, increase mobility of the trunk, improve reaching and symmetrical activities of the upper extremity, increase weight shifting to the right side of the body, and facilitate prolonged expiration during movement. Other goals for Jason for the three month period will be worked on at other times.

Activities for Jason include the following:

1. In supine, the knees are bent to the chest with the hips slightly raised from the supporting surface. The therapist applies deep pressure as she slides her hands down his arms to facilitate arm extension bilaterally to enable Jason to place his hands on his bottom. As she rotates his legs from side to side in this position, she asks Jason to "hold" his bottom.

2. In supine, with the knees still bent to the chest, the therapist asks Jason to reach with both arms for an 8" diameter ball that is held above his head. Assistance is given to the right arm for the reaching, as necessary. Jason is asked to bring the ball to the therapist. Emphasis is placed on getting Jason to make the "b" sound for ball.

3. Jason rolls from his back onto his right side and practices "one arm" push-ups into side sitting.

4. Jason is assisted into a straddling position on a bolster that allows his hips and knees to be approximately at a 90 degree position. The therapist is positioned on her knees in front of the bolster, facing Jason while she stabilizes the bolster. The therapist plays "boat" with him and tilts Jason from side to side to stimulate weight shifting. Faster tilting can be used to facilitate lateral protective reactions during "falling off the boat."

5. From the straddled position on the bolster, Jason is assisted as necessary to rise to standing with equal weight on both feet to blow bubbles from a wand that is held by the mother. Repeated squatting to standing is used for grading of movements.

6. In standing, Jason reaches with his right hand for a dowel shaped toy that is held on his left side, which he can then drop into a bucket placed on the floor on the right. He repeats the same activity using the left hand and reaching to the right. The activity can be repeated until it loses its novelty.

CASE NO. 2 — JILL
Cerebral Palsy, Spastic Quadriparesis, Mental Retardation, 7 Years

Goal: Increase tolerance to movement.

Objective: Tolerate swinging in a hammock in anterior/posterior direction for 2 minutes.

Objective: Express no displeasure during a 5 minute (bumpy) ride outside in her wheelchair.

Goal: Decrease general rigidity and increase mobility, particularly of the upper trunk and proximal joints.

Objective: Independently roll a distance of 10 feet in 5 minutes.

Objective: Maintain for one minute, prone on elbows position without collapsing while turning her head from right to left.

Goal: Facilitate righting reactions with head and trunk.

Objective: In supported sitting, right head to vertical 2 out of 3 times when tilted laterally.

Objective: In supported sitting, maintain a "chin tuck" for 10 seconds when placed in that position.

Goal: Improve eye tracking and downward gaze.

Objective: Spontaneously track the teacher as she walks in front of Jill.

Objective: Two out of 3 times, attempt to follow the trajectory of an object as it is dropped from above her head to the floor.

Goal: Facilitate reach, grasp, and release of objects.

Objective: In the wheelchair, reach above 60 degrees to bat a suspended object on command.

Objective: With the classroom aide stabilizing a dowel, successfully grasp and release on command, 2 of 5 times.

Goal: Improve oral motor control.

Objective: Initiate vowels without trunk and neck extension on command.

Objective: During feeding, close lips on bowl of spoon 25% of the time to remove the food.

Treatment Session Goals

Jill receives indirect services from the school physical therapist in her classroom for 30 minutes each week. General IEP goals that relate to physical therapy consultation include decreasing sensitivity to sensory and tactile input, increasing general mobility, facilitating reaching, and improving oral motor function.

The physical therapist works with the teacher and classroom aide on the following activities:

1. During a ten minute music session, Jill is swaddled in a cotton blanket and placed supine in the hammock. Initially, she lays motionless and watches a teddy bear suspended in a hammock above her swing from side to side (eye tracking). Then, Jill is swung gently in anterior/posterior direction for 15 seconds. She and the teddy bear take turns swinging for a few minutes.

2. Jill is removed from the hammock and placed sidelying on the floor. The classroom aide administers the slow passive trunk rotation to facilitate generalized relaxation.

3. Prone over a roll, Jill is encouraged to play with a classmate with a battery operated toy. While propping on one elbow, she reaches with the other arm to activate the toy by hitting a large plate switch.

4. With the classroom aide sitting in a rocking chair and with Jill on her lap, firm pressure is applied around the face and within the mouth. This is followed by feeding Jill an animal cracker and having her drink a thickened liquid from a cup during snack time.

5. At recess, Jill is given a "piggy back" ride by the classroom aide to the playground.

6. On the playground, Jill takes turns with her classmates in rolling down a large incline. The classroom aide assists Jill in initiating the rolling by using control at the legs.

CASE NO. 3 — TAYLOR
Myelomeningocele, Repaired L 1-2, 4 Years

Goal: Increase strength and endurance in trunk and upper extremities.

Objective: Perform 10 push-ups independently.

Objective: Perform 10 push-up shoulder depression exercises sitting in the wheelchair, while the therapist stabilizes his legs.

Goal: Increase variety of movement transitions and transfers.

Objective: Move from sitting to quadruped and back to sitting independently.

Objective: In new orthosis, will push from prone to standing with minimal assistance.

Goal: Facilitate visual motor integration.

Objective: Successfully complete 5 object obstacle course in his wheelchair, 2 of 3 times.

Objective: In standing, pull correctly shaped or numbered stickers off mirror on command.

Goal: Maintain good skin care program.

Objective: Correctly don socks and shoes without creating potential pressure areas, 100% of the time.

Objective: Call adults' attention to reddened areas, if they occur.

Goal: Improve balance reactions in sitting and in standing with orthosis.

Objective: Maintain independent balance for one minute while moving head in various directions.

Objective: Maintain sitting position on tilt table when tilted 30 degrees in any direction.

Goal: Achieve independent ambulation with orthosis and crutches.

Objective: Balance in orthosis with only one crutch for 30 seconds.

Objective: Ambulate with crutches and orthosis for 10 feet with assistance.

Treatment Session Goals

The treatment session goals were set for Taylor based on a one hour therapy session at school. Treatment will take place in the physical therapy room. Goals for the treatment session include increasing strength and endurance of upper extremities and trunk, facilitating motor planning and visual motor integration, practicing transitions of movement, and improving balance reactions in standing.

Activities to be done are:

1. Taylor pushes his wheelchair from the classroom to the therapy room following a circuitous route (obstacle course).

2. Seated in his wheelchair, Taylor completes a series of shoulder girdle strengthening exercises using pulleys and wheelchair push-ups. He records his number of repetitions on a chart on the wall.

3. Taylor actively transfers from the wheelchair to the floor. He and the therapist take turns imitating each other in various transitions of movement, i.e., rolling, side sitting, sitting, quadruped.

4. Therapist places Taylor prone over a large ball and Taylor uses upper back extension to look up at the ceiling and to bat at a suspended ball.

5. On the floor, Taylor completes several active exercises including bridging, reverse sit-ups, and push-ups. He records his number of repetitions on the chart on the wall.

6. Taylor assists in undressing, with attention paid to skin condition, and is assisted into his long leg braces and into standing.

7. In standing, a number of balance activities are attempted. These include lifting one crutch momentarily and attempting to place the crutch on a specific location on the floor.

8. Taylor is assisted in ambulation for a distance of 5 feet.

9. With assistance, Taylor transfers to the floor and removes the orthosis and dresses for return to the classroom.

10. Before wheeling himself back to the classroom, Taylor receives a sticker for every 20 repetitions recorded on his chart.

CASE NO. 4 — ASHLEY
Down Syndrome, 15 Months

Goal: Increase overall postural tone and stability.

Objective: Maintain an appropriate alignment in quadruped for 30 seconds with no more than one verbal cue from the therapist.

Objective: Move in and out of sidelying to side sitting without locking elbow in extension, 3 out of 6 times attempted.

Goal: Increase tolerance for handling and increase interest in movement.

Objective: Creep into therapist's lap at least once during the 45 minute treatment session.

Objective: Get on and off a tyke bike with assistance.

Goal: Improve strength and stability at shoulders, hips and knees.

Objective: Maintain an upright kneeling position with adequate trunk and hip extension for one minute.

Objective: Maintain standing position without knee hyperextension 25% of the time.

Goal: Improve grasp and release skills.

Objective: Release an object, without flinging the object, 50% of the time.

Objective: Pick up a small object without raking, 3 of 10 attempts.

Goal: Develop postural reactions in sitting, quadruped, and standing.

Objective: Maintain sitting balance when legs are lifted one at a time in a diagonal movement, 3 out of 5 times.

Objective: Maintain balance in quadruped when creeping on and off cushions placed on the floor.

Goal: Improve oral motor functioning.

Objective: Move tongue laterally to touch solids placed on side gums/teeth, 3 of 5 presentations.

Objective: Produce vocalization 3-5 seconds in length with less nasality and greater loudness on command.

Treatment Session Goals

Ashley is seen for physical therapy consultation for 45 minute sessions with the teacher and parents. Demonstration of appropriate activities are done at each session. The following treatment session goals were developed for such a session. The goals include increasing postural tone, strength, and stability; facilitating weight shifting and grading of movements; increasing tolerance for handling; improving grasp and release; and facilitating tongue movement.

Activities to be done during the session include:

1. Therapist greets Ashley by lifting her up and holding her in a hugging position while the therapist turns in a circle (vestibular and proprioceptive input).

2. Ashley sits on the therapist's lap, while her legs are extended as she faces the therapist. Ashley reaches for a hat placed on the therapist's head while the therapist's legs are moved up and down to shift Ashley's weight.

3. Ashley is rocked in all fours with approximation through the head and pelvis, through the long axis of the spine.

4. In the hands and knees position, Ashley reaches forward with one hand to grasp an object, alternating reach with the arms.

5. Creeping up and over a series of three pillows placed on the floor is accomplished with therapist assistance, if needed.

6. Ashley maintains half-kneeling at a small bench, and works on placing one inch blocks in and out of a container. Having the right and left leg forward is alternated.

7. Ashley stands at a chair, stoops to get a toy on the floor and then returns to standing.

8. Before snack time, Ashley self administers an electric tooth brush for oral desensitization.

9. During a snack, crunchy cereal is placed between the teeth on either side of the mouth.

CONCLUSION

Not all goals, objectives, or therapeutic techniques for each of the children were addressed in this chapter. Setting goals and objectives provides a framework for administering treatment. A variety of techniques often can be used to meet the same objective or several objectives simultaneously. Although repetition is important in treatment, a variety of activities makes the sessions enjoyable and motivating for the child and the therapist. Creativity, therefore, is the art of pediatric therapy. ❑

CHAPTER 15

RESEARCH TECHNIQUES FOR THE CLINICIAN

Susan R. Harris, Ph.D., PT, FAPTA

◆

During the past decade, increased emphasis has been placed on conducting clinical research in physical therapy. The American Physical Therapy Association (APTA) has defined clinical research as "a systematic process for formulating and answering questions about the uses of, the bases for, and the effectiveness of physical therapy practice." [1] With the passage of Public Law 94-142 (PL 94-142) in 1975,[2] physical therapists and other "related services" providers working in the public schools were required to participate in assessing and assuring the effectiveness of their treatment strategies in enabling children with disabilities to benefit from special education. Only through measurement and collection of objective and quantifiable data on children's gross motor, fine motor, and self-help skills is it possible to establish accountability" for our intervention strategies. [3]

IMPORTANCE OF CLINICAL RESEARCH IN PEDIATRIC PHYSICAL THERAPY

For physical therapists who work with children with developmental disabilities, the use of clinical research strategies in documenting the efficacy of treatment is vital. Not only is such documentation required by law, [2]

but it is necessary also to answer a variety of important clinical questions. For example, is this particular treatment approach making positive changes in the child's functional abilities? Will the child get worse if I continue treatment? Will the child improve more quickly if I increase therapy from one hour/week to two hours/week? Only through systematic clinical research is it possible to reliably answer such questions. There is great temptation among physical therapists, particularly those who are recent graduates, to assume that their treatment is creating a beneficial change for the child. Even seasoned clinicians who have recently completed continuing education courses, such as in the neurodevelopmental treatment (NDT) approach or sensory integration (SI) approach, have vested interests in "believing" that their newly-acquired intervention techniques are affecting positive change in their clients. Because we have all chosen to work in a helping profession, our desire to "help" may overshadow our abilities to objectively define and measure our successes or our failures. We owe it to the children, as well as to their parents, teachers, and physicians, to reliably document the effects of our treatment. Such documentation can be accomplished through carefully formulated clinical research plans.

Applied vs. Basic Research

Many clinicians are "turned off" by the term "research" because to them it implies esoteric laboratory experiments, which have little functional relevance to the day-to-day practice of physical therapy. Common misconceptions about research are that it requires large numbers of subjects (not readily available in the average clinical setting), an inordinate amount of time (which will detract from treatment time), a large amount of money, and an advanced knowledge of statistics and complex data analysis. While it is true that some types of research encompass the foregoing requirements, there are also simpler and less sophisticated types of research which have functional relevance for physical therapists.

Research is often classified as either basic or applied. Basic research examines questions which are apt to be abstract and which may be used to generate new theories. Generally, applied research is directed at answering questions of practical significance.[4] Much of basic research is conducted in a tightly controlled laboratory setting. Applied research is more appropriate for the clinical setting. The research strategies presented in this chapter are of an applied nature, i.e. relevant to an individual or society. There is a need for both basic and applied research in the area of developmental disabilities.

Reliability and Validity

Reliability and validity are important components of both applied and basic research. To demonstrate accountability, physical therapists must ensure that their evaluation tools, as well as their treatment outcomes, are both reliable and valid. Reliability refers to the consistency between measurements.[5] Consistency may be assessed between two different raters (inter-rater reliability) or across a series of measures conducted by one rater (intra-rater reliability). A common measurement tool used in physical therapy is the goniometer. If two therapists independently measured hip range of motion (ROM) in three children with myelomeningocele, recorded their measurements independently, and agreed perfectly in all planes of ROM measured, we could conclude that they have achieved perfect inter-rater reliability. If one of the therapists continued to measure hip ROM on one child across several different therapy sessions and the scores were compared, we would be examining intra-rater reliability.

Once reliability of a measurement tool is established within the clinical setting, this tool can be used to evaluate treatment outcomes. For example, if the therapist wanted to examine the effects of passive stretching of the hip flexor muscles on decreasing hip flexor tightness in a child with myelomeningocele, a series of baseline or pre-treatment measures and a series of ROM measures both during and after the intervention phase (stretching procedures) would be collected. Only through a systematic and reliable series of measures is it possible to document the efficacy of passive stretching.

In actual practice, little research has been published on the reliability of goniometry for use with children with developmental disabilities. A recent clinical research study examining goniometric reliability of upper extremity measurements for a child with spastic quadriplegia concluded that "there was wide variability in measurements both within and between raters."[6, p. 348] Even with this lack of documented reliability of goniometry, many clinicians continue to use this measurement tool to make claims about the effectiveness of their treatment.

Another important component of clinical research is validity or the extent to which an instrument measures what it is supposed to measure. A goniometer is designed to clinically measure joint angle or the angle between two or more bones which form a joint. We infer from palpating bony landmarks that we are measuring the angle of the bones to one another. One method for establishing the validity of this clinical technique is to take x-rays of the joint angle. For example, if we were to measure an elbow flexion contracture through goniometry and then x-ray the arm to measure the actual angle of the humerus to the radius, we could assess the validity of our clinical measure. Physical therapists working with children with developmental disabilities use a variety of standardized tests to assess areas such as gross motor, fine motor, and visual-perceptual development. These tools are used both in qualifying a child to receive special services as well as in measuring developmental change as a result of treatment. It is crucial that these instruments are both reliable and valid in accomplishing their aims. Therapists are advised to read the reliability and validity data published in the test administration manuals before assuming that the test is acceptable. Even though a test has been published and distributed widely, it may not possess acceptable levels of reliability and validity. It is our responsibility as clinicians to assure that the measures we are using for assessment and documentation of treatment outcome are both reliable and valid. Refer to Chapter 2 for information on the reliability and validity of currently used pediatric assessment tools.

Research Terminology

There are a number of terms, common to all types of research, which the physical therapist should be able to understand and use when reading about or conducting clinical research. Some of these terms, such as reliability and validity, have been defined in the preceding section. Two common terms, used in both experimental and correlational research, are independent and dependent variables. In experimental research, the independent variable is the variable which is manipulated by the experimenter, and is known also as the treatment variable. The dependent variable, known also as the outcome variable, is used to evaluate the influence of the independent variable on treatment. Referring back to our example of measuring the effects of passive stretching of the hip flexor muscles on decreasing hip flexor tightness, the independent variable is the passive stretching and the dependent variable is the range of hip extension. In correlational research, the relationship of two or more variables is examined, but none of the variables are manipulated by the investigator, as in experimental research. Research on reliability and validity of measures is usually correlational research. In the example in which the validity of goniometric measures of an elbow flexion contracture is evaluated through subsequent x-rays, the goniometric measures would comprise the independent variable and the ROM as measured on x-ray would be the dependent variable. In addition to using widely-accepted measurement tools, such as goniometry and standardized developmental assessment instruments, therapists may rely on practical, functional measures developed within their own clinical settings to serve as dependent variables. The advantage of such measurement strategies is that they may be "individualized" for each child in the caseload. Such measures are frequently developed as part of the goals and objectives required in the individual education program (IEP) mandated by PL 94-142.[2,3]

One type of dependent measure commonly used in pediatric therapy settings is frequency or the number of times a behavior occurs.[7] Perhaps you have written an objective to decrease the number of tongue thrusts which occur during a 30-minute feeding session. By simply counting the number of tongue thrusts which occur, you can measure the frequency of this behavior.

Another type of measurement appropriate to clinical settings is percentage occurrence or the number of occurrences of the behavior divided by the number of opportunities in which the behavior can occur, multiplied times 100.[7] For example, if the goal is to increase heel strikes in the involved foot of a child with spastic hemiplegia you would begin by taking baseline data on this behavior. By having the child walk down a 50-foot hallway, you could count the number of heelstrikes during the total number of steps on the involved side. If the child shows heelstrike on 5 occasions out of 20 possible steps, you would compute $5/20 \times 100 = 25\%$.

Duration is another common type of measurement in which the length or amount of time the behavior occurs during a given observation period is assessed.[7] For example, the duration of independent sitting or independent standing is an important functional measure for many children with developmental disabilities. Children with mental retardation often show delays in their response time to a given stimulus. To assess the effects of intervention on improving such behaviors, a measure of latency would be used. If you are working on undressing skills for a child with Down syndrome, for example, you may decide to measure the latency or length of time between giving the command, such as "shoe off!" and the child's initiation of the behavior.

These represent four of the more common types of dependent measures used in clinical research. For a more extensive description of these and other types of behavioral measures, refer to the textbook by Tawney and Gast.[7]

A MODEL FOR CLINICAL RESEARCH: THE SINGLE SUBJECT RESEARCH DESIGN

Physical therapists in clinical settings have many questions about the efficacy of their treatment strategies and yet usually do not have sufficient numbers of similar patients to conduct large group experimental research. The necessity of having a control group to compare the effects of treatment vs. no treatment also raises ethical issues about withholding treatment, even if its efficacy is unproven. The single subject research design offers clinicians a method for empirically evaluating treatment effectiveness for individual clients or small groups of clients without the need for a control group.[8] Instead, subjects serve as their own control.

Single subject research design involves carefully controlled manipulation of the treatment variable and analysis of its effects on the outcome variable.[9] Target behaviors or outcome variables must be clearly specified and operationally defined with continuous measures of these variables taken throughout each phase of the study. Data collection methods must be reliable and extraneous variables must be carefully controlled.

Single subject research design should not be confused with the case study approach.[10] Whereas single subject research involves continuous and systematic data collection with careful manipulation of the treatment variable, the case study is usually a subjective description of an individual's behavior, which lacks the experimental control of the true research design.[9,10] Although case studies can be used to generate hypotheses for future research, they cannot be used to document efficacy of treatment because of their lack of experimental control. Nonetheless, case studies are still important in physical therapy because they may stimulate research ideas in which cause-and-effect relationships can be examined. Two such case studies using children with cerebral palsy have appeared in the recent physical therapy literature.[11,12] Single subject research designs are particularly appropriate for use with children with developmental disabilities. Because of the great heterogeneity of diagnostic categories, it is virtually impossible to find enough similar subjects for a large group study. Even within each specific disability, such as cerebral palsy, there are a variety of subtypes, i.e. spastic diplegia, athetosis, and ataxia. There are justifiable ethical concerns about withholding treatment to any person with a disability, as is often necessary in group comparison research.

Single subject research designs may be incorporated directly into an ongoing clinical program. There is no need for elaborate, expensive equipment or sophisticated data analysis techniques. Changes in behavior may be graphed on simple graph paper and visually analyzed.[13] Another benefit is the collection of repeated measures throughout each phase of the study, a more powerful control for within-subject variability than a pretest/posttest design. Finally, in applied research such as this, changes must be clinically significant to be meaningful. In large group research, it is possible to effect changes which are statistically significant, but may have little value clinically to individual patients.

Measurement In Single Subject Research Design

To ensure reliability, the dependent measures or target behaviors in single subject research must be carefully defined. A clear operational definition for the behavior being measured will enhance both reliability and replicability of the design. For example, if your goal is to improve a child's upper extremity strength you must carefully define how you plan to measure strength. To use a frequency type of measure, you might define upper extremity strength as the number of wheelchair push-ups a child with myelomeningocele can accomplish in a given period of time. The types of clinical, behavioral measures defined in the foregoing section are those frequently used in single subject research: frequency, percent, duration, and latency.

It is important to assess inter-rater reliability of your dependent measures during each phase of the study. In the foregoing example, it would be important to have a colleague or physical therapist assistant also count the number of wheelchair push-ups the child can achieve during at least one or two measurement sessions in each phase of the study. To increase reliability, you might need to carefully define that a complete wheelchair push- up includes full extension of both elbows with the child's buttocks clearing the seat of the wheelchair.

One potential problem encountered in behavioral measurement is examiner bias. Because of the need to believe that our treatment is effective, our objectivity may be threatened in counting behaviors which we seek to increase (or decrease) as a result of treatment. By using a colleague who is "blind" to the phase of the study in which the child is involved to collect inter-rater reliability data, we can increase the believability of our results.

One common criticism of single subject research design is its lack of generalizability or external validity.

To increase the power or generalizability of the single subject design, it must be replicated across different children, in different settings, and by different therapists.[9,10]

Types of Experimental Designs

The simplest type of single subject design is the A-B design simple baseline design.[8-10] During the A-phase or baseline period, the target behavior is measured in its naturally occurring state (prior to introducing the intervention or treatment variable). This phase is then used as the "control" against which the frequency of behaviors in the other phases are compared. During the B-phase, the treatment variable is introduced and measurement of the target behavior continues. A minimum of three data points during each phase of treatment is desirable. Because of its inability to control for the effects of confounding variables, such as maturation, the A-B design is not considered a true experimental design. It may be useful, however, in conjunction with a case study approach to generate ideas for future research.

The A-B-A or withdrawal design allows for control of extraneous variables in the environment in that the third phase provides for a return to baseline conditions through withdrawal of the treatment variable. One limitation of this design is that it can be used only with behaviors which are reversible. Much of what we teach in therapy ultimately will be retained, even after the specific intervention is removed, either through environmental reinforcers or the child's delight in accomplishing a new task. A second drawback of this design is the ethical issue of terminating the study in a no treatment phase, thus lessening the positive gains from treatment. To counter this drawback, the A-B-A-B design is proposed. Known also as the withdrawal-reinstatement design, the A-B-A-B design concludes with a second B-phase in which the treatment is reinstated. This is more desirable ethically than the A-B-A design but is limited by the need to target a behavior which is reversible. Another type of single subject design is the alternating treatments design.[14] While less commonly used than some of the foregoing designs, the alternating treatments design has been used to evaluate the effects of lower extremity orthoses on improving standing balance in a child with cerebral palsy.[15] This design is used to investigate the effects of two or more interventions on a single behavior of a client. Following a baseline phase, two or more treatments are introduced and rapidly alternated. The final phase usually involves implementation of only the most effective treatment.[16] There are a number of other single subject designs which are also appropriate for use with children with developmental disabilities such as the multiple baseline, the multiple probe, the changing criterion, and the parallel treatments design. These designs are more complex and will not be described in this chapter. For further information on descriptions and uses of these designs with exceptional children, refer to the text by Wolery, Bailey, and Sugai.[16] To provide further clarification of the four designs that have been described above, each will be used in the four case studies of the children described in Chapter 4.

CASE STUDIES

CASE NO. 1 — JASON (A-B DESIGN)
Cerebral Palsy, Right Hemiparesis, 18 Months

For Jason, the following goal was developed: Jason will increase the use of the right upper extremity during play activities. The specific objective is: Jason will increase the frequency with which he uses his right hand during a five-minute free play session. To set up an A-B design, the treatment and outcome variables must first be operationally defined. Based on Jason's case study which includes a history of tactile defensive behavior to light touch, sensory disregard, and neglect of the right upper extremity, the following therapy plan was proposed: joint approximation through the right shoulder and into the open hand with Jason in quadruped; tactile desensitization activities which Jason can do on himself using the left hand to gently rub the right upper extremity; and positive reinforcement (praise) by the therapist

when Jason uses the right hand in play activities. This therapy plan encompasses the independent or treatment variable. The target behavior or outcome variable is increased use of the right hand during play activities. Because Jason is treated in the home, his mother will be instructed in assisting with data collection for frequency of right hand use.

During baseline (A-phase), the therapist collects frequency data on the number of times Jason uses his right hand during a five-minute free play session after therapy. She collects data on three successive days and notes the following pattern of right hand use: Day 1 — three occasions; Day 2 — four occasions; Day 3 — two occasions. She plots these data on regular graph paper and notes a fairly stable baseline pattern (Figure 1). Therefore, it is an appropriate time to introduce the new treatment plan. It is important to realize that baseline does not have to mean total absence of therapy. It is possible that Jason has been getting some generalized PT for some time, but the previous therapy has not focused on use of the right upper extremity.

On Day 4, the therapist introduces the new therapy plan which includes joint approximation, tactile desensitization, and praise for use of the right hand during play in therapy. She then continues to collect data during the five-minute free play session after therapy. Jason's mother, who is "blind" to the phases of treatment,

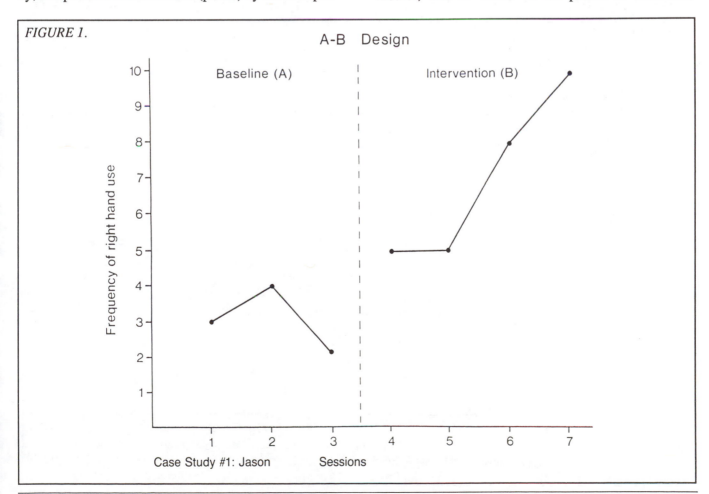

FIGURE 1.

A-B Design

Baseline (A)   Intervention (B)

Frequency of right hand use

Case Study #1: Jason   Sessions

collects inter-rater reliability data once during each phase of the study. Jason's use of his right hand increases: Day 4 — five occasions; Day 5 — five occasions; Day 6 — eight occasions; Day 7 — ten occasions (Figure 1). While it is tempting to conclude that the new therapy plan has accounted for this improvement, it is important to realize that the A-B design does not allow for such conclusions because it does not control for outside variables. Perhaps developmental maturation has influenced Jason's use of his right hand more than the therapy itself. To counter these limitations, an A-B-A or A-B-A-B design would be preferable.

CASE NO. 2 — JILL (A-B-A DESIGN):
Cerebral Palsy, Spastic Quadriparesis, Mental Retardation, 7 Years

Jill can raise her head in prone but only momentarily. Since head raising in prone is important both developmentally and functionally, the following goal was written: Jill will improve head control in prone. The specific objective reads: Jill will increase duration of head-raising in prone over a wedge. Thus the target behavior or dependent measure is increased head-raising in prone.

Jill has not responded to more naturally occurring stimuli, such as tactile and vestibular input for facilitation of her prone head righting. Since there is both neurophysiological[17] and clinical evidence[18] that vibra-tory stimulation will facilitate contraction of weak agonist muscles while inhibiting spasticity in the antagonist muscles, it was decided that a therapeutic vibrator would be used as the treatment modality. Since the facilitatory effect of vibration is relatively brief (approximately 30 minutes),[18] this type of intervention could be expected to produce a reversible pattern of behavior once it was removed. Thus, the treatment variable for this A-B-A study was operationally defined as two minutes of vibratory stimulation to the posterior neck muscles using a small mechanical vibrator which vibrates at a frequency of 100-200 Hz and an amplitude of 1.5mm. [19]

Baseline data were taken with Jill positioned in prone over a wedge for a 5-minute period while in the classroom. A stopwatch was used to measure the total duration of head raising during the observation period. Head raising was further defined as lifting the head to an angle where the nose was perpendicular with the floor. Inter-rater reliability data were collected during each phase of the study by a PT assistant who was unaware of the treatment plan.

During the B-phase, vibration was applied for two minutes in a cephalo-caudal direction while Jill was prone on the wedge. Data were collected on duration of head raising for a 5-minute period immediately following vibration. Dramatic improvement was noted as evidenced by changes in both level and trend of the data

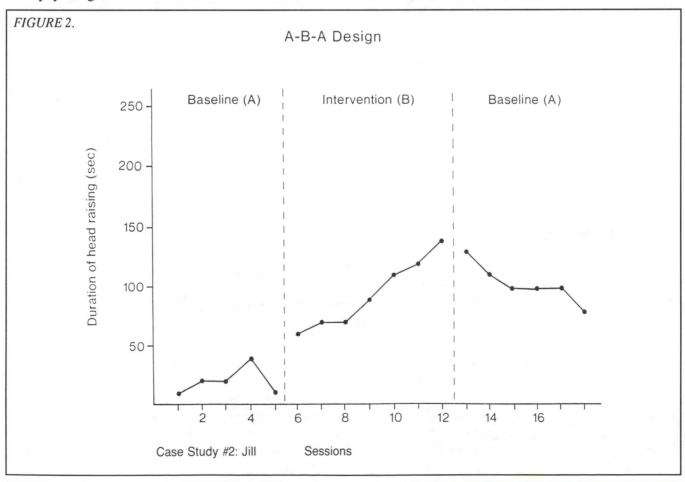

FIGURE 2.

A-B-A Design

Baseline (A) | Intervention (B) | Baseline (A)

Duration of head raising (sec)

Case Study #2: Jill   Sessions

(Figure 2). When treatment was withdrawn during the second A-phase, the duration of head raising decreased but not to the initial baseline level. Such change implies that Jill may have been reinforced intrinsically by the head raising such that she desired to continue this newly learned behavior. For ethical reasons, it would be desirable to proceed to a second B-phase, thus converting to an A-B-A-B or withdrawal-reinstatement design.

CASE NO. 3 — TAYLOR (A-B-A-B DESIGN)
Myelomengocele, Repaired L 1-2, 4 Years

Taylor lacks the upper extremity muscle strength and endurance necessary to use ambulation aids effectively. The following goal and objective are proposed. *Goal:* Taylor will increase his upper extremity muscle strength and endurance. *Objective:* While wearing his lower extremity orthoses, Taylor will ambulate 10 consecutive lengths of the parallel bars, without rest breaks, using a swing-to gait for three consecutive days. Thus, ambulation in the parallel bars is the target behavior or dependent measure.

The treatment variable is composed of a three-part therapy plan: wheelchair push-ups, quadruped push-ups, and positive reinforcement through a bar graph monitoring Taylor's progress. During baseline, Taylor was introduced to the parallel bars and instructed in how to accomplish a swing-to gait. A complete length of the parallel bars was defined as one in which Taylor required no physical assist from the therapist. Baseline data were plotted in Figure 3. The ambulation routine was part of Taylor's overall therapy program but was not emphasized or strongly reinforced during baseline.

During intervention, Taylor was taught to do both wheelchair push-ups and push-ups in quadruped. Following these activities, the therapist showed him a sticker-chart made up like a bar graph and told him he could put on one sticker for each length of the parallel bars he could walk without sitting down. As can be seen from Figure 3, Taylor's success in the parallel bars improved dramatically. An attempt to return to baseline conditions (second B-phase), however did not result in a reversal of the behavior. Instead, Taylor's progress continued although the trend was not as marked as during the intervention.

It is not surprising that this behavior did not reverse itself. First of all, muscle strength and endurance will not diminish appreciably immediately upon discontinuing exercises. Secondly, the ambulation in the parallel bars, although the dependent measure in this study, will serve to increase and maintain upper extremity strength. Thirdly, even though the overt reinforcer (the sticker chart) was removed during the second phase, Taylor probably continued to feel intrinsic reinforcement for his success.

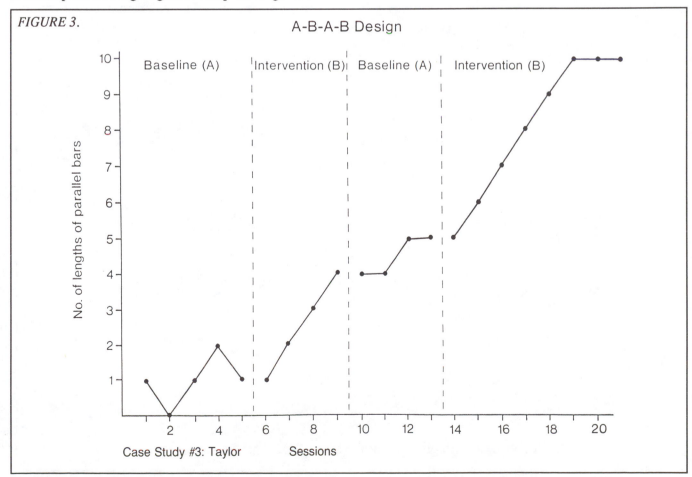

FIGURE 3.

A-B-A-B Design

Case Study #3: Taylor   Sessions

When intervention was reinstated during the second B-phase, the trend of the earlier B-phase continued and Taylor achieved his objective of 100% success for three consecutive days by Session 21. Due to the failure of the data to reverse during withdrawal of the intervention, it is impossible to definitely conclude that the exercise and reinforcement package "caused" the improvements noted. Taylor's success was no doubt due, in part, to intrinsic reinforcers as well as to strength acquired from the walking activity itself. By visually analyzing trends in the data during each phase, it is obvious that the steepest slopes of improvement occurred during the two B-phases, however lending support to the efficacy of the intervention package.

CASE NO. 4 — ASHLEY
(ALTERNATING TREATMENTS DESIGN):
Down Syndrome, 15 Months

Ashley tends to keep her mouth open, a typical problem of infants with generalized hypotonia. Not only does the open mouth contribute to feeding problems, as in Ashley's case, but it is often a source of concern for parents who think that it contributes to making the child "look" retarded. Since Ashley is capable of closing her mouth, but does so infrequently, it is unclear whether the persistent mouth opening is a behavioral or a neurophysiological problem. In an effort to answer this question, two different treatment approaches were compared using an alternating treatment design. *Goal:* Ashley will decrease open mouth behavior. *Objective:* Ashley will close her mouth within 2 seconds of behavioral or neurophysiological cues.

This initial study is directed at the latency of Ashley's response. Based on the success of either or both interventions, a subsequent objective would be geared toward increasing the duration of mouth closure to improve the functional relevance of this behavior. The two treatment variables consist of a verbal cue to Ashley to "close mouth, Ashley," and a behavioral cue of chin tapping based on Mueller's approach to oral-motor facilitation.[20,21] During baseline, Ashley was seated in an adaptive chair in front of the examiner and was engaged in fine motor play activities. The examiner collected data on the number of times Ashley closed her mouth during a 3-minute period (using a golf counter). No verbal cues or reinforcers were provided.

During the intervention phase, the two treatment strategies were rapidly alternated in random order. With Ashley again seated in a special chair engaged in fine motor play, the examiner applied one treatment for a 3-minute period, took a 1-minute break, then applied the second treatment for a 3-minute period. For the verbal/behavioral intervention, the examiner verbally cued Ashley to close her mouth and then demonstrated this

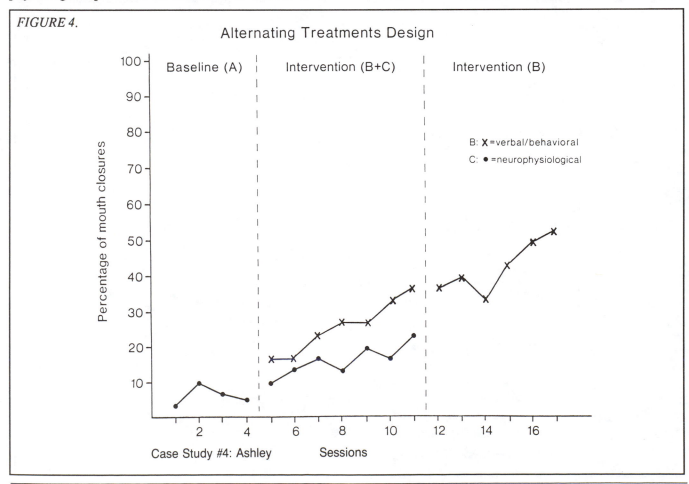

FIGURE 4.

Alternating Treatments Design

behavior. Each time Ashley closed her mouth within two seconds the data recorder (the parent) made a "+." Failure to close her mouth within two seconds resulted in a "—" mark. Successful completion of the behavior resulted in a smile from the examiner combined with praise such as "Good closing your mouth, Ashley!" Failure to comply resulted in the examiner looking away and ignoring Ashley for five seconds.

For the neurophysiological intervention, the examiner introduced five rapid "chin taps" each time the mouth was open and waited two seconds (from the final chin tap) for a response. Chin tapping was done with the dorsum of the fingers in a quick upward motion underneath the mandible. No verbal cues or behavioral reinforcement were given during this intervention. Both successes and failures were recorded

Treatments were randomly alternated during each session to control for possible order effects. Due to the complexity of counting behaviors which occur within a given time period (two seconds), a second person was needed to count and record data. This was a good opportunity to involve the parent in the child's therapy program. A third person was needed to collect inter-rater reliability data at least once during each phase. Data were recorded as number of successful trials/total number of trials x 100 (percentage data).

In Figure 4, it can be seen that the verbal/behavioral intervention was slightly more successful than the neurophysiological approach. Thus the final phase of the study used the verbal/behavioral intervention as the treatment variable. Since both intervention approaches yielded some positive changes, it is logical to conclude that combining both approaches might bring about even quicker changes. Such a study might be attempted following completion of this study.

This hypothetical single subject study with Ashley was based, in part, on an actual series of single-subject studies conducted on five young children with Down syndrome.[22] Readers are referred to the study by Purdy, Deitz, and Harris for further information on this topic.[22]

SUMMARY AND CONCLUSIONS

The primary goal of this chapter is to demonstrate that research techniques for the clinician can be relatively simple, inexpensive, and require little additional time and effort. Secondly, systematic measurement and accountability of the efficacy of our treatment strategies are both ethical and legal responsibilities of all physical therapists working with children with developmental disabilities, particularly those in public school settings. Through the use of such behavioral measurement strategies as individualized therapy goals and objectives and single subject research designs, it is possible for each of

us to examine the effectiveness of a variety of treatment strategies with individual children in our clinical practices.

Not only do we, as clinicians, have the responsibility to demonstrate treatment efficacy, we also have the responsibility to share results with professional colleagues. Through oral dissemination at inservice sessions and in presentations at local, state, and national meetings, as well as through publication of research in scholarly journals and professional newsletters, we must share not only our successes, i.e. those treatment modalities which were efficacious, but also our failures. For example, if replications of a study within our own setting repeatedly have shown a particular treatment not to be effective, we owe it to our colleagues to share this information as much as we are required to share results of successful treatments. Both the new graduate and experienced physical therapist have responsibilities to expand our knowledge base in physical therapy through carefully controlled clinical research. It is hoped that this chapter will encourage physical therapists at all levels of experience to conduct clinical research within their own settings and to share their results with their colleagues.

For readers interested in pursuing single subject research in greater depth, two excellent, recent references are suggested: a text by Ottenbacher for physical and occupational therapists[23] and a descriptive article by Gonella.[24] ❏

REFERENCES

1. Plan to Foster Clinical Research in Physical Therapy. Goals adopted by American Physical Therapy Association House of Delegates, 1980 (Revised: November, 1984)

2. Education for All Handicapped Children Act, Public Law 94-142. U.S. Congress, Senate, 94th Congress, first session, 1975

3. O'Neill DL, Harris SR: Developing goals and objectives for handicapped children. Phys Ther 62:295-298, 1982

4. Cox RC, West WL: Fundamentals of Research for Health Professionals. Laurel, MD, Ramsco, 1982

5. Isaac S, Michael WB: Handbook on Research and Evaluation. San Diego, CA, Edits, 1971, p 87

6. Harris SR, Smith LH, Krukowski L: Goniometric reliability for a child with spastic quadriplegia. J Pediatri Orth 5:348-351, 1985

7. Tawney JW, Gast DL: Single Subject Research in Special Education. Columbus, OH, Merrill, 1984

8. Martin JE, Epstein LH: Evaluating treatment effectiveness in cerebral palsy. Phys Ther 56:285-294, 1976

9. Hersen M, Barlow DH: Single Case Experimental Designs: Strategies for Studying Behavior Change. New York, NY, Pergamon Press, 1976

10. Hacker B. Single subject research strategies in occupational therapy: Part 1. Am J Occ Ther 34:103-108, 1980

11. Hallum A: Subject-induced reinforcement of head-lifting in the prone position: A case report. Phys Ther 64:1390-92, 1984

12. Smith LH, Harris SR: Upper extremity inhibitive casting for a child with cerebral palsy. Phys Occ Ther Pediatri 5:71-79, 1985

13. Wolery M, Harris SR: Interpreting results of single-subject research designs. Phys Ther 62:445-452,1982

14. Barlow DH, Hayes SC: Alternating treatments design: One strategy for comparing the effects of two treatments in a single subject. J Appl Beh Anal 12:199-210, 1979

15. Harris SR, Riffle K: Effects of inhibitive ankle-foot orthoses on standing balance in a child with cerebral palsy: A single subject design. Phys Ther 66:663-667, 1986

16. Wolery M, Bailey DB, Sugai GM: Effective Teaching: Principles and Procedures of Applied Behavior Analysis. Boston, MA, Allyn & Bacon,1988

17. Bishop B: Vibratory stimulation: Possible applications of vibration in treatment of motor dysfunctions. Phys Ther 55:139-143, 1975

18. Hagbarth KE, Eklund G: The muscle vibrator-A useful tool in neurologic therapeutic work. Scand J Rehab Med 1:26-34, 1969

19. Eklund G, Steen M: Muscle vibration therapy in children with cerebral palsy. Scand J Rehab Med 1:33-37, 1969

20. Mueller HA: Facilitating feeding and prespeech. In Pearson PH, Williams CE (eds): Physical Therapy Services in the Developmental Disabilities. Springfield, IL, Charles C Thomas, 1972, pp 283-310

21. Mueller HA: Feeding. In Finnie NR: Handling the Young Cerebral Palsied Child at Home. New York, NY, EP Dutton, 1976, pp 113-132

22. Purdy AH, Deitz JC, Harris SR: Efficacy of two treatment approaches to reduce tongue protrusion of children with Down syndrome. Dev Med Child Neurol 29:469-476, 1987

23. Ottenbacher KJ: Evaluating Clinical Change: Strategies for Occupational and Physical Therapists. Baltimore, MD, Williams & Wilkins, 1986

24. Gonella C: Single-subject experimental paradigm as a clinical decision tool. Phys Ther 70:601-609, 1989

Index